Trends in Critical Care Medicine

Edited by Theodoros Aslanidis

Published in London, United Kingdom

Trends in Critical Care Medicine
http://dx.doi.org/10.5772/intechopen.1008094
Edited by Theodoros Aslanidis

Contributors
Ahmad M. Obeidat, Ashish Kumar, Aurelio Rodríguez-Pérez, Daniel Pethers, Daolin Tang, David Merle, Fernando Ruiz Gonzalez, Francisco Merced-Ortiz, Hana Elamin, Hussain Ayyaz, Héctor Trujillo-Morales, Ingrid Bonilla-Mercado, Jiao Liu, Mertcan Sevgi, Mohammad Ataur Rahman, Mojahid Mohammed Khalid Alhussein, Muhammad Saqib, Nazario Ojeda-Betancor, Negin Sanadgol, Norhan Attia Ahmed, Pedro Yasfir González-Noris, Prabu Bhuvanendran, Raúl Vega-Rodríguez, Sanghamitra Padhy, Saskin Vitaly Alexandrovich, Sohel M.G. Ahmed, Sonia I. Vicenty-Rivera, Theodoros Aslanidis, Wanrong Wu, Yichun Wang, Yuanhang Fan, Zhenhui Zhang, Zia Mahmood, Ángel Becerra-Bolaños

First published in London, United Kingdom, 2025 by IntechOpen
IntechOpen is the global imprint of INTECHOPEN LIMITED, registered in England and Wales, registration number: 11086078, 167-169 Great Portland Street, London, W1W 5PF, United Kingdom

For EU product safety concerns: IN TECH d.o.o., Prolaz Marije Krucifikse Kozulić 3, 51000 Rijeka, Croatia, info@intechopen.com or visit our website at intechopen.com.

British Library Cataloguing-in-Publication Data
A catalogue record for this book is available from the British Library

Trends in Critical Care Medicine
Edited by Theodoros Aslanidis
p. cm.
Print ISBN 978-1-83634-227-4
Online ISBN 978-1-83634-226-7
eBook (PDF) ISBN 978-1-83634-228-1

If disposing of this product, please recycle the paper responsibly.

Meet the editor

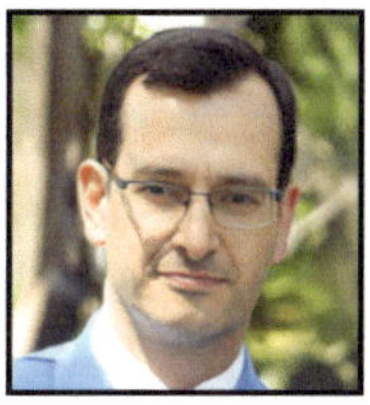

Dr. Theodoros K. Aslanidis has extensive clinical experience in prehospital and in-hospital anesthesia, emergency care, and critical care. His primary expertise in clinical fields is critical care and prehospital emergency medicine, while his Ph.D. was focused on electrodermal activity monitoring in the ICU. He is currently working as a consultant-researcher at the Intensive Care Unit of Agios Pavlos General Hospital of Thessaloniki, Greece. He also served as Head of Postgraduate Studies at the College of Offshore and Remote Medicine in Pretty Bay, Malta, where he remains a faculty member.

Contents

Preface **IX**

Chapter 1 **1**
Introductory Chapter: Critical Thinking for Critically Ill Versus or with Guidelines and Artificial Intelligence?
by Theodoros Aslanidis

Chapter 2 **7**
Cardiogenic Shock: A Phenotype-Based Approach – A Crucial Advancement in Tailored Management
by Ingrid Bonilla-Mercado, Francisco Merced-Ortiz and Sonia I. Vicenty-Rivera

Chapter 3 **35**
Ferroptosis in Sepsis-Induced Acute Lung Injury
by Yuanhang Fan, Wanrong Wu, Jiao Liu, Daolin Tang, Zhenhui Zhang and Yichun Wang

Chapter 4 **53**
Challenges in Critical Care Lung Ultrasound
by Pedro Yasfir González-Noris

Chapter 5 **63**
Intensive Care Management of Stroke
by Hussain Ayyaz and Saskin Vitaly Alexandrovich

Chapter 6 **79**
Eye Care in the Intensive Care Unit
by Negin Sanadgol, Daniel Pethers, David Merle and Mertcan Sevgi

Chapter 7 **107**
Pharmacological Safety in Neonatal Care: A Focus on Clinical Pharmacy Intervention
by Norhan Attia Ahmed

Chapter 8 **115**
Withdrawal/Withholding of Life-Sustaining Therapies in the Intensive Care Unit
by Ángel Becerra-Bolaños, Raúl Vega-Rodríguez, Héctor Trujillo-Morales, Nazario Ojeda-Betancor and Aurelio Rodríguez-Pérez

Chapter 9 **147**
Brain Stem Death
by Hana Elamin, Ahmad M. Obeidat, Ashish Kumar, Mojahid Mohammed Khalid Alhussein, Mohammad Ataur Rahman, Zia Mahmood, Fernando Ruiz Gonzalez, Sanghamitra Padhy, Prabu Bhuvanendran and Sohel M.G. Ahmed

Chapter 10 **179**
Trends in Critical Care Medicine: Innovations Shaping the Future
by Muhammad Saqib

Preface

With over 52,000 articles indexed in the PubMed NLM database for the term "Critical care" in the last 12 months (June 2024-June 2025), it is challenging to keep up with the current trends in the evolution of intensive care medicine.

The general trend follows that of the rest of the medical fields, with a focus on patient-centered care and a more personalized approach to medicine. The tremendous technological progress, driven by the integration of digital health, clinical informatics, advanced monitoring, clinical decision support systems, and artificial intelligence, has further enhanced the dynamic of this evolution.

Within the framework of guidelines development, and especially in clinical thinking about daily clinical problems, there appears to be a struggle to adapt to a shifting landscape. New ethical considerations and questions arise, and the answers are anything but easy.

The current IntechOpen book aims to gather and synthesize information and updates on selected topics in critical care. Neither the editor nor the authors have the illusion or the expectation that every subject in the current intensive care medicine can or will be covered. Still, with chapters focusing on issues like cardiogenic shock, stroke, lung ultrasound, sepsis-related lung injury, or brain death, the present book will hopefully provide valuable insights and information about contemporary care for the critically ill.

Moreover, it will contribute to our better understanding of the changing environment in our intensive care unit.

Theodoros Aslanidis
Agios Pavlos General Hospital,
Intensive Care Unit,
Thessaloniki, Greece

Chapter 1

Introductory Chapter: Critical Thinking for Critically Ill Versus or with Guidelines and Artificial Intelligence?

Theodoros Aslanidis

1. Critical thinking: The challenges remain

Albert Einstein once said: "In theory, theory and practice are the same. In practice, they are not". Medicine is an applied science: it applies knowledge of basic sciences in order to maintain and promote health. Thus, basic science knowledge is necessary for clinical practice, yet not sufficient [1]. Knowledge in a clinical setting is also gained by evidence-based medicine: "the conscientious, explicit and judicious use of current best evidence in making decisions about the care of individual patients. It means integrating individual clinical expertise with the best available external clinical evidence from systematic research" [2].

The golden bridge between knowledge and patient outcomes, however, is critical thinking. Critical thinking (CrT) is defined as "purposeful self-regulatory judgment which results in interpretation, analysis, evaluation and inference, as well as explanation of the evidential, conceptual, methodological, criteriological, or contextual considerations upon which that judgement is based" [3].

Especially in highly dynamic and complex settings such as intensive care units (ICU), critical thinking becomes essential. The latter fact is currently starting to shift medical training focus from clinical to critical thinking. The challenges, though, remain: What is the nature of critical thinking? There is no definite consensus about that: some use several cognitive skills [3] (such as observation, analysis, inference) as content of CrT. On the other hand, there is the view that CrT is a skill or a learning process specific to a given body of knowledge (e.g., intensive care medicine, emergency medicine, oncology, etc.) [4].

How do you measure it then? Though there are a lot of critical thinking assessment tools (CTA) (**Table 1**), their application in clinical practice is limited.

Adoption of such tools in clinical settings can help us understand our thought process, its strengths and its weaknesses, improve it and monitor our change over time.

What can you do to develop it further? There are a lot of strategies that are suggested to promote CrT. Discussing biases (i.e., deviation of typical thinking process due to, e.g., stress or time-constraint) and de-biasing strategies—such as feedback and accountability, or teaching inductive reasoning are some of them [6, 7].

Furthermore, CrT is not only an individual's skill. Team cognition, which refers to the relationship and interaction among ICU team members to augment their CrT in real

Watson-Glaser critical thinking appraisal (WGCTA)	Halpern critical thinking assessment (HCTA)
California Critical Thinking Skills Test (CCTST)	The Health Science Reasoning Test (HSRT)
Cornell Critical Thinking Test (CCTT)	California Critical Thinking Disposition Inventory (CCTDI)
Professional Judgment Rating Form (PJRF)	Holistic Critical Thinking Scoring Rubric
Argumentative writing	Dialog CA coding scheme
Script concordance test (SCT)	

Table 1.
Critical thinking assessment tools and methods [4, 5].

environment (also known as macrognition), is something that can be used to increase patient safety and transparent decision-making in multi-disciplinary teams [8].

2. Guidelines: Critical thinking inhibitor?

However, the existence of guidelines for nearly everything seems to get in the way of critical thinking. Guidelines are the link between the best available evidence and clinical practice [9], they are recommendations that help to plan a strategy and they often are used as a "safety net" or even soft-law rules to judge our decisions. So, "What's the point of thinking? It's all there" [10]. Or even worse: clinicians are to blame when they are not following guidelines, and they are criticized for relying solely on them!

The answer about the usefulness of guidelines is paradoxically ... critical thinking. Despite the evolution both in clinical research and guidelines development, many current guidelines suffer from limitations and biases, related to panel composition (which may not consider possible conflicts of interest), disease or population focus (too narrow), low or medium level of available evidence and lack of formal procedures for their update [11]. As Allan S. Detsky said, "In all cases, opinions that convert data into recommendations require subjective judgments. Since these judgments are human endeavour, they naturally leave room for error and bias" [12, 13].

Besides guidelines' documents development, guidelines application poses an additional challenge and area for critical thinking. Currently, there is no mention of how guidelines should be applied in clinical practice, in combination with a physician's clinical experience, in the case of a specific patient [14]. Nevertheless, experience plays a significant role in medical practice. Apart from that, guidelines are disease-focused and not patient-focused. In the era of personalized medicine, where we all accept biological fluidity of normality, guidelines cannot adapt to every possible scenario. There is a lot of research regarding overcoming implementation challenges of clinical practices in different settings [15] and the use of tools to evaluate usefulness of guidelines, such as the G-TRUST tool [16]. However, this is a dynamic process that is far from ending.

3. Artificial intelligence: A game changer or a disruption?

Artificial intelligence (AI) and Machine Learning (ML) can enhance patient care and have been increasingly used in ICU settings, as an invaluable tool for data analysis, pattern recognition, diagnostics and therapy decisions aid [17]. Still, it is not devoid of limitations such as data transparency, bias in database origin and model validation—especially in a highly dynamic environment, lack of sufficient number of clinical trials and experiments for safety and efficacy, lack of empathy or ethics consideration, AI systems sustainability needs, limited education and understanding of the model input-output process by physicians, patients and even designers [18, 19].. And above all… it is a human product.

4. Solution?: Skeptical medicine

No matter how good the tools that current medical progress provides us are, we should always keep in mind that science is an ongoing process. Critical thinking is the procedure that integrates and combines patient data, doctor's knowledge, experience and motivation, recommendations from guidelines or AI systems, ethics and interpersonal relationships with all engaged in patient care to reach the best possible decision for the given framework. And even then, our decision will still be human, prone to error or bias. This is normal…that is the nature of medicine.

Conflict of interests

The author has no conflict of interest.

Author details

Theodoros Aslanidis
Intensive Care Unit, "Agios Pavlos" General Hospital, Thessaloniki, Greece

*Address all correspondence to: thaslan@hotmail.com

References

[1] Byrne J. Skeptical Medicine. 2019. Available from: https://sites.google.com/site/skepticalmedicine/

[2] Sackett DL, Rosenberg WM, Gray JA, Haynes RB, Richardson WS. Evidence based medicine: What it is and what it isn't. BMJ. 1996;**312**(7023):71-72. DOI: 10.1136/bmj.312.7023.71

[3] Facione PA. Critical Thinking: A Statement of Expert Consensus for Purposes of Educational Assessment and Instruction: "The Delphi Report". The California Academic Press, University of California; 1990

[4] Rickles ML, Zimmer SR, Slusser SR, Williams DM, Zipp JF. Assessing change in student critical thinking for introduction to sociology classes. Teaching Sociology. 2013;**41**:271-281. DOI: 10.1177/0092055X1347912

[5] Cui R, Zhao L. Assessing students' critical thinking in dialogue. Journal of Intelligence. 2024;**12**(11):106. DOI: 10.3390/jintelligence12110106

[6] Hayes MM, Chatterjee S, Schwartzstein RM. Critical thinking in critical care: Five strategies to improve teaching and learning in the intensive care unit. Annals of the American Thoracic Society. 2017;**14**(4):569-575. DOI: 10.1513/AnnalsATS.201612-1009AS

[7] Ho YR, Chen BY, Li CM. Thinking more wisely: Using the Socratic method to develop critical thinking skills amongst healthcare students. BMC Medical Education. 2023;**23**(1):173. DOI: 10.1186/s12909-023-04134-2

[8] Jagpal SK, Alismail A, Lin E, Blackwell L, Ahmed N, Lee MM, et al. Beyond the individual: A multidisciplinary model for critical thinking in the intensive care unit. Advances in Medical Education and Practice. 2024;**15**:409-417. DOI: 10.2147/AMEP.S429982

[9] Brihcko L, Mitra B, Cameron P. When guidelines guide us to harm. Emergency Medicine Australasia: EMA. 2018;**30**(6):740-742. DOI: 10.1111/1742-6723.13189

[10] McCann SR. Can guidelines inhibit innovation and critical thinking? Bone Marrow Transplantation. 2020;**55**:1217-1219. DOI: 10.1038/s41409-020-0825-5

[11] Guerra-Farfan E, Garcia-Sanchez Y, Jornet-Gibert M, Nuñez JH, Balaguer-Castro M, Madden K. Clinical practice guidelines: The good, the bad, and the ugly. Injury. 2023;**54**(Suppl 3):S26-S29. DOI: 10.1016/j.injury.2022.01.047

[12] Franco JVA, Arancibia M, Meza N, Madrid E, Kopitowski K. Clinical practice guidelines: Concepts, limitations and challenges. Medwave. 2020;**20**(3):e7887. DOI: 10.5867/medwave.2020.03.7887

[13] Detsky AS. Sources of bias for authors of clinical practice guidelines. CMAJ. 2006;**175**(9):1033-1035. DOI: 10.1503/cmaj.061181

[14] Geleris P, Boudoulas H. Problems related to the application of guidelines in clinical practice: A critical analysis. Hellenic Journal of Cardiology. 2011;**52**(2):97-102

[15] Salari H, Najm F, Yazdankhahfard M, Esfandiari A. Challenges, barriers and solutions for implementing clinical practice guidelines: A qualitative study in southern Iran. BMJ Open Quality.

2024;**13**(3):e002595. DOI: 10.1136/bmjoq-2023-002595

[16] Pereira VC, Silva SN, Carvalho VKS, et al. Strategies for the implementation of clinical practice guidelines in public health: An overview of systematic reviews. Health Research Policy and Systems. 2022;**20**:13. DOI: 10.1186/s12961-022-00815-4

[17] Suresh V, Singh KK, Vaish E, Gurjar M, Ambuli Nambi A, Khulbe Y, et al. Artificial intelligence in the intensive care unit: Current evidence on an inevitable future tool. Cureus. 2024;**16**(5):e59797. DOI: 10.7759/cureus.59797

[18] Gonzalez FA, Santonocito C, Lamas T, Costa P, Vieira SM, Ferreira HA, et al. Is artificial intelligence prepared for the 24-h shifts in the ICU? Anaesthesia Critical Care & Pain Medicine. 2024;**43**(6):101431. DOI: 10.1016/j.accpm.2024.101431

[19] Barea Mendoza JA, Valiente Fernandez M, Pardo Fernandez A, Gómez ÁJ. Current perspectives on the use of artificial intelligence in critical patient safety. Medicina Intensiva (English Edition). 2025;**49**(3):154-164. DOI: 10.1016/j.medine.2024.04.002

Chapter 2

Cardiogenic Shock: A Phenotype-Based Approach – A Crucial Advancement in Tailored Management

Ingrid Bonilla-Mercado, Francisco Merced-Ortiz and Sonia I. Vicenty-Rivera

Abstract

Cardiogenic shock is a circulatory failure characterized by low cardiac output, leading to inadequate blood flow to organs and ultimately tissue hypoxia. Current definitions, pathophysiological principles, and management strategies reveal significant knowledge gaps that must be addressed for personalized shock therapy and the ethical use of modern technologies and resources. Invasive hemodynamic assessment has become increasingly crucial in managing cardiogenic shock, particularly in determining the need for acute and chronic mechanical circulatory support. Different phenotypes of cardiogenic shock exhibit unique hemodynamic profiles, requiring tailored treatment approaches. Phenotyping cardiogenic shock enables timely therapeutic interventions, and evaluating patients' hemodynamic responses to therapy can guide decisions on whether to escalate or de-escalate treatment, including the use of mechanical circulatory support. Additionally, risk modifiers can enhance mortality risk stratification, offering a more reliable approach to patient care that goes beyond merely evaluating shock severity. Continuous reassessment in managing cardiogenic shock is crucial, as it keeps healthcare professionals engaged and proactive.

Keywords: cardiogenic shock, percutaneous coronary intervention, temporary mechanical circulatory support, acute MI, acute HF, cardiac critical care

1. Introduction

Cardiogenic shock (CS) is a heterogeneous critical state characterized by reduced cardiac output, leading to cellular tissue hypoxia due to insufficient oxygen delivery that fails to meet cellular metabolic needs and oxygen consumption requirements [1]. Therefore, this leads to insufficient tissue perfusion and subsequent organ dysfunction. CS is a complex syndrome that can arise from various etiologies, mostly known to be caused by acute myocardial infarction (AMI), but it could be triggered by both cardiac and non-cardiac etiologies and is associated with high mortality rates. CS is the leading cause of morbidity and mortality in patients with cardiac diseases [1]. Despite significant advancements in percutaneous coronary interventions (PCI), the availability of temporary mechanical circulatory support (MCS), and the widespread acknowledgment that early revascularization is crucial for survival, the improvement in acute CS mortality has been stagnant for the past 20 years since the seminal SHOCK (Should we emergently revascularize Occluded Coronaries for cardiogenic shock) trial was published [2]. This pivotal study significantly influenced our understanding and management of CS. The effects of shock are initially reversible but can quickly become irreversible, resulting in multiorgan failure (MOF) and death. When a patient presents with undifferentiated shock, it is essential for the clinician to immediately initiate therapy while rapidly identifying the etiology to ensure that definitive treatment can be administered to reverse shock, prevent MOF, and prevent death. Traditional management of CS has relied on generalized protocols that may not adequately address the diverse underlying pathophysiological mechanisms. CS management can be challenging because of heterogeneous presentation and a complex hemodynamic profile. Despite novel technologies for treating shock patients, CS mortality remains high.

Additionally, the changes in patient demographics and comorbidities, along with improvements in medical therapy, have contributed to an increase in the prevalence of non-AMI-CS and a subsequent decline in the incidence of AMI. This shift underscores the need for a different focus in treatment. The change from AMI-related CS to other causes, such as heart failure decompensation with cardiogenic shock (HF-CS), right ventricular failure, valvular disease, arrhythmias, myocarditis, and post-cardiotomy cardiogenic shock, is significant as it reflects the evolving nature of CS and the need for a more comprehensive approach to treatment (**Figure 1**). As our

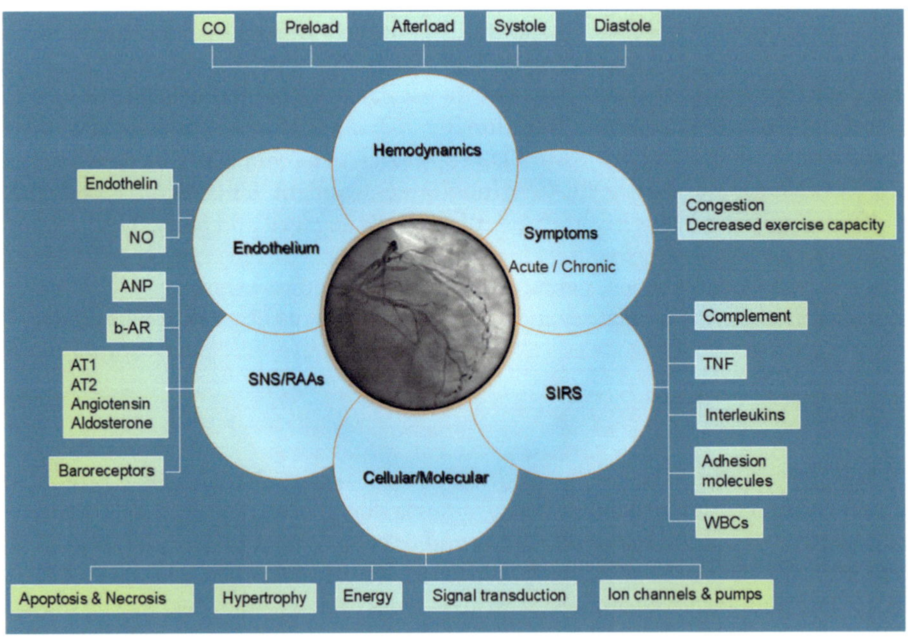

Figure 1.
Cardiogenic shock pathophysiology.

understanding of CS evolves, a shift toward a phenotype-based approach promises to enhance patient outcomes by tailoring interventions to the specific characteristics of the individual patient.

2. Epidemiology

The prevalence of CS is increasing, partly due to the aging population and the rising incidence of coronary artery disease (CAD) and heart failure. There is an increasing recognition of CS occurring in non-ischemic contexts, including severe heart failure, myocarditis, and post-cardiac surgery. CS is the leading cause of morbidity and mortality in patients with cardiac diseases. It has been reported that it accounts for about 15% of the intensive care unit admissions, with a 30-day mortality of 40–80%, with AMI and acute decompensated heart failure as main causative etiologies. The condition is seen in 5–10% of the patients hospitalized for AMI, 10–12% with ST-elevation myocardial infarction (STEMI), and in 5% of all acute decompensated heart failure. Therefore, timely recognition, treatment, and stabilization are paramount, including decision-making for mechanical support devices and early revascularization strategies. Advances in medical and interventional therapies have changed the landscape of CS. The long-term prognosis in survivors of CS often faces long-term complications, including persistent heart failure and reduced quality of life. Discerning the epidemiology of CS is crucial for healthcare providers to identify at-risk populations, implement preventive measures, and develop effective treatment strategies.

3. Pathophysiological changes leading to CS

Development of CS is preceded by a cascade of events that leads to myocardial damage and subsequent hypoperfusion. In AMI, the preceding event is typically an acute obstruction of a coronary artery. In contrast, in acute heart failure (AHF), the preceding event can arise from an acute event (de novo) or from the deterioration of chronic heart failure (**Figure 1**). In both scenarios, there will be decreased cardiac output secondary to myocardial damage, limiting the heart's oxygen supply required to meet the metabolic demands, resulting in systemic hypoperfusion and tissue hypoxia [3]. The pathophysiology of CS involves multiple interconnected mechanisms that interact and may lead to clinical deterioration. As myocardial demand increases, an imbalance develops between oxygen supply and delivery to various organs, resulting in myocardial ischemia, exacerbating cardiac dysfunction. Compensatory mechanisms responding to reduced cardiac output can trigger excessive sympathetic nervous system activation (SNS). This results in an increased heart rate and contractility that aims to restore cardiac output. The Renin-Angiotensin-Aldosterone system is also activated, leading to vasoconstriction, fluid retention, increased blood volume, and elevated blood pressure. However, this overactivity can worsen fluid overload and negatively impact cardiac output. The activation of the SNS, along with excessive release of catecholamines such as norepinephrine and epinephrine, increases heart rate and intensifies peripheral vasoconstriction to maintain perfusion to vital organs [4]. Nonetheless, this exaggerated activation of the SNS can lead to increased afterload and systemic vascular resistance, creating a detrimental cycle of systemic vasoconstriction, tissue hypoperfusion, and ischemia. On its own,

CS at its later stages may also trigger a systemic inflammatory response, characterized by reduced systemic vascular resistance and elevated cytokines, secondary to tissue damage. Systemic vascular resistance varies significantly among patients with acute myocardial infarction and cardiogenic shock (AMI-CS). It is typically near normal but can be inappropriately low during vasopressor administration. Mechanistic studies show that inducible nitric oxide synthase production and cytokine cascades from myocardial necrosis can lead to systemic inflammatory responses and vasodilation. End-organ injuries, like ischemic hepatopathy, can also cause vasodilation even without myocardial ischemia. Furthermore, factors such as vasodilatory medications administered in the ICU and heightened infection risks can influence distributive physiology in CS. This may result in coronary hypoperfusion and myocardial depression, particularly in patients with prior heart conditions [5]. Multiple studies have also demonstrated the presence of various inflammatory cytokines, including IL-1β, IL-6, IL-8, TNF-α, and C-reactive protein (CRP), as well as the activation of soluble adhesion molecules and the complement system, during AMI-CS [6–8]. Additionally, the degree of inflammatory markers and lactate levels is strongly associated with the extent of tissue hypoperfusion and the shock duration [9–11]. Moreover, a retrospective evaluation of patients with CS who received MCS found a strong association between the CRP concentrations and 30-day in-hospital mortality, with elevated CRP levels associated with higher mortality regardless of the shock severity [9]. This underlying tissue ischemia and hypoxia can cause endothelial injury, leading to increased vascular permeability, edema, impaired circulation, gut edema with bacterial translocation, and mesenteric ischemia, among the multiple possible pathologies associated with systemic inflammation.

4. Cardiogenic shock clinical features and diagnostic process

The patient presenting with CS exhibits a combination of signs and symptoms indicative of reduced perfusion, including altered mental status, dyspnea, peripheral edema, orthopnea, low blood pressure or hypotension, cold and clammy extremities, and delayed capillary refill, among others. A heightened clinical suspicion is essential, as it can significantly influence management and patient outcomes (**Table 1**). Thus, integrating clinical findings with imaging studies and laboratory results can enhance the assessment of a patient's underlying perfusion status. CS is defined by a sustained decline in cardiac output, resulting in clinical and biochemical evidence of tissue hypoperfusion. The diagnostic process begins with an increased clinical suspicion in patients who display signs or symptoms suggesting

Initial evaluation (SUSPECT)			
Symptoms & signs	Diaphoresis, altered mental status, dyspnea, chest pain, JVD/HJR/Kussmaul, rales/wheezes, lower extremity swelling, etc.		
Urine output [12]	KDIGO 1	KDIGO 2	KDIGO 3
	< 30 ml/h (0.5 ml/kg•h) for 6 consecutive hours	< 30 ml/h (0.5 ml/kg•h) for 12 consecutive hours	<0.3 ml/kg•h for 24 hrs. Or anuria in 12 hrs
Sustained hypotension	SBP <90 mm Hg, MAP <65 mm Hg for>30 minutes or vasopressor need		

Initial evaluation (SUSPECT)				
Perfusion (Abnormalities in renal function [13], liver function test, Troponin, ABG, lactate level [14], and mixed venous saturation)	pH <7.2, metabolic acidosis w/ a lactic acid >2 mmol/L			
	Lactate ≥5 and pH < 7.2	Lactate ≥ 5 and pH > 7.2	Lactate <5 and pH < 7.2	Lactate <5 and ≥ pH 7.2
	ALT >200 U/L or > 3× upper limit of normal			
	Mixed venous oxygen saturation < 50% or Δ- change in arterial saturation 20–30%			
	KDIGO 1	KDIGO 2	KDIGO 3	
	↑SCr ≥1.5–2 from baseline Or ↑SCr ≥ 26 μmol/L in 48 hrs	↑SCr ≥ 2–3 from baseline	↑SCr ≥ 3 from baseline Or ↑SCr ≥ 354 μmol/L Or Need for RRT	
ECG/ECHO (POCUS)	12-Lead ECG		ECHO (POCUS)	
	STT elevations STT depressions RV STT elevations		Ventricular dysfunction (RV, LV, BiV) New wall motion abnormalities	
Congestion (physical evaluation or invasive hemodynamics)	LH-predominant	BiV-predominant	RV-predominant	
	CI < 2.2 CVP <14 mm Hg PCWP >18 mm Hg CVP/PWPC <0.86 PAPi >1.5 LV-CPO < 0.6 RV-CPO > 0.3	CI < 2.2 CVP >14 mm Hg PCWP *Variable* CVP/PWPC >0.86 PAPi >1.5 LV-CPO <0.6 RV-CPO *Variable*	CI < 2.2 CVP >14 mm Hg PCWP <18 mmHg CVP/PWPC >0.86 PAPi <1.5 LV-CPO *Variable* RV-CPO <0.3	
Triage (Shock team activation and/or transfer to higher level of care)	Level 3 Centers capable of initial CS diagnosis, available general cardiology evaluation. However, no PCI or tMCS availability.	Level 2 Centers with onsite interventional and general cardiologist and STEMI and/or PCI with tMCS availability Percutaneous tMCS (Intra-Aortic Balloon Pump (IABP) ± LVAD ±Right Ventricular Assist Device (RVAD))	Level 2 Centers with onsite interventional, general cardiologist, critical care medicine and heart failure cardiologists STEMI and/or PCI with tMCS availability Advanced percutaneous and surgical tMCS	

JVD: jugular vein distention; HJR: hepatojugular reflux; KDIGO: Kidney Disease Improving Global Outcomes; SCr: serum creatine; ALT: alanine transferase; POCUS: point of care ultrasound; CVP: central venous pressure; PCWP: pulmonary capillary wedge pressure; PAPi: pulmonary artery pulsatility index; LV-CPO: left ventricle cardiac power output; RV-CPO: right ventricle cardiac power output; PCI: percutaneous cardiac intervention; tMCD: temporary mechanical cardiac assist device; IABP: Intra-aortic balloon pump LVAD: left ventricular assist devise; RVAD: right ventricular assist devise.

Table 1.
CS initial evaluation.

hypoperfusion or inadequate cardiac output unresponsive to intravascular volume expansion. Key clinical indicators of hypotension include a systolic blood pressure (SBP) of less than 90 mmHg, a mean arterial pressure of less than 60 mmHg, or a drop in SBP of more than 30 mmHg from baseline for at least 30 minutes. Supportive management aims to maintain a 90 mmHg or higher systolic blood pressure. Signs such as narrow pulse pressure (less than 25% of the systolic blood pressure) and oliguria or anuria, with urine production below 30 mL/hour (or 0.5 mL/kg/h), are also significant. Additionally, patients may present subtle clinical manifestations, such as decreased appetite, early satiety, abdominal pain, nausea, or vomiting, which may stem from mesenteric ischemia due to inadequate gastrointestinal perfusion. Supraventricular tachycardia with heart rates exceeding 100 bpm should also raise concern as an early indication of CS.

Regarding physical findings in CS, patients will appear with classic signs and symptoms and new or worsening hypotension, tachypnea, and tachycardia. Most patients will demonstrate a combination of various physical findings, including distended neck veins, coolness of the skin, rales, gallop rhythm, or new heart murmur on examination, and decreased volume and intensity of the distal pulses. The absence of pulmonary congestion at clinical evaluation does not exclude CS and is not associated with a better prognosis in this population. Complicating the situation, the SHOCK trial registry showed that up to a third of the patients failed to demonstrate pulmonary congestion, and 5.2% of patients were normotensive with systolic blood pressures above 90 mm Hg and signs of peripheral hypoperfusion. This cohort of patients showed similar cardiac indices, pulmonary wedge capillary pressures, and left ventricular ejection fractions but demonstrated increased systemic vascular resistance when compared to hypotensive patients with cardiogenic shock. These findings defined "euvolemic CS," underscoring the danger of relative hypotension and the possibility of hypoperfusion occurring without marked hypotension [15]. Euvolemic CS is commonly observed in diuretic-responsive patients with chronic heart failure (HF) experiencing subacute decompensation. In invasive cardiac monitoring, significantly low pulmonary capillary wedge pressure will be observed. This clinical presentation is commonly seen in up to 28% of patients with prior myocardial infarction associated with CS and/or chronic kidney disease. Physical evaluation findings can be variable and will provide insight into which ventricle is primarily involved in cardiogenic shock. For instance, a patient with findings suggestive of right heart failure (isolated hypoperfusion) can arrive with lower extremity swelling, scrotal edema, hepatomegaly, increased jugular vein distention, and regurgitant murmurs in the tricuspid valve area. On the other hand, patients with left-heart failure findings (isolated pulmonary congestion) can present a lung auscultatory combination of rales/crackles/wheezes, displaced cardiac apex, and left-sided heart murmurs. Other patients can demonstrate a combination of right- and left-sided heart failure findings (congestion with hypoperfusion) with cool extremities, cyanosis, orthopnea, and delayed capillary refill, better known as "Mixed-CS."

Laboratory evaluation will substantiate the clinical findings of end-organ hypoperfusion through a comprehensive metabolic panel and arterial blood gases, which will reveal metabolic acidosis (pH < 7.2), elevated lactate levels (>2.0 mmol/L), elevated liver enzymes exceeding three times their upper limit, and elevated renal parameters. Furthermore, additional laboratory data, such as decreased serum sodium levels and elevated cardiac biomarkers like NT-pro-BNP or high-sensitivity troponin, can provide insight into an acute coronary event and clinical prognosis. Other laboratories that require close monitoring in these patients include CBC and CRP. Multiple studies have demonstrated that leukocytosis is a consequence of physical stress; hence, high serum catecholamine levels correlate with the degree of leukocytosis. Moreover, studies evaluating the utility of CRP and white blood cell counts (WBC) retrospectively demonstrate that both markers are equally suitable for prognosis in patients with cardiogenic shock at initial stages [16, 17]. Furthermore, the higher the WBC count (>11.6 × 106/mL) and CRP levels, the higher the 30-day mortality rate from all causes, each becoming an independent predictor of all-cause mortality [18].

All patient signs and symptoms suggestive of shock/hypoperfusion should undergo a baseline 12-lead electrocardiogram to rule out the possibility of an acute coronary event that might warrant interventional cardiology evaluation and early triage by cardiac catheterization evaluation. Besides ECG, which helps diagnose AMI-HF, point-of-care ultrasound (POCUS) has gained popularity recently as an effective diagnostic modality in patients with suspected cardiogenic shock. Both will evaluate and exclude evidence of acute ischemia by 12-lead electrocardiographic changes of ST-segment elevation or echocardiographic evidence of wall motion abnormalities (**Table 1**). In the case of POCUS, it can aid in narrowing the myriad diagnoses that can mimic CS, such as septic shock, massive pulmonary embolism, cardiac tamponade, pneumothorax, severe asthma, or COPD exacerbation. POCUS can be used to determine the overall right and left ventricular (LV) function, presence of pericardial effusions, and noninvasive status. It is easily accessible at the bedside, providing real-time imaging and allowing serial examinations to assess dynamic responses to treatment. Moreover, a meta-analysis of literature reviews to assess the diagnostic accuracy of POCUS for each type of shock concluded that the identification of the etiology of each kind of shock using POCUS was characterized by high sensitivity and positive likelihood ratios, especially for obstructive shock [19]. Furthermore, there have been reports on POCUS's utility in preserving cardiac function and determining the appropriate timing for weaning from ECPELLA management in patients with COVID-19-related myocarditis [20]. On the other hand, invasive procedures are not typically required early in diagnosing and managing patients with an initial suspicion of CS; however, they provide valuable insight into elucidating the congestive profile, ventricular involvement, and differentiating among the various phenotypes to guide treatment. Nevertheless, the utilization of complete hemodynamic data obtained by timely placement of PACs before MCS initiation has been associated with lower mortality in patients with advanced stages of CS [21].

5. Understanding cardiogenic shock, phenotypes, and profiles

CS is an heterogenous condition that manifests through a wide array of clinical presentations with some key critical features: (1) Hemodynamic instability leading to reduced cardiac output and signs of tissue hypoperfusion (e.g., cool extremities, altered mental status); (2) signs and symptoms during presentation may include shortness of breath, chest pain, fatigue, and signs of fluid overload (e.g., edema, jugular venous distention); (3) high mortality rate despite aggressive management (e.g., inodilators, vasopressors, and temporary mechanical assist devices) making prompt recognition and treatment crucial. Furthermore, the heterogeneous presentation, with diverse etiologies, severity, hemodynamic patterns, and clinical profiles, makes diagnosing and staging the condition challenging. Therapeutic options in patients with CS will depend on their comorbidities, underlying disease pathology, disease severity, and type of shock. Over the past two to three decades, significant advances have been made in revascularization strategies and the availability of temporary mechanical assist devices. Nevertheless, inpatient and 30-day hospital mortality in this population has remained high. There is increasing interest in categorizing patients' risk based on observable traits and clinical presentation. Evaluating clinical characteristics to determine phenotypes, combined with staging, is essential for prognostic insights, as phenotypes can be linked to different outcomes. Contemporary data suggest that phenotyping characterization should be based on the underlying etiology, CS pathophysiology, CS severity/acuity, and clinical profiles.

5.1 Phenotyping by CS etiology

The presentation of CS is heterogeneous, with multiple clinical conditions that lead to hemodynamic and biochemical changes that lead to tissue hypoperfusion. The Scientific Expert Panel from the Shock Academic Research Consortium (SHARC). They considered four main factors, such as the underlying cause, setting, timing of the event, and other considerations (e.g., ventricular predominance, hemodynamic subtype, post-cardiac arrest) that would affect or contribute to the clinical scenario. Using these parameters, they defined the etiological profiles or phenotypes into AMI-CS, HF-CS, secondary CS, and post-cardiotomy-CS (**Figure 2**). The AMI-CS will include patients with CS due to AMI with evidence of myocardial ischemia, regardless of whether it is accompanied by electrocardiographic evidence of ST elevations (STEMI vs. NSTEMI), if it complies with the Task Force Universal Definition of myocardial infarction. This definition will include patients developing post-myocardial complications such as symptomatic bradycardias, tachyarrhythmias, mechanical complications, and cardiac arrest. In AMI-CS, clinical presentation and physical exam findings can indicate which ventricle is primarily affected (e.g., as shown in **Figure 3**, LH-CS, Mixed-CS, and RH-CS) [22].

On the other hand, the etiology of heart failure-CS (HF-CS) is related to myocardial dysfunction, which could be ischemic or non-ischemic in etiology. An event can be distinguished as a new onset versus an acute exacerbation in patients with chronic disease based on the patient's baseline hemodynamic status. As in AMI-CS, patients with HF-CS clinical presentation and physical examination findings can provide clues about the ventricle that is primarily involved (e.g., LH-CS, Mixed-CS, and RH-CS) [22].

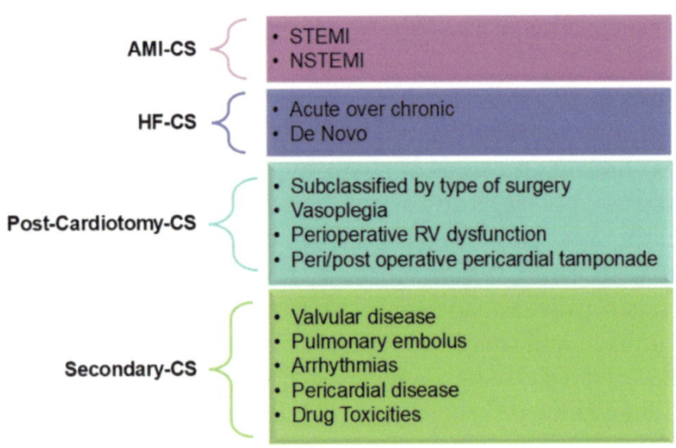

Figure 2.
Cardiogenic shock phenotype by etiology.

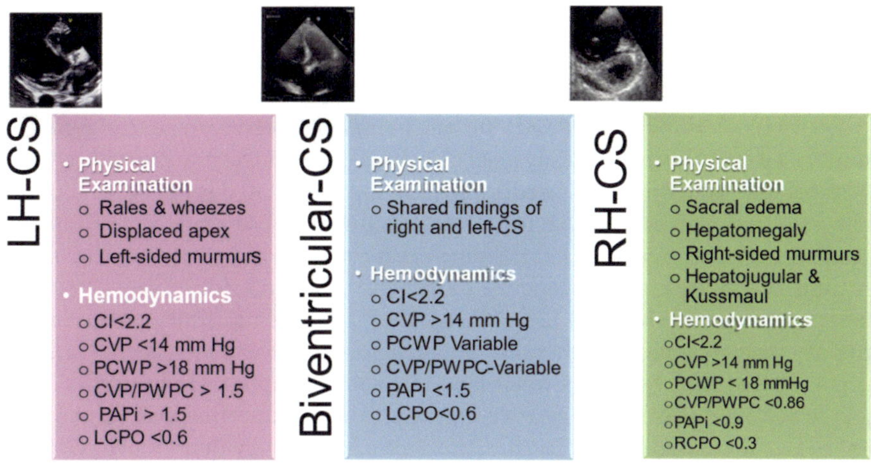

Figure 3.
Cardiogenic shock phenotype by ventricular involvement or pathophysiology.

However, little is known about cardiogenic shock from etiologies other than AMI-CS. Recently, there has been a growing recognition of distinct etiologies related to AMI-induced cardiogenic shock, which are increasingly acknowledged in CS. One of these studies is the Shock Academic Research Consortium (SHARC). This trial evaluated 8974 patients who met shock criteria; 65% experienced CS, 17% had mixed shock, 12% had hypovolemic shock, and 3% had other types of shock. From the patients meeting the CS criteria, distinct phenotypes were observed, each demonstrating unique pathophysiologic characteristics. Furthermore, these phenotypes included different etiologies other than acute myocardial infarction but also persistent left ventricular dysfunction, decompensated heart failure, and shock secondary to arrhythmias or valvular heart disease. In terms of inpatient hospital mortality, the trial demonstrated that the highest inpatient mortality was seen in mixed-CS (48%), followed by AMI-CS (41%), similar in de novo HF-CS (31%) and secondary CS (31%), with the lowest observed in acute-on-chronic HF-CS (25%) [23].

Another condition that could lead to CS is post-cardiotomy syndrome, observed in postoperative patients who show an inability to be weaned from cardiopulmonary bypass after cardiac surgery, resulting in poor perfusion and a low cardiac output state. Clinically, patients exhibit persistent hypotension (SBP < 90 mm Hg), cardiac index (CI) <2.2 L/min/m^2, unresponsiveness to intravascular volume replacement, and signs of impaired end-organ perfusion occurring immediately or within several hours after cardiac surgery. This condition can occur in 0.5–1.5% of cardiac surgeries, with an in-hospital mortality rate of 67% [22, 24, 25].

Finally, the Shock Academy Consortium included the last category as secondary or non-myocardial causes of CS, encompassing many heterogeneous conditions leading to low-output states and poor tissue perfusion. This category includes conditions such as severe valvular heart disease, pericardial diseases, pulmonary hypertension with right ventricular failure, and ongoing refractory incessant arrhythmias not related to tachycardia-induced cardiomyopathy. Nevertheless, it does not include toxic (drug-induced) or septic causes as primary drivers of CS; similarly, it excludes pulmonary hypertension secondary to left-sided heart failure.

5.2 Phenotyping by CS hemodynamic pathophysiology

Traditionally, CS has been classified based on hemodynamic parameters, focusing on measuring cardiac output and systemic vascular resistance. However, this approach often overlooks the underlying mechanisms contributing to the syndrome. For multiple years, the most widely used classification was the one created by Killip and Kimball for stratifying and predicting mortality after 30 days of AMI. It divided patients into four classes based on the clinical findings and severity of pulmonary congestion, presence of a third heart sound, and evidence of hypotension (SBP lower than 90 mm Hg) and evidence of peripheral vasoconstriction (e.g., cyanosis, oliguria, acute mental changes) [26]. In his cohort of patients, 32% were in class 1 (no pulmonary congestion or peripheral hypoperfusion), 38% were in class 2 (isolated pulmonary congestion), 10% were in class 3 (isolated peripheral hypoperfusion), and 19% were in class 4 (both pulmonary congestion and hypoperfusion). Their 30-day mortality rate increased as the classification increased, with values of 6%, 17%, 38%, and 81%, respectively. Another study similarly categorizes the patient's clinical status and invasive hemodynamic findings according to evidence of heart failure after an AMI. The patients were divided into four groups based on both pulmonary capillary wedge pressure (PCWP) and cardiac index (CI). Group 1, labeled "warm-dry," is characterized by CI > 2.0 L/min/m2 and PCWP <20 mmHg. Group 2, termed "cold-dry," includes those with CI ≤ 2.0 L/min/m2 and PCWP <20 mmHg. Group 3, called "warm-wet," is defined by CI > 2.0 L/min/m2 and PCWP ≥20 mmHg. Finally, Group 4, known as "cold-wet," consists of patients with CI ≤ 2.0 L/min/m2 and PCWP ≥20 mmHg [27–29]. However, the patient's clinical presentation can vary significantly, influenced by the underlying etiology, patient comorbidities, and shock duration. Additionally, there has been a recent recognition of the mortality associated with hypoperfusion, regardless of the presence of hypotension, which may be worse than the mortality related to isolated hypotension. In the SHOCK trial, the mortality among the study population varied depending on their groups, with Group A (no pulmonary congestion/no hypoperfusion) and B (isolated pulmonary congestion) showing the lowest inpatient mortality, 21% and 22%, respectively, when compared to groups C (isolated hypoperfusion) and D (congestion with hypoperfusion), which had the in-hospital mortality of 70% and 60% respectively [7, 11, 15].

However, the different etiologies leading to CS can be further subdivided as LV-dominant (LV-CS), RV-dominant (RV-CS), or biventricular shock (BiV-CS) based on clinical presentation and hemodynamic data obtained through direct pulmonary catheterization. By using this classification framework, each type can be treated optimally with different management strategies, which can ultimately improve perfusion (**Figure 2**). LV-CS is characterized by elevated PCWP, normal or reduced central venous pressure (CVP), and reduced LV function. On the other hand, RV-CS is characterized by elevated CVP, normal to low PCWP, and near-normal LV systolic performance. Finally, BiV-CS is characterized by elevated CVP, elevated PCWP, and reduced LV performance. Besides the direct PAC hemodynamic measures, there are other PAC-derived measures like the pulmonary artery pulsatility index (PAPi), the right atrial pressure, the pulmonary capillary wedge pressure ratio (CVP/PCWP ratio), and the cardiac power output. These measures have been instrumental in refining the acute management and decision-making process for the use of transient MCD (**Table 2**). The PAPi provides a hemodynamic measure of the right ventricular function. PAPi is derived from the formula: (systolic pulmonary arterial pressure – diastolic pulmonary pressure)/right atrial pressure. It serves as a prognostic

PAC-derived hemodynamic parameters		
Systemic Vascular Resistance (SVR) SVR = (MAP-CVP)/(CO*80)		• Normal range: 800–1200 dyne-s/cm5.
Pulmonary Vascular Resistance (PVR) PVR = 80(mPAP-PCWP)/(CO)		• Normal range: 24–160 dyne-sec/cm5. • Normal range: 0.3–2.0 Wood units (=PVR/80).
Pulmonary artery pulsatility index PAPi = (PA pulse pressure)/CVP	• Provides a more specific measure for RV dysfunction than the ratio of filling pressures (CVP/PCWP >0.86). • A strong predictor of severe RV failure after MI. • A potential indicator of benefit from right ventricular support.	• Normal PAPi is >2. • PAPi of 1–2 is worrisome. • PAPi <0.9 Overt RV failure.
CVP/PCWP	• Provides an idea of RV function.	• CVP ≈ ½PCWP (normal CVP/PCWP ratio < 0.5). • CVP/PCWP >0.6–0.8 suggests predominant RV failure.
Cardiac power output LV-CPO = (MAP*CO)/451 RV-CPO = (mean PAP-CVP)(CO)/451	• LV-CPO is an index of LV function. • LV-CPO is a strong predictor of mortality in CS.	• Normal CPO: ~0.8–1.1 Watts. • LV-CPO <0.6 (predictor of in-hospital mortality and need for mechanical support). • RV-CPO <0.3 Watts. • The optimal RCPO may vary depending on the context CS phenotype.

CVP: central venous pressure; PCWP: pulmonary capillary wedge pressure; PAPi: pulmonary artery pulsatility index; LV-CPO: left ventricle cardiac power output; RV-CPO: right ventricle cardiac power output.

Table 2.
Pulmonary arterial catheter derived hemodynamic parameters.

marker to determine the risk of all-cause mortality, major adverse cardiac events, and heart failure hospitalization. Additionally, it has been shown to be useful in predicting right ventricular failure in patients with acute inferior wall infarction and patients undergoing left ventricular assist device (LVAD) implant [28, 30]. Another PAC-derived measure is the CVP/PCWP ratio, which is also used as a clinical indicator of right ventricular function. In a patient with preserved RV systolic performance, the CVP/PCWP ratio is 1:2; however, when RV dysfunction ensues, the RAP will start to rise slowly, leading to a change in the 1:2 ratio, suggesting progressive dysfunction [31]. An increased CVP/PWCP is associated with reduced RV performance and higher pulmonary vascular resistance, thus leading to adverse outcomes [32]. Furthermore, it has also been associated with impaired renal function and can be used as a preoperative predictor surrogate to determine postoperative outcomes in patients with advanced heart failure referred for left ventricular assist device (LVAD) implant [33]. Lastly, the cardiac power output (CPO) and cardiac output index (CPI) are crucial hemodynamic parameters used in the management of patients with CS. They reflect the hydraulic energy delivered by the ventricles. The LV-CPO is derived from the mean arterial pressure (MAP) and cardiac output (CO), and the RV-CPO is derived from mean pulmonary arterial pressure (mPAP) minus the right atrial pressures (CVP) multiplied by the CO. In the Shock trial registry, the LV-CPO showed a strong correlation with inpatient mortality, patient age, and females, demonstrating a higher mortality among this cohort of patients with CPO values of <0.6 [34].

5.3 Phenotyping by hemodynamic and severity profile

In 2019, the Society for Cardiovascular Angiography and Interventions (SCAI) multidisciplinary committee formulated an expert consensus statement to create a standardized classification using vasopressors, inotropes, and acute mechanical circulatory support devices during CS hospitalization. This scheme categorizes patients into five stages (A to E), ranging from "at risk" to "in extremis" with CS (**Figure 4**). Early stages of shock, like pre-shock and shock, are generally more amenable to treatment than late-stage shock, linked to irreversible organ failure and death. This classification scheme is a straightforward tool requiring no calculations and enhances communication among clinicians and researchers regarding patients with CS. The SCAI Shock Classification also establishes a management framework for patients with or at risk for CS. For each SCAI shock stage, specific assessment and management strategies can be tailored to the severity of the condition. This framework enhances clarity in discussing patient status, offers new insights into the trajectories of hospitalized CS patients, and allows clinical trials to differentiate subsets of patients with CS appropriately. The CS Working Group plays a crucial role in this research, substantially enhancing our understanding of CS. Their registry has clarified SCAI clinical profiles using data from seventeen hospitals that enrolled CS patients between 2016 and 2021 [29]. The registry documented clear indicators of hypotension, hypoperfusion, and treatment intensity, verifying their link to mortality. It also established formal criteria for each stage, improving our capability to assess the relationship between baseline and maximum stages and mortality outcomes. Out of 3455 patients involved during the study, heart failure (52%) and myocardial infarction (32%) were the primary causes of CS. The overall mortality rate for the cohort was 35%, notably higher among those with myocardial infarction, out-of-hospital cardiac arrests, and those receiving multiple drugs and devices. Since 2019, this classification has been widely utilized in the management of patients with CS in order to determine their risk across the disease spectrum. Furthermore, the combination of different staging with pH and lactic acid levels and laboratory data can provide insight into the CS severity and inpatient mortality prediction, serving as a risk modifier for the SCAI classification [35].

5.4 Machine-based learning clinical profile

CS heterogeneity encompasses more than illness severity and mortality risk factors, even with various staging and risk assessment systems for stratifying patients with similar SCAI classification. Machine-based learning (MBL) can enhance precision and unbiased medicine by matching treatment to patients based on six (6) distinct baseline variables: Glomerular filtration rate (GFR), Alanine aminotransferase (ALT), lactate, bicarbonate (HCO3), platelets, and WBC count, as seen in **Figure 5** [36]. By evaluating whether CS phenotypes possess distinctive clinical profiles using MBL, following a consensus clustering analysis, clear clusters of hospitalized CS were identified. This parameter identified three clinical phenotypes

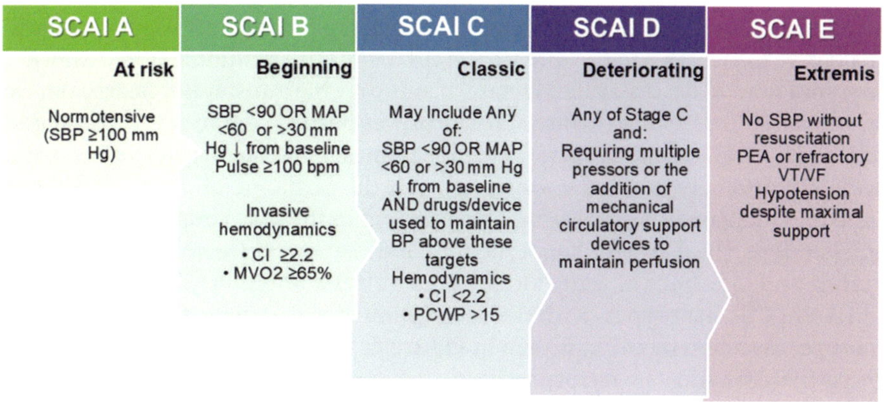

Figure 4.
Cardiogenic shock phenotype according to severity and hemodynamic profile.

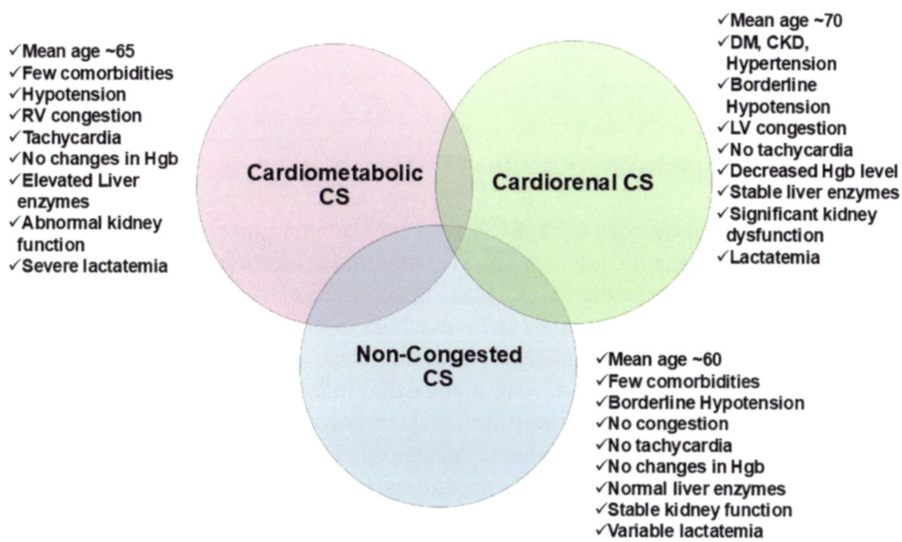

Figure 5.
Cardiogenic shock phenotype using clinical profile and machine-based learning.

(non-congested, cardiorenal, and cardiometabolic or hemometabolic shock) with specific clinical characteristics and associated outcomes, regardless of whether the event was AMI-CS or HF-CS, acute vs. chronic. Key features used to differentiate the phenotypes of CS upon admission included blood pressure (SBP, MBP, and DBP), kidney function (creatinine, BUN, and eGFR), electrolytes (potassium and bicarbonate), liver function (total protein and albumin), RBC-associated indicators (RBC count and RDW), and several scoring systems (SOFA, APS III, and APACHE IV). The non-congested phenotype exhibited lower heart rate, filling pressures (right atrial and pulmonary capillary wedge pressures), and a higher blood pressure relative to the other phenotypes, representing a stable profile. The cardiorenal-CS phenotype includes older patients with multiple comorbidities. These patients will exhibit a lower heart rate, elevated pulmonary arterial and pulmonary capillary wedge pressures, and a lower glomerular filtration rate, suggesting renal involvement from shock, and are less likely to be referred for temporary mechanical supports requiring palliative measures. On the other hand, patients with cardiometabolic shock phenotypes tend to have elevated lactate, alanine aminotransferase, heart rate, right atrial pressure, low blood pressure, cardiac power output, and index. This suggested a multiorgan involvement, featured by transaminases and lactic acidosis in a patient with CS. Additionally, it was demonstrated that the cardiometabolic CS phenotype had a 4-fold increase in mortality when compared to the non-congested CS phenotype. Therefore, the distinct phenotypes of CS show varying hospital mortality, ICU mortality, and incidence of acute kidney injury after admission [37]. A diagram with the different CS phenotypes, with the description of the patients that fall in each phenotype, as shown by MBL, is seen in **Figure 4**. Further studies were also able to replicate these findings by retrospectively analyzing patients admitted with CS and providing their CS phenotypes. Concluding that MBL could help identify phenotypes in a mixed-CS population, showing good discrimination of in-hospital all-cause mortality. Furthermore, using this cohort of patients demonstrates that MBL CS phenotypes are compatible with SCAI CS classification and provide an additional predictive value when both methods are used together. Moreover, it has been shown that different phenotypes can be associated with varying choices of acute mechanical assist devices [38].

6. Tailoring management strategies

Clinical factors, laboratory tests, ECG, and cardiac imaging should supplement patients' initial hypotension assessment. This should include evaluating signs/symptoms, assessing urine output, confirming evidence of sustained hypotension for >30 minutes, and evaluating perfusion markers of end-organ hypoperfusion [39]. Once the phenotype is established, treatment can be tailored accordingly. For example, patients with CS secondary to myocardial infarction may be managed with percutaneous coronary intervention (PCI) or coronary artery bypass grafting (CABG). In contrast, patients with heart failure-related CS might respond better to pharmacological therapies, such as vasodilators or inotropes like dobutamine. Furthermore, some patients might require a combination of pharmacological and mechanical interventions, depending on the CS pathophysiology and hemodynamics. Despite the increasing use of invasive therapies in CS, evidence-based treatment regimens that are known to improve outcomes are limited, and these patients require palliative care evaluation for further support and management. **Figure 6** shows a summary of the information discussed in the section below.

6.1 Pharmacotherapy

The management of CS should be tailored to the individual patient, considering the underlying cause and overall clinical condition. Early recognition and prompt treatment are critical for improving outcomes in patients with this life-threatening condition. Pharmacologic medical management is essential for stabilizing the patient while reducing pulmonary congestion, if present, and improving cardiac output and tissue perfusion. This management aims to optimize the determinants of cardiac output, including preload, afterload, contractility, and heart rate. In CS medical therapy management, inotropes and vasopressors serve as the primary cornerstone

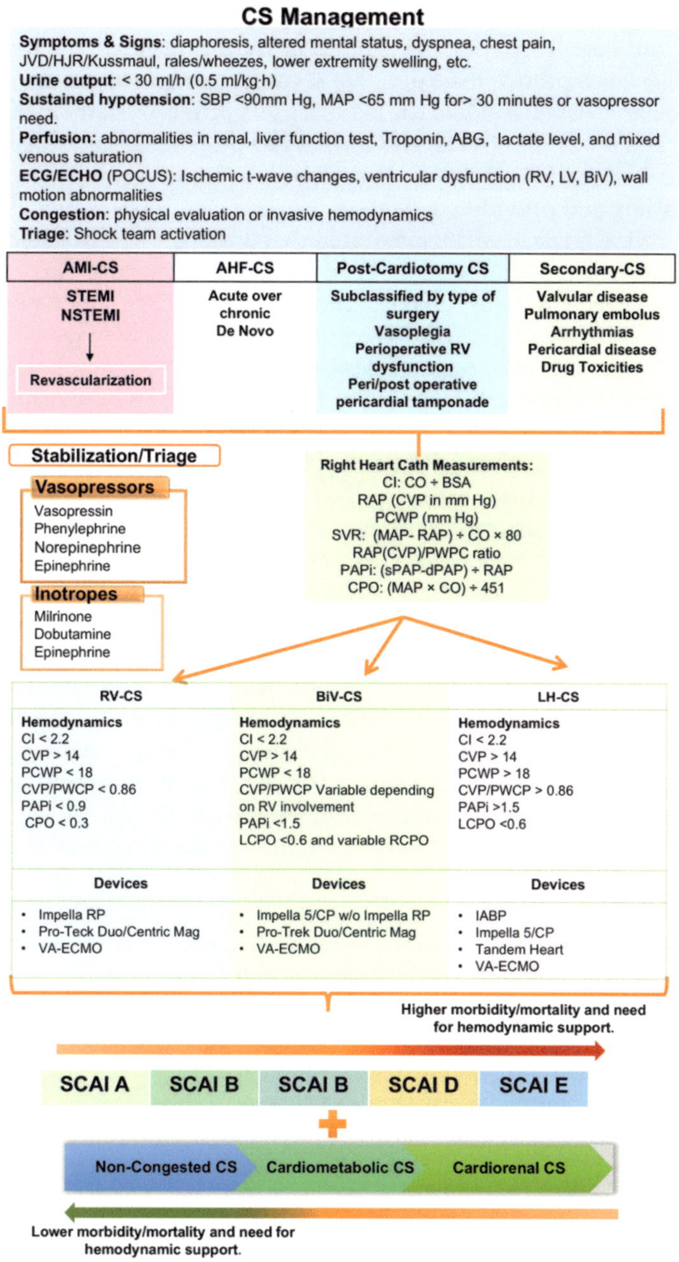

Figure 6.
Cardiogenic shock clinical management.

therapies. The indication for their use will depend highly on the patient's clinical status, degree of organ hypoperfusion, and disease progression. The most used agents are the cardiac calcitropes (catecholamines and PDE3 inhibitors); these medications are known to increase myocardial force production by altering the concentration of intracellular Ca^{2+} [40]. They are characterized mainly by their action on specific myocardial receptors rather than their effect on vascular tone, chronotropic response, and cardiac performance. The catecholamine calcitropes are dobutamine, dopamine, epinephrine, and norepinephrine, all exhibiting varying degrees of α and β receptor activity. The α receptors induce peripheral vasoconstriction, thereby increasing systemic vascular resistance, while the β-1 receptors primarily demonstrate positive chronotropic and inotropic effects, and the β-2 receptors act as vasodilators. These drugs alleviate symptoms and may be beneficial in acute shock, facilitating bridging to transplantation, and providing palliation. Nevertheless, observational cohorts and randomized clinical trials have demonstrated that prolonged use of catecholamines and phosphodiesterase-3 inhibitors is linked to increased mortality in patients with CS, believed to be secondary to enhanced intracellular calcium concentration [40]. Thus, the AHA/ACC/HFSA guidelines recommendations for management of CS provided a class 1 indication [41]. Nevertheless, ESC's main recommendations stressed the early CS identification and treatment of inciting events and the management of organ dysfunction and considered inotropes/vasopressors if organ hypoperfusion deteriorates despite management (Class 2b) [42].

Dobutamine is one of the most prescribed agents for increasing contractility during CS. This intravenous drug is a synthetic catecholamine that primarily stimulates β1 and α1 receptors, showing a weak affinity for β2 receptors. It directly regulates mean arterial pressure by enhancing cardiac output, albeit at the cost of stroke volume and heart rate. Low doses (5 mcg/kg/min) can trigger a mild vasodilatory effect through α1-receptors but can cause intense vasoconstriction at higher doses [40, 43].

Milrinone is a non-catecholamine calcitropic that works through inhibition of PDE3, thus decreasing cAMP degradation, mimicking β1 and β2 effects with increased intracellular calcium. Milrinone and dobutamine are used as inotropes to improve myocardial contractility. However, the DOREMI trial showed no significant differences in cardiovascular or renal outcomes between the two inotropes [44]. Nevertheless, a subsequent meta-analysis demonstrated a substantial benefit of milrinone over dobutamine in patients with AHF with or without CS [45, 46]. However, in the OPTIME-CHF trial, milrinone showed a deleterious impact in patients with ischemic etiology and no clear evidence of hypoperfusion, with worse outcomes on the composite of death and 60-day rehospitalization (42 vs. 36%, $P = 0.01$) [47]. Another type of inodilator commonly used in Europe is Levosimendan. This medication works by increasing the sensitivity of troponin C to calcium, thus facilitating the interaction between actin and myosin without affecting the myocardial oxygen consumption. Furthermore, Levosimendan causes vasodilation by stimulating the ATP-sensitive potassium channels in the mitochondria [48]. In multiple meta-analyses, Levosimendan demonstrated a trend toward improved survival compared to other inotropes [49].

In cases where patients with CS show intractable hypotension or mixed type-CS, a vasopressor effect is required. The AHA/ACC and ESC guidelines recommend Norepinephrine (NE) as a first-line agent for maintaining blood pressure in shock states [41, 42]. NE is an endogenous catecholamine synthesized, stored, and released from sympathetic neurons [50]. This drug has strong alpha-1 and beta-1 adrenergic effects. It is infused at 0.02–1 micrograms/kg/min with tapering starting at 0.1 micrograms/kg/min with a half-life of 5–10 minutes. It is associated with side effects such as tachycardia, myocardial ischemia, and tachyarrhythmias. Nevertheless, because of its short half-life, symptoms can be easily controlled by lowering the dose. When compared to dopamine, norepinephrine showed potential vasopressor advantages as seen in a meta-analysis of multiple randomized controlled trials; norepinephrine was associated with a lower 28-day mortality, a lower risk of cardiac arrhythmias (e.g., atrial fibrillation, ventricular tachycardia, ventricular fibrillation), and gastrointestinal side effects. Furthermore, this effect was not associated with the type of cardiogenic shock (AMI-CS vs. AHF-CS) [51].

Epinephrine is a naturally occurring catecholamine that binds to β1, β2, and α1 adrenergic receptors, causing increased cardiac output and peripheral vasoconstriction. This drug is especially crucial in cardiac arrest situations and is linked to a high 30-day survival rate among this cohort of patients. Nevertheless, its utility in CS is mainly as a rescue medication for intractable hypotension, which is poorly responsive to other drugs when additional cardiac output and blood pressure support are needed [40]. The recommended dosages in CS range from 0.01 to 0.3 micrograms/kg/min. However, it has been shown to have deleterious effects due to its α1-mediated increase in systemic vascular resistance through its effect on the right ventricular and pulmonary pressures. Moreover, it increases the myocardial oxygen demand with an increase in heart rate through its β1-effect. High, prolonged doses (>0.3–0.05 micrograms/kg/min) have been associated with direct cardiac toxicity, arterial wall damage, and myocyte apoptosis stimulation [52].

While diuretics are not a primary treatment for cardiogenic shock, they may be used to manage fluid overload and pulmonary congestion, particularly in patients with a congestive phenotype. Failure to address congestion will lead to microcirculatory ischemia and multiple organ failure. Hesitation and concern usually arise when the use of diuretics in conjunction with vasopressors is being contemplated, mostly due to the risk vs. benefit effects of the combination therapy. However, a recent study using a population of critically ill patients admitted to the ICU receiving >6 hours of vasopressor therapy and treated with diuretics for management of volume overload demonstrated that the use of diuretics is effective to increase urine output, without increasing the vasopressor dose, potentially reducing hospital mortality [52]. Furthermore, the patients receiving diuretics did not have an increased risk of developing acute kidney injury or requiring more renal replacement therapies. Therefore, highlighting the positive effects, the addition of diuretics to the critically ill patients who meet the criteria for diuretic therapy [52].

6.2 Temporary mechanical assist device

Temporary mechanical assist devices are employed to manage patients experiencing severe heart failure or CS or to provide support during high-risk procedures that necessitate short-term hemodynamic assistance. They are designed to improve cardiac output, stabilize hemodynamic parameters, and afford sufficient time for recovery or implement additional durable interventions, especially when managing patients with a classification of CS SCAI B and above. The choice of device indications depends on the clinical scenario, patient characteristics, and the underlying cause of cardiogenic shock or heart failure. The decision on the appropriate tMCD will depend on the type (LV-CS, BiV-CS, and RV-CS) and phenotypic presentation. The decision process will involve a combination of findings depending on the patient's clinical condition, laboratory data, hemodynamic parameters, echo (POCUS) findings, and goals of care (**Figure 5**).

In cases where left ventricular support is needed, it is indicated when there is evidence of a cardiac index (CI) less than 2.2, a central venous pressure (CVP) greater than 0.86, and a pulmonary artery pulsatility index (PAPi) of less than 1.5. The choice of the most appropriate device will depend on the patient's SCAI staging, phenotypic presentation, and the degree of hypoperfusion. The most universally known temporary mechanical device is the Intra-Aortic Balloon Pump (IABP), which reduces the workload through a balloon that inflates and deflates in coordination with the cardiac cycle, thus supporting the patient hemodynamically and also decreasing the ischemic burden in patients with refractory ischemia and severe coronary artery disease. This device has been researched for acute myocardial infarction with cardiogenic shock (AMI-CS). Studies, including the Gusto 1 trial, indicate that early intra-aortic balloon pump (IABP) placement can reduce mortality at 30 days and 12 months. However, more recent studies have not demonstrated the same benefits and have shown no significant advantages in mortality rates at the 30-day or 12-month mark [53]. Multiple meta-analyses and old National Registry of Myocardial Infarction studies have further substantiated these findings. Thus, the AHA/ACC guideline recommendations for AMI-CS provided a recommendation class 2a, and the ESC guidelines provided a 2b recommendation of IABP on this population [41, 42].

Two types of temporary ventricular assist devices (VADs) are also used for LV-CS whenever higher LV support is required: pulsatile or continuous-flow devices. The Impella® is a short-term VAD with a micro axial flow pump built into the tip of a catheter and uses the Archimedes screw theory to mimic the natural blood flow through the blood vessels [54]. When used for left ventricular support, it is inserted percutaneously through the femoral artery and passed retrogradely through the aortic valve to provide LV support. Previous trials comparing Impella® and IABP in AMI-CS patients have demonstrated better hemodynamic parameters, including cardiac index, cardiac output, and mean arterial pressure in Impella® patients; however, acute mortality rates were similar between the two devices [55–57].

On the other hand, another type of transient MCD required in patients with severe hemodynamic deterioration of LV parameters or whenever escalation of hemodynamic support is required is the Tandem Heart®. This device is a percutaneously implanted centrifugal pump capable of providing a flow of 5 L/min at a maximum rate of 7500 rpm through a transeptal cannula that provides left atrial blood to the systemic circulation (femoral artery), effectively unloading the left ventricle. The THEME registry showed that using Tandem Heart® is associated with early lactate clearance, improvement in cardiac index, and favorable 30-day (74%) and 180-day (66%) survival [58]. In a retrospective analysis of the National Inpatient Sample 2017 database, a comparison of both temporary ventricular assist devices (Impella® and Tandem Heart®) found that cardiogenic shock mortality remains high despite using these devices. Nevertheless, the mortality was higher in the cohort of patients who received mechanical support with Impella® [59].

Finally, Veno-arterial Extracorporeal Membrane Oxygenation (VA ECMO) circuits comprise a venous (inflow, drainage) cannula, a pump, an oxygenator, and an arterial (outflow, return) cannula [60]. This configuration can be initiated using either peripheral or central access. It offers cardiac and respiratory support by pumping blood through an artificial lung (membrane oxygenator) outside the body and returning it to the patient. It is primarily used for patients in SCAI E, providing oxygenation and support for those with severe cardiac and respiratory failure. It is indicated for patients experiencing refractory cardiogenic shock, severe respiratory failure, or as a temporary solution while awaiting recovery, transplantation, or other definitive therapies. A large meta-analysis with 12,756 patients with CS demonstrated that using ECMO can prolong the therapeutic window, thus allowing the heart to recover. In this cohort of patients, the inpatient mortality was 62%, with age, presence of infection, and shorter duration of ECMO support directly associated with in-hospital mortality [60]. ECMO-treated patients often develop complications, some of them serious, like renal failure requiring renal replacement therapy and bleeding. Conversely, a systematic review and meta-analysis of propensity-matched/adjusted observational trials of Impella® versus VA ECMO in CS suggest that Impella® is associated with better short-term survival and results in fewer bleeding events requiring transfusions [61].

On the other hand, in patients with RV-CS (*CI < 2.2, CVP/PWPC < 0.86, and PAPi < 0.9)*, in which additional support for the right ventricle is required, other devices need to be used. One of those is the Impella-RP®, which is indicated in scenarios of CS with a main profile of right heart failure, such as in acute inferior MI and acute pulmonary embolism, among others [62]. This device is inserted percutaneously into the femoral vein with its inlet port in the right atrium-inferior vena cava junction. The impeller will displace the blood through the outflow cannula in the pulmonary artery, allowing an output of 4 L/min. A sub-analysis of the IMP-IT Registry revealed that the Impella® device demonstrates favorable survival outcomes in patients with right ventricular-predominant cardiogenic shock [63]. Nonetheless, complications associated with the device are typical and must be thoughtfully evaluated when opting to escalate care to the Impella®. Another device when higher RV support is required is the Protek Duo Right Ventricular Assist Device (RVAD) [64]. It is an extracorporeal continuous-flow pump that provides a centrifugal flow of up to 4.5 L/min. It is indicated when there is higher RV support for management of RV-CS in acute inferior MI with right ventricular involvement, post-cardiotomy with right ventricular failure, s/p left ventricular assist device placement (LVAD) with RV failure after implant, and heart transplant patients.

The CentriMag Circulatory Support System is designed for use with a cardiopulmonary or other extracorporeal bypass circuit. It provides temporary circulatory support for up to 30 days for the support of LV, RV, or both sides of the heart. This system is intended for post-cardiotomy patients who are unable to wean off cardiopulmonary bypass, serving as a bridge to help determine whether the patient's heart will recover or if alternative, long-term therapy will be necessary. A meta-analysis of the CentriMag device has shown that it offers effective temporary cardiac and cardiopulmonary support for patients experiencing cardiogenic shock (CS). The use of this device has been linked to improved survival rates in various conditions: 82% for patients with pericardiotomy-related CS, 63% for postcardiotomy-related CS, 62% for transplant rejection or failure, and 83% for right ventricular failure following left ventricular assist device (LVAD) placement [65].

ECMO is reserved for patients with a potentially reversible underlying etiology in cases with refractory RV-CS. This device can help manage hypoxemia from pulmonary failure while supporting the right ventricle, reducing preload and RV wall tension while delivering oxygenated blood flow to the coronary circulation [66]. However, clinical studies failed to demonstrate differences in clinical outcomes between ECMO use and conservative management. ECMO demonstrated a significant reduction in 30-day mortality rates, with a rate of 38.5% compared to 47.9% for Levosimendan. The risk ratio (RR) was calculated at 0.76, accompanied by a 95% confidence interval of 0.63–0.90 ($p < 0.001$). However, ECMO was linked to a higher incidence of complications, including bleeding (23.4% versus 12.7%) and infections (18.9% compared to 10.5%) [14].

Finally, in patients with BiV-CS *(CI < 2.2, variable CVP/PWPC, and PAPi < 1.5)*, a combination of devices that will provide support on both ventricles will be used, depending on their clinical, hemodynamic, and perfusion status. Furthermore, each device has potential complications, including infection, bleeding, vascular injury, and malfunction. Patients with these devices require close monitoring in an intensive care setting to assess hemodynamic status and manage complications.

6.3 Cardiogenic shock teams

The management of cardiogenic shock focuses on restoring adequate cardiac output, improving tissue perfusion, and addressing the underlying cause of the shock. For instance, patients with CS due to acute myocardial infarction may benefit from immediate revascularization, while those with heart failure may require diuretics and inotropic support. In 2019, the National Shock Initiative demonstrated that using shock protocols to manage patients admitted with AMI-CS improved clinical outcomes, emphasizing their use as best clinical practice for early transient MCS in patients presenting with AMI-CS treated with PCI [13, 14]. Nevertheless, CS mortality has not been significantly impacted despite the multiple advances seen in previous years with reperfusion therapies and temporary mechanical assist devices. One approach is to utilize a shock team with protocols that facilitate and guide multidisciplinary team interactions, allowing for earlier diagnosis and management of a patient with hypotension. To date, the use of cardiac shock care centers to improve outcomes in CS is well established [67].

If cardiogenic shock is the primary diagnosis, this team will include or obtain support from providers specializing in heart failure, interventional cardiology, critical care, cardiovascular surgery, and perfusion services [68]. This team serves as a backbone, offering emergency consultation to healthcare providers offering direct care to critical patients. This type of management may encompass early pharmacological interventions (e.g., inotropes, vasopressors), mechanical support (e.g., intra-aortic balloon pump, ventricular assist devices), and revascularization procedures (e.g., angioplasty, coronary artery bypass grafting) as appropriate, based on the patient's diagnosis. The phenotype-based approach to managing CS consists of multiple key components: accurate diagnosis, targeted interventions, and continuous reassessment of the patient's condition [69].

6.4 Continuous reassessment

The dynamic nature of cardiogenic shock needs continuous monitoring and reassessment of the patient's condition. Regular evaluation of hemodynamic parameters, clinical symptoms, and laboratory values is crucial for assessing the effectiveness of interventions and making timely adjustments to the management plan. Clinical examination, laboratories, and hemodynamic measures should be performed as often as 2–4 hours during the critical phase and may be spaced out to 6–8 hours once patients stabilize. This interactive process ensures that care remains aligned and updated to meet the patient's evolving needs and requirements, bearing in mind decisions to escalate or de-escalate treatment as needed, including the possibility of palliative care and/or hospice. Close attention should be kept on complications related to device lines and access that might suggest limb ischemia, bleeding, etc.

7. Implications for patient outcomes

Adopting a phenotype-based approach to CS management can significantly improve patient outcomes. For example, examination of the rates of MCS utilization, associated factors, and clinical outcomes in patients with HF-CS and AMI-CS using data from the National Inpatient Sample spanning 2016 to 2020 revealed increased MCS utilization during the study period, with variations across devices and CS phenotypes. Among this patient cohort, AMI-CS exhibited higher rates of IABP (32.4 vs. 8.9%), VA ECMO (2.8 vs. 2.4%), and percutaneous ventricular assist device usage (14.5 vs. 8.1%) when compared to HF-CS ($p < 0.01$). Notably, factors associated with lower MCS utilization included being female, aged over 60 years, black patients, having atrial fibrillation, chronic obstructive pulmonary disease, diabetes mellitus, cirrhosis, a history of stroke, or prior myocardial infarction. After adjusting for various factors, patients with HF-CS had significantly better outcomes compared to those with AMI-CS, experiencing fewer adverse events such as inpatient death, stroke, tracheostomy, mechanical ventilation, and blood transfusion. However, HF-CS was associated with higher odds of acute renal failure requiring dialysis. Patients with AMI-CS had shorter hospital stays (8.8 vs. 15.0 days, $p < 0.001$), incurred lower charges ($251,580 vs. $294,792, $p < 0.001$), and were less likely to be discharged home. Overall, the study indicated that CS patients continue to face high rates of morbidity and mortality. The underlying etiology of shock significantly influences outcomes, with AMI cases showing more severe complications. This underscores the necessity for a standardized approach that accounts for etiology, individual patient factors, care availability, and equitable access [64]. By personalizing treatment strategies, clinicians can target specific mechanisms contributing to shock, enhance interventions' efficacy, and minimize adverse effects. Furthermore, this approach fosters a more comprehensive understanding of the disease, facilitating better communication among healthcare providers and improving interdisciplinary collaboration.

Research indicates that tailored management strategies can reduce mortality rates, shorten hospital stays, and improve the quality of life for patients recovering from cardiogenic shock. As healthcare systems increasingly emphasize value-based care, implementing phenotype-based approaches aligns with delivering high-quality and patient-centered care.

8. Conclusion

Cardiogenic shock remains a daunting challenge in clinical practice, given its complexity and the variability in patient presentations. A phenotype-based approach to management offers a promising strategy for enhancing patient care by tailoring interventions to the specific characteristics of individual patients. The CS phenotypes do not provide a one-size-fits-all but are rather interactive and supplement one another. As we strengthen our comprehension of cardiogenic shock and its core mechanisms, adopting this new paradigm is crucial for better outcomes and more effective management of this critical condition. By progressing beyond conventional, one-size-fits-all treatment protocols, we can develop a more nuanced and practical approach to cardiogenic shock, benefiting patients and healthcare systems.

Conflict of interest

The content of this publication does not represent the views of the VA Healthcare System, the Department of Veterans Affairs, or the United States. The authors declare no conflict of interest.

Author details

Ingrid Bonilla-Mercado[1], Francisco Merced-Ortiz[2] and Sonia I. Vicenty-Rivera[2*]

1 VA Caribbean Healthcare System, San Juan, Puerto Rico

2 Bruce W. Carter, Miami VA Healthcare System, Miami, FL, United States

*Address all correspondence to: sonia.vicentyrivera@va.gov

References

[1] van Diepen S, Katz JN, Albert NM, et al. Contemporary management of cardiogenic shock: A scientific statement from the American Heart Association. Circulation. 2017;**136**(16):e232-e268. DOI: 10.1161/CIR.0000000000000525

[2] Jentzer JCA, Baran DA. The changing face of cardiogenic shock: Definitions, epidemiology, and severity assessment. Current Opinion in Critical Care. 2023;**29**(4):363-370. DOI: 10.1097/MCC.0000000000001065

[3] Stavrou VT, Vavougyios GD, Tsirimona G, Boutlas S, Santo M, Hadjigeorgiou G, et al. The effects of 4-week respiratory muscle training on cardiopulmonary parameters and cognitive function in male patients with OSA. Applied Sciences. 2025;**15**(5):2532. DOI: 10.3390/app15052532

[4] Riese H, Oosterom E, Ormel J, Altemus M, Benjamini Y, Bouma E, et al. No associations between single nucleotide polymorphisms in corticoid receptor genes and heart rate and cortisol responses to a standardized social stress test in adolescents: The TRAILS study. Behavior Genetics. 2011;**41**:253-261. DOI: 10.1007/s10519-010-9385-6

[5] Wildhirt SM, Dudek RR, Suzuki H, Bing RJ. Involvement of inducible nitric oxide synthase in the inflammatory process of myocardial infarction. International Journal of Cardiology. 1995;**50**:253-261

[6] Shpektor A. Cardiogenic shock: The role of inflammation. Acute Cardiac Care. 2010;**12**(4):115-118. DOI: 10.3109/17482941.2010.523705

[7] Hochman JS, Sleeper LA, Webb JG, Sanborn TA, White HD, Talley JD, et al. Early revascularization in acute myocardial infarction complicated by cardiogenic SHOCK. SHOCK investigators. Should we emergently revascularize occluded coronaries for cardiogenic shock. The New England Journal of Medicine. 1999;**341**:625-634. DOI: 10.1056/NEJM199908263410901

[8] Kohsaka S, Menon V, Lowe AM, Lange M, Dzavik V, Sleeper LA, et al. SHOCK investigators systemic inflammatory response syndrome after acute myocardial infarction complicated by cardiogenic shock. Archives of Internal Medicine. 2005;**165**(14):1643-1650. DOI: 10.1001/archinte.165.14.1643

[9] Dettling A, Weimann J, Sundermeyer J, Beer BN, Besch L, Becher PM, et al. Association of systemic inflammation with shock severity, 30-day mortality, and therapy response in patients with cardiogenic shock. Clinical Research in Cardiology: Official Journal of the German Cardiac Society. 2024;**113**(2):324-335. DOI: 10.1007/s00392-023-02336-8

[10] Frangogiannis NG, Smith CW, Entman ML. The inflammatory response in myocardial infarction. Cardiovascular Research. 2002;**53**(31):47

[11] Hochman JS. Cardiogenic shock complicating acute myocardial infarction: Expanding the paradigm. Circulation. 2003;**107**(24):2998-3002. DOI: 10.1161/01.CIR.0000075927.67673.F2

[12] Hilton R. Defining acute renal failure. CMAJ. 2011;**183**(10):1167-1169. DOI: 10.1503/cmaj.081170

[13] Basir MB, Kapur NK, Patel K, et al. Improved outcomes associated with the

use of shock protocols: Updates from the National Cardiogenic Shock Initiative. Catheterization and Cardiovascular Interventions. 2019;**93**(7):1173-1183. DOI: 10.1002/ccd.28307

[14] Pereira S, Santos M. ECMO vs. Levosimendan in the treatment of cardiogenic shock: A Meta-analysis with perspectives for Latin America. Journal of the Society for Cardiovascular Angiography and Interventions. 2025;**4**(5):2772-9303. DOI: 10.1016/j.jscai.2025.102868

[15] Menon V, White H, LeJemtel T, Webb JG, Sleeper LA, Hochman JS. The clinical profile of patients with suspected cardiogenic shock due to predominant left ventricular failure: A report from the SHOCK trial registry. Journal of the American College of Cardiology. 2000;**36**(3):1071-1076. DOI: 10.1016/S0735-1097(00)00874-3

[16] Dudda J, Schupp T, Rusnak J, et al. C-reactive protein and White blood cell count in cardiogenic shock. Journal of Clinical Medicine. 2023;**12**(3):965. Published 2023 Jan 27. DOI: 10.3390/jcm12030965

[17] Field CJ, Gougeon R, Marliss EB. Circulating mononuclear cell numbers and function during intense exercise and recovery. Journal of Applied Physiology. 1991;**71**(1089):1097. DOI: 10.1152/jappl.1991.71.3.1089

[18] Sasmita BR, Zhu Y, Gan H, Hu X, Xue Y, Xiang Z, et al. Leukocyte and its subtypes as predictors of short-term outcome in cardiogenic shock complicating acute myocardial infarction: A cohort study. Shock. 2022;**57**:351-359. DOI: 10.1097/SHK.0000000000001876

[19] Yoshida T, Yoshida T, Noma H, et al. Diagnostic accuracy of point-of-care ultrasound for shock: A systematic review and meta-analysis. Critical Care. 2023;**27**:200. DOI: 10.1186/s13054-023-04495-6

[20] Kato S, Kurosaka E, Nakata K. Point-of-care ultrasound (POCUS)-guided management of cardiogenic shock in COVID-19 fulminant myocarditis with combined Veno-arterial extracorporeal membrane oxygenation and Impella (ECPELLA): A case report. Cureus. 2024;**16**(5):e60665. DOI: 10.7759/cureus.60665

[21] Garan A, Kanwar M, Thayer K, et al. Complete hemodynamic profiling with pulmonary artery catheters in cardiogenic shock is associated with lower in-hospital mortality. Journal of the American College of Cardiology Heart Failure. 2020;**8**:903-913. DOI: 10.1016/j.jchf.2020.08.012

[22] Sinha SS, Morrow DA, Kapur NK, Kataria R, Roswell RO. 2025 concise clinical guidance: An ACC expert consensus statement on the evaluation and management of cardiogenic shock: A report of the American College of Cardiology Solution set Oversight Committee. Journal of the American College of Cardiology. 2025;**85**(16):1618-1641. DOI: 10.1016/j.jacc.2025.02.018

[23] Berg DD, Bohula EA, Patel SM, et al. Epidemiology of cardiogenic shock using the shock academic research consortium (SHARC) consensus definitions. European Heart Journal Acute Cardiovascular Care. 2024;**13**(10):709-714. DOI: 10.1093/ehjacc/zuae098

[24] Waksman R, Pahuja M, van Diepen S, et al. Standardized definitions for cardiogenic shock research and mechanical circulatory support devices: Scientific expert panel from the shock academic research consortium (SHARC).

Circulation. 2023;**148**(14):1113-1126. DOI: 10.1161/CIRCULATIONAHA.123

[25] Corujo Rodriguez A, Richter E, Ibekwe SO, Shah T, Faloye AO. Postcardiotomy shock syndrome: A narrative review of perioperative diagnosis and management. Journal of Cardiothoracic and Vascular Anesthesia. 2023;**37**(12):2621-2633. DOI: 10.1053/j.jvca.2023.09.011

[26] Killip T 3rd, Kimball JT. Treatment of myocardial infarction in a coronary care unit. A two-year experience with 250 patients. The American Journal of Cardiology. 1967;**20**(4):457-464. DOI: 10.1016/0002-9149(67)90023-9

[27] Forrester JS, Diamond G, Chatterjee K, Swan HJC. Medical therapy of acute myocardial infarction by application of hemodynamic subsets. The New England Journal of Medicine. 1976;**295**:1404-1413

[28] Korabathina R, Heffernan KS, Paruchuri V, et al. The pulmonary artery pulsatility index identifies severe right ventricular dysfunction in acute inferior myocardial infarction. Catheterization and Cardiovascular Interventions. 2012;**80**(4):593-600. DOI: 10.1002/ccd.23309

[29] Kapur N, Kanwar M, Sinha S, et al. Criteria for defining stages of cardiogenic shock severity. JACC. 2022;**80**(3):185-198. DOI: 10.1016/j.jacc.2022.04.049

[30] Zern EK, Wang D, Rambarat P, et al. Association of pulmonary artery pulsatility Index with adverse cardiovascular events across a hospital-based sample. Circulation. Heart Failure. 2022;**15**(2):e009085. DOI: 10.1161/CIRCHEARTFAILURE.121.009085

[31] Labrada L, Vaidy A, Vaidya A. Right ventricular assessment in pulmonary hypertension. Current Opinion in Pulmonary Medicine. 2023;**29**(5):348-354. DOI: 10.1097/MCP.0000000000000980

[32] Drazner MH, Vélez-Martinez M, Ayers CR, et al. Relationship of right- to left-sided ventricular filling pressures in advanced heart failure: Insights from the ESCAPE trial. Circulation. Heart Failure. 2013;**6**(2):264-270. DOI: 10.1161/CIRCHEARTFAILURE.112.000204

[33] Grodin JL, Drazner MH, Dupont M, et al. A disproportionate elevation in right ventricular filling pressure, in relation to left ventricular filling pressure, is associated with renal impairment and increased mortality in advanced decompensated heart failure. American Heart Journal. 2015;**169**(6):806-812. DOI: 10.1016/j.ahj.2015.02.017

[34] Fincke R, Hochman JS, Lowe AM, et al. Cardiac power is the strongest hemodynamic correlate of mortality in cardiogenic shock: A report from the SHOCK trial registry. Journal of the American College of Cardiology. 2004;**44**(2):340-348. DOI: 10.1016/j.jacc.2004.03.060

[35] Jentzer JC, Schrage B, Patel PC, Kashani KB, Barsness GW, Holmes DR Jr, et al. Association between the academia, lactic acidosis, and shock severity with outcomes in patients with cardiogenic shock. Journal of the American Heart Association. 2022;**11**(9):e024932. DOI: 10.1161/JAHA.121.0249

[36] Wang L, Zhang Y, Yao R, et al. Identification of distinct clinical phenotypes of cardiogenic shock using machine learning consensus clustering approach. BMC Cardiovascular Disorders. 2023;**23**(1):426. Published 2023 Aug 29. DOI: 10.1186/s12872-023-03380-y

[37] Zweck E, Kanwar M, Li S, et al. Clinical course of patients in cardiogenic shock stratified by phenotype. Journal of the American College of Cardiology Heart Failure. 2023;**11**(10):1304-1315. DOI: 10.1016/j.jchf.2023.05.007

[38] Polyzogopoulou E, Bezati S, Karamasis G, Boultadakis A, Parissis J. Early recognition and risk stratification in cardiogenic shock: Well, begun is half done. Journal of Clinical Medicine. 2023;**12**(7):2643. Published 2023 Apr 1. DOI: 10.3390/jcm12072643

[39] Psotka MA, Gottlieb SS, Francis GS, Allen LA, Teerlink JR, Adams KF, et al. Cardiac calcitropes, myotropes, and mitotropes: JACC review topic of the week. Journal of the American College of Cardiology Heart Failure. 2019;**73**(18):2345-2353. ISSN 0735-1097. DOI: 10.1016/j.jacc.2019.02.051

[40] Riccardi M, Pagnesi M, Chioncel O, et al. Medical therapy of cardiogenic shock: Contemporary use of inotropes and vasopressors. European Journal of Heart Failure. 2024;**26**(2):411-431. DOI: 10.1002/cjhf.3162

[41] Heidenreich PA, Bozkurt B, Aguilar D, et al. AHA/ACC/HFSA guideline for the Management of Heart Failure: A report of the American College of Cardiology/American Heart Association joint committee on clinical practice guidelines. Circulation. 2022;**145**(18):e1033. DOI: 10.1161/CIR.0000000000001073

[42] McDonagh TA, Metra M, et al. 2021 ESC guidelines for the diagnosis and treatment of acute and chronic heart failure: Developed by the task force for the diagnosis and treatment of acute and chronic heart failure of the European Society of Cardiology (ESC). With the special contribution of the Heart Failure Association (HFA) of the ESC. European Journal of Heart Failure. 2022;**24**(1):4-131. DOI: 10.1002/ejhf.2333

[43] Kislitsina ON, Rich JD, Wilcox JE, et al. Shock - classification and pathophysiological principles of therapeutics. Current Cardiology Reviews. 2019;**15**(2):102-113. DOI: 10.2174/1573403X15666181212125024

[44] Mathew R, Di Santo P, Jung RG, et al. Milrinone as compared with dobutamine in the treatment of cardiogenic shock. The New England Journal of Medicine. 2021;**385**(6):516-525. DOI: 10.1056/NEJMoa2026845

[45] Lozada Martinez ID, Bayona-Gamboa AJ, Meza-Fandiño DF, et al. Inotropic support in cardiogenic shock: Who leads the battle, milrinone or dobutamine? Annals of Medicine and Surgery. 2022;**82**:104763. Published 2022 Sep 22. DOI: 10.1016/j.amsu.2022.104763

[46] Abraham WT, Adams KF, Fonarow GC, et al. In-hospital mortality in patients with acute decompensated heart failure requiring intravenous vasoactive medications: An analysis from the acute decompensated heart failure National Registry (ADHERE). Journal of the American College of Cardiology. 2005;**46**(1):57-64. DOI: 10.1016/j.jacc.2005.03.051

[47] Felker GM, Benza RL, Chandler AB, et al. Heart failure etiology and response to milrinone in decompensated heart failure: Results from the OPTIME-CHF study. Journal of the American College of Cardiology. 2003;**41**(6):997-1003. DOI: 10.1016/s0735-1097(02)02968-6

[48] Guarracino F, Zima E, Pollesello P, Masip J. Short-term treatments for acute cardiac care: Inotropes and inodilators. European Heart Journal Supplements: Journal of the European Society of

Cardiology. 2020;**22**(Suppl. D):D3-D11. DOI: 10.1093/eurheartj/suaa090

[49] Pollesello P, Parissis J, Kivikko M, Harjola VP. Levosimendan meta-analyses: Is there a pattern in the effect on mortality? International Journal of Cardiology. 2016;**209**:77-83. DOI: 10.1016/j.ijcard.2016.02.014

[50] Francis GS, Bartos JA, Adatya S. Inotropes. Journal of the American College of Cardiology. 2014;**63**(20):2069-2078. DOI: 10.1016/j.jacc.2014.01.016

[51] Rui Q, Jiang Y, Chen M, Zhang N, Yang H, Zhou Y. Dopamine versus norepinephrine in the treatment of cardiogenic shock: A PRISMA-compliant meta-analysis. Medicine (Baltimore). 2017;**96**(43):e8402. DOI: 10.1097/MD.0000000000008402

[52] Bandak G, Sakhuja A, Andrijasevic NM, Gunderson TM, Gajic O, Kashani K. Use of diuretics in shock: Temporal trends and clinical impacts in a propensity-matched cohort study. PLoS One. 2020;**15**(2):e0228274. DOI: 10.1371/journal.pone.0228274

[53] Thiele H, Zeymer U, Thelemann N, et al. Intraaortic balloon pump in cardiogenic shock complicating acute myocardial infarction: Long-term 6-year outcome of the randomized IABP-SHOCK II trial. Circulation. 2019;**139**(3):395-403. DOI: 10.1161/CIRCULATIONAHA.118.038201

[54] Zein R, Patel C, Mercado-Alamo A, Schreiber T, Kaki A. A review of the Impella devices. Interventional Cardiology. 2022;**17**:e05. Published 2022 Apr 8. DOI: 10.15420/icr.2021.11

[55] Mebazaa A, Combes A, van Diepen S, et al. Management of cardiogenic shock complicating myocardial infarction. Intensive Care Medicine. 2018;**44**(6):760-773. DOI: 10.1007/s00134-018-5214-9

[56] Ouweneel DM, Engstrom AE, Sjauw KD, et al. Experience from a randomized controlled trial with Impella 2.5 versus IABP in STEMI patients with cardiogenic pre-shock. Lessons learned from the IMPRESS in STEMI trial. International Journal of Cardiology. 2016;**202**:894-896. DOI: 10.1016/j.ijcard.2015.10.063

[57] Seyfarth M, Sibbing D, Bauer I, et al. A randomized clinical trial to evaluate the safety and efficacy of a percutaneous left ventricular assist device versus intra-aortic balloon pumping for treatment of cardiogenic shock caused by myocardial infarction. Journal of the American College of Cardiology. 2008;**52**(19):1584-1588. DOI: 10.1016/j.jacc.2008.05.065

[58] Megaly M, Gandolfo C, Zakhour S, et al. Utilization of TandemHeart in cardiogenic shock: Insights from the THEME registry. Catheterization and Cardiovascular Interventions. 2023;**101**(4):756-763. DOI: 10.1002/ccd.30582

[59] Khalid Y, Dasu N, Dasu K, et al. Impella versus tandemheart In cardiogenic shock nationwide database analysis 2017. JACC. 2021;**77**(18_Suppl. 1):818. DOI: 10.1016/S0735-1097(21)02177-X

[60] Rajsic S, Treml B, Jadzic D, et al. Extracorporeal membrane oxygenation for cardiogenic shock: A meta-analysis of mortality and complications. Annals of Intensive Care. 2022;**12**(1):93. Published 2022 Oct 5. DOI: 10.1186/s13613-022-01067-9

[61] Rao P, Khalpey Z, Smith R, Burkhoff D, Kociol RD. Venoarterial extracorporeal membrane oxygenation for cardiogenic shock and cardiac

arrest. Circulation. Heart Failure. 2018;**11**(9):e004905. DOI: 10.1161/CIRCHEARTFAILURE.118.004905

[62] Stub D, Chan W, Ball J, et al. Impella compared to venoarterial extracorporeal membrane oxygenation In cardiogenic shock: A systematic review and meta-analysis of propensity score-matched studies. Shock. 2025;**63**(4):512-519. DOI: 10.1097/SHK.0000000000002540

[63] Botti G, Gramegna M, Burzotta F. et al. Impella RP for patients with acute right ventricular failure and cardiogenic shock: A subanalysis from the IMP-IT registry. Journal of Personalized Medicine. 2022;**12**(9):1481. Published 2022 Sep 9. DOI: 10.3390/jpm12091481

[64] John KJ, Nabzdyk CGS, Chweich H, Mishra AK, Lal A. ProtekDuo percutaneous ventricular support system-physiology and clinical applications. Annals of Translational Medicine. 2024;**12**(1):14. DOI: 10.21037/atm-23-1734

[65] Borisenko O, Wylie G, Payne J, Bjessmo S, Smith J, Yonan N, et al. Thoratec CentriMag for temporary treatment of refractory cardiogenic shock or severe cardiopulmonary insufficiency: A systematic literature review and meta-analysis of observational studies. ASAIO Journal (American Society for Artificial Internal Organs: 1992). 2014;**60**(5):487-497. DOI: 10.1097/MAT.0000000000000117

[66] Grant C Jr, Richards JB, Frakes M, Cohen J, Wilcox SR. ECMO and right ventricular failure: Review of the literature. Journal of Intensive Care Medicine. 2021;**36**(3):352-360. DOI: 10.1177/0885066619900503

[67] Montisci A, Panoulas V, Chieffo A, et al. Recognizing patients as candidates for temporary mechanical circulatory support along the spectrum of cardiogenic shock. European Heart Journal Supplements: Journal of the European Society of Cardiology. 2023;**25**(Suppl. I):I3-I10. Published 2023 Dec 13. DOI: 10.1093/eurheartjsupp/suad127

[68] Rab T, Ratanapo S, Kern KB, et al. Cardiac shock care centers: JACC review topic of the week. Journal of American College of Cardiology. 2018;**72**(21):2685. DOI: 10.1016/j.jacc.2018.10.028. J Am Coll Cardiol. 2018;72(16):1972-1980. doi:10.1016/j.jacc.2018.07.074

[69] Alhuneafat L et al. Temporary mechanical circulatory support utilization and outcomes in cardiogenic shock phenotypes: A comparative analysis of heart failure and acute myocardial infarction. Cardiovascular Revascularization Medicine: Including Molecular Interventions. 20 Jan 2025:S1553-8389(25)00021-1. DOI: 10.1016/j.carrev.2025.01.007

Chapter 3

Ferroptosis in Sepsis-Induced Acute Lung Injury

Yuanhang Fan, Wanrong Wu, Jiao Liu, Daolin Tang, Zhenhui Zhang and Yichun Wang

Abstract

Sepsis is a life-threatening medical condition that arises when the body's response to an infection becomes dysregulated, resulting in widespread organ dysfunction and failure. Approximately 50% of septic patients in intensive care units develop acute lung injury (ALI), a condition that significantly increases mortality rates. Therefore, gaining a deeper understanding of the pathophysiological mechanisms underlying sepsis-induced ALI is crucial for the development of effective prevention and treatment strategies for infected individuals. Ferroptosis is a type of oxidative cell death characterized by the accumulation of iron and uncontrolled lipid peroxidation. Recent research has emphasized the connection between ferroptosis and sepsis-induced organ dysfunction, particularly in the context of lung injury. In sepsis-induced ALI, disruptions in iron homeostasis lead to the accumulation of intracellular iron. This process is intricately linked with various key regulatory elements, such as glutathione peroxidase 4 (GPX4), solute carrier family 7 member 11 (SLC7A11), acyl-CoA synthetase long-chain family member 4 (ACSL4), arachidonate 15-lipoxygenase (ALOX15), as well as ferritin and ferroportin. This comprehensive review will explore recent advancements in understanding ferroptosis mechanisms in sepsis-induced acute lung injury (ALI) and discuss the potential of targeting ferroptosis as a novel therapeutic approach, along with associated challenges.

Keywords: sepsis, acute lung injury, ferroptosis, oxidative stress, inflammation

1. Introduction

Sepsis, a common complication resulting from severe trauma, burns, infections, and major surgeries, is a life-threatening condition defined by multi-organ dysfunction due to an inadequate or dysregulated host response to infection [1–3]. It stands as a leading cause of mortality among ICU patients [4, 5]. In the United States, sepsis results in approximately 300–400 hospitalizations per 100,000 people, with an overall mortality rate of roughly 20% [6]. In mainland China, a comprehensive study across 44 hospitals reported a sepsis incidence of 20.6 cases per 100 ICU admissions, accompanied by a daunting 90-day mortality rate of 35.5% [7].

IntechOpen

Key factors contributing to higher 90-day mortality include advanced age, lower body weight, elevated Sequential Organ Failure Assessment (SOFA) scores, and the site of infection, notably in the lungs [7].

Regrettably, timely and effective sepsis treatment remains a challenge, with the lungs often being one of the first organs affected [8]. Sepsis is the leading risk factor for acute lung injury (ALI) and a significant contributor to the high mortality rate in septic patients [9]. Research indicates that up to 50% of ICU patients with sepsis develop ALI [10, 11], and epidemiological studies reveal that the lungs are the most common infection site in sepsis patients, accounting for 68.2% of cases [7]. Despite its significant clinical implications, the molecular mechanisms responsible for sepsis-induced ALI remain incompletely understood. Therefore, gaining a comprehensive understanding of the pathophysiological mechanisms behind sepsis-induced ALI is vital for the development of effective prevention and treatment strategies.

This review emphasizes the role of ferroptosis, a non-apoptotic form of regulated cell death involving iron and lipid peroxide accumulation, in sepsis-induced acute lung injury (ALI). We briefly overview the pathology of sepsis-induced ALI, establish cell death pathways, and delve into the mechanisms and modulation of ferroptosis in this context. Lastly, we discuss the therapeutic potential of targeting ferroptosis for sepsis-induced ALI.

2. Pathology of sepsis-induced ALI

ALI is a complex and severe pulmonary condition triggered by systemic inflammatory response syndrome (SIRS) in response to sepsis [8, 12, 13]. It is characterized by intense lung inflammation, increased pulmonary vascular permeability, and subsequent alveolar damage [14, 15]. Key pathogenic mechanisms include overwhelming inflammation, oxidative stress, and coagulation dysfunction. During sepsis, a dysregulated immune response leads to the excessive release of pro-inflammatory cytokines, often referred to as a "cytokine storm," causing widespread tissue damage, especially in the pulmonary system [16]. Concurrently, oxidative stress results from an imbalance between the production of reactive oxygen species (ROS) and the body's antioxidant defenses, further exacerbating cellular and tissue injury in the lungs [17, 18]. Additionally, sepsis can disrupt normal coagulation pathways, leading to either localized clotting within lung vasculature or disseminated intravascular coagulation, both of which impair gas exchange and contribute to respiratory failure [19, 20]. Collectively, these dysfunctions result in impaired gas exchange, reduced lung compliance, and severe respiratory distress, defining features of ALI.

2.1 Inflammation in sepsis-induced ALI

Excessive inflammatory response and immune suppression are key mechanisms in sepsis [21]. Research suggests that dysregulation of pro-inflammatory and anti-inflammatory pathways is a pivotal pathological mechanism in sepsis-induced ALI [22, 23]. The ongoing recruitment and activation of various inflammatory cells, coupled with the release of large quantities of inflammatory mediators, trigger an uncontrolled inflammatory response, leading to a systemic inflammatory response syndrome [24].

During immune hyperactivation, macrophage activation releases inflammatory mediators, such as tumor necrosis factor-alpha (TNF-α) and interleukins, triggering a cascade that recruits additional inflammatory cells [25]. This accumulation in lung tissue disrupts the alveolar-capillary barrier, increases vascular permeability, and impairs gas exchange, compromising lung function [26]. Studies highlight that early in sepsis-induced acute respiratory distress syndrome (ARDS), capillary function deteriorates due to neutrophil retention, and inhibiting pro-inflammatory cytokines can mitigate ALI [27–29]. Inhibiting inflammatory signaling pathways such as nuclear factor kappa-B (NF-κB) pathway also protects against structural damage and inflammatory cell infiltration, alleviating lung and liver injury in sepsis [30].

2.2 Oxidative stress in sepsis-induced ALI

During sepsis, neutrophils in lung tissue release a large number of inflammatory mediators and produce ROS [31]. Excessive ROS can damage cellular structures and functions, impair mitochondrial membranes, and create oxidative byproducts, such as malondialdehyde, which reduces the active substance on the alveolar surface, increases surface tension, and decreases alveolar compliance [32]. In animal models, the rapid and excessive production of inflammatory cytokines and ROS disrupts the endothelial barrier, leading to microvascular leakage and subsequent lung injury [15, 33]. Furthermore, upregulating antioxidant enzymes and inhibiting mitogen-activated protein kinase (MAPK)/NF-κB activation may prove effective therapeutic strategies for sepsis-induced ALI [34], underscoring the potential of targeting oxidative stress in the treatment of sepsis-induced ALI.

2.3 Coagulation in sepsis-induced ALI

Sepsis-induced ALI is also associated with coagulation dysfunction. In this condition, the coagulation system is activated, and anticoagulation mechanisms are inhibited [35, 36]. The excessive release of coagulation factors hampers fibrinolysis and induces pulmonary interstitial fibrosis. Pathogen stimulation damages endothelial cells and exacerbates coagulation dysfunction [37, 38]. Disrupted coagulation cascades lead to microthrombus formation, impaired fibrinolysis, and activation of platelets and endothelial cells, resulting in vascular occlusion and impaired pulmonary oxygenation [39]. Additionally, the dysregulated coagulation cascade may contribute to the release of pro-inflammatory mediators and the recruitment of inflammatory cells, further exacerbating lung injury [40].

3. Mechanisms of ferroptosis in sepsis-induced ALI

3.1 Overview of ferroptosis

Regulated cell death (RCD) is a fundamental biological process characterized by the orderly and regulated elimination of cells, playing a pivotal role in both the development and maintenance of organismal homeostasis [41, 42]. This process differs from accidental cell death, which is unregulated. Traditionally, RCD mainly encompasses apoptosis. However, in recent years, new types of non-apoptotic RCD, such as necroptosis and pyroptosis, have been discovered. Additionally, ferroptosis, an iron-dependent RCD pathway, has emerged as relevant in sepsis and associated organ damage, underscoring the evolving understanding of cell death's role in disease processes.

In 2012, Dixon first proposed the term of ferroptosis, a non-apoptotic form of cell death that is iron-dependent and characterized by the accumulation of lipid ROS [43, 44]. The occurrence of ferroptosis is iron-dependent, and pro-oxidant factors can directly or indirectly affect glutathione peroxidase 4 (GPX4), leading to decreased antioxidant capacity and accumulation of lipid ROS, ultimately resulting in oxidative cell death [44, 45].

In ferroptosis, iron accumulates due to dysregulation of iron homeostasis. This may involve increased iron uptake mediated by transferrin receptor 1 (TfR1) or reduced iron export facilitated by ferroportin (Fpn). Furthermore, impaired iron storage by ferritin can contribute to iron overload [46]. Conversely, ferroportin is the sole iron transporter capable of reducing cellular iron levels and mitigating ferroptosis. Overexpressing TfR1 or disrupting Fpn can trigger intracellular ferroptosis, while ferrostatin-1 can upregulate Fpn, lower cellular iron levels, ameliorate lipid peroxidation, and reduce the occurrence of ferroptosis [47].

Lipid peroxidation is a critical step in ferroptosis, involving the oxidative damage of polyunsaturated fatty acids (PUFAs) within cellular membranes. Elevated iron levels and the presence of ROS can trigger lipid peroxidation [48]. Iron participates in the Fenton reaction, generating lipid hydroperoxides from PUFAs, a process mediated by enzymes like arachidonate 15-lipoxygenase (ALOX15) and enhanced by acyl-CoA synthetase long-chain family member 4 (ACSL4). These lipid hydroperoxides propagate through a chain reaction, leading to the formation of phosphatidylethanolamine (PE) containing arachidonic acid (AA) or its derivative, adrenaline, causing widespread membrane damage and dysfunction. Ferroptosis is often accompanied by a breakdown of the GSH-dependent lipid repair system [49]. Disruption of the cellular antioxidant defense system, including GSH levels and decreased activity of GPX4, further amplifies lipid peroxidation and promotes ferroptosis [50, 51]. This process is associated with solute carrier family, such as solute carrier family 7 member 11 (SLC7A11)/xCT/system xc-system, which sustains GSH production. Therefore, factors such as ferritin, ACSL4, and ALOX15 act as inducers of ferroptosis, whereas ferroportin-1, GPX4, and SLC7A11 act as suppressors of ferroptosis (**Figure 1**).

3.2 Ferroptosis and sepsis-induced ALI

In sepsis-induced ALI, ferroptosis is also activated. Excessive iron accumulation and the resulting lipid peroxidation are believed to contribute to oxidative stress, membrane damage, and cell death in both epithelial and immune cells within lung tissues, further exacerbating the development of ALI. The regulation of this process is typically governed by the aforementioned ferroptotic regulators.

3.2.1 Iron metabolism and lipid peroxidation in sepsis-induced ALI

Dysfunction of iron metabolism is the most important feature and the first step of ferroptosis. In sepsis-associated ALI, sepsis causes the accumulation of iron ions in both alveolar epithelial cells and immune cells. Iron promotes lipid peroxidation, leading to abnormal cell death, as well as activation of immune cells such as neutrophil migration and macrophage inflammatory polarization. The accumulated iron can also induce fibroblast proliferation, which may exacerbate the inflammatory response and lead to pulmonary fibrosis [27]. As reported by Li et al., sepsis-induced the release of a large amount of iron. Cytoplasmic Fe^{2+} further led to the expression of spliced mitochondrial membrane protein (SFXN1), which transports cytoplasmic Fe^{2+} into the mitochondria,

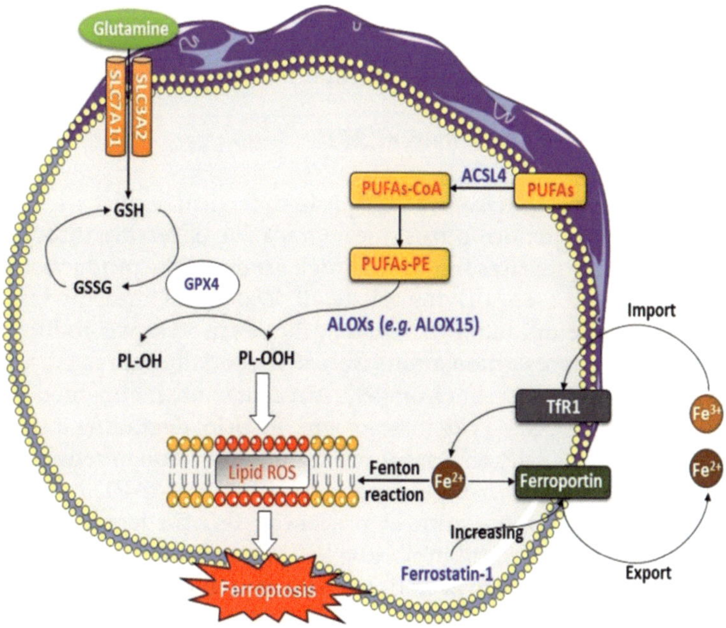

Figure 1.
Regulators in ferroptosis. TfR1 mediated import of iron uptake while ferroportin exports iron, which can be upregulated by ferrostatin-1. ACSL4 and ALOX15 contribute to the oxidation of PUFAs within cellular membranes. Excessive iron levels and the presence of ROS can initiate lipid peroxidation. Iron participates in the Fenton reaction, generating lipid hydroperoxides from PUFAs, leading to widespread membrane damage and dysfunction. The impairment of the GSH-dependent lipid repair system, such as the dysfunction of GPX4 and SLC7A11/SLC32A1, further amplifies lipid peroxidation and promotes ferroptosis.

resulting in mitochondrial ROS and ferroptosis [52]. He et al. also found that ferroptosis was a key mechanism in sepsis-induced ALI. Both 4-octyl itaconate (4-OI), which inhibited GPX4-dependent lipid peroxidation by increasing nuclear factor erythroid 2-related factor 2 (NRF2) accumulation and activation [53]. Treatment with protectin conjugates in tissue regeneration 1 (PCTR1) reduces the levels of Fe^{2+}, prostaglandin-endoperoxide synthase 2(PTGS2), and lipid ROS, increases the levels of GSH and GPX4 and improves mitochondrial ultrastructure damage, thus alleviating sepsis-induced ALI [54].

As another key factor of ferroptosis, lipid peroxidation is usually activated by disrupted iron homeostasis. Iron serves as a crucial cofactor for various cellular processes and can generate ROS through Fenton and Haber-Weiss reactions [55]. In sepsis, bacterial infections require iron for growth, and the release of intracellular iron from shedding cells provides excess iron for bacterial utilization. The shed intracellular iron becomes a feast for the infected bacteria [56, 57]. Meanwhile, bacterial infection provides various materials for lipid peroxidation, including reactive oxygen species and fatty acids, forming a vicious cycle that exacerbates infection, leading to sepsis and multi-organ dysfunction [56]. Ferroptosis exacerbates infection by introducing multiple bacterial growth sources, which in turn facilitate lipid peroxidation in sepsis [58].

3.2.2 Ferroptosis biomarkers and their functions in sepsis-induced ALI

As previously mentioned, ferroptotic regulators, including inducers like ACSL4 and ALOX15, and suppressors such as ferroportin-1, GPX4, and SLC7A11, play pivotal roles in sepsis-induced ferroptosis in ALI. Their expressions, as inducers or suppressors, partially dictate the activation or inactivation of the ferroptotic pathway, thereby influencing the extent of lung tissue damage and the progression of ALI.

3.2.2.1 Ferroptosis inducers in sepsis-induced ALI

As the primary intracellular iron storage protein, ferritin regulates iron availability under normal conditions. In ferroptosis, the degradation of ferritin through a process known as ferritinophagy releases free iron, which catalyzes the production of ROS and lipid peroxidation, thereby driving cell death. Wang et al. measured the levels of ferroptosis-related factors and inflammatory factors in 50 sepsis-induced ALI patients and found ferroptosis biomarkers were differentially expressed, with significantly higher ferritin and serum iron [59]. A recent study highlighted that nuclear receptor coactivator 4 (NCOA4) can interact with ferritin, degrading it in an iron-dependent manner, which releases a substantial amount of iron in sepsis-induced ALI [52]. Conversely, overexpression of yes-associated protein 1 (YAP1) inhibits ferroptosis-mediated eosinophil proliferation by preventing ferritin degradation, thereby reducing Fe^{2+} in the cytoplasm and inhibiting Fe^{2+} transport into mitochondria via mitochondrial membrane protein SFXN1, thereby reducing mitochondrial ROS production and alleviating sepsis-induced ALI [60]. Additionally, prior exposure to the ferritin light chain has been shown to restrain a dysregulated response to infection, with myeloid ferritin light chain deficiency resulting in improved organ functions and attenuated damage in the liver, lungs, and kidneys in a sepsis mouse model [61].

ACSL4 is a key enzyme involved in regulating lipid composition, which enhances the generation of lipid hydroperoxides from PUFAs in ferroptosis [62, 63]. As a biomarker of ferroptosis, the increase of ACSL4 is a signal of the activation of ferroptosis. In sepsis-induced ALI, the expression of ACSL4 is upregulated in lung tissues, alveolar epithelial cells, and macrophages [64, 65]. Wang et al. observed enhanced ferroptosis levels in sepsis-induced ALI models, marked by increased ROS and ACSL4 and decreased GPX4, regulated by circRNA exocyst complex component 5 (EXOC5) [64]. Meanwhile, the stability of ACSL4 mRNA was regulated by the RNA-binding protein PTBP1. Suppressing ACSL4 could be a potential strategy to inhibit ferroptosis and improve ALI in sepsis. Lai et al. found that uridine significantly alleviated lung injury, inflammation, tissue iron levels, and lipid peroxidation in sepsis-induced ALI mice, partially through ACSL4 downregulation and SLC7A11, GPX4, and heme oxygenase 1 (HO-1) upregulation. Additionally, these effects were also observed in LPS-induced macrophages, indicating that ACSL4 facilitates ferroptosis in immune cells. Activating the NRF2 signaling pathway to react with ASCL4 could improve sepsis-induced ALI [65].

ALOX15 is a member of ALOX family which mediates catalyzes the peroxidation of PUFAs in lipid membranes during ferroptosis. An increased level of ALOX15 was observed in sepsis patients on days 1 and 8 in the ICU [66]. However, a recent preprint study indicated that endothelial ALOX15 might have a protective effect in mild lung thrombosis during sepsis-induced ALI [67], suggesting the possible multiple roles of ALOX15 in sepsis-induced ALI. Overall, research on ALOX15's connection to ferroptosis in sepsis-induced ALI is limited, necessitating further studies for validation.

3.2.2.2 Ferroptosis suppressors in sepsis-induced ALI in sepsis-induced ALI

Ferroportin is a crucial iron-exporter protein that helps maintain iron homeostasis by transporting iron out of cells, reducing iron accumulation, and consequently mitigating lipid peroxidation and cell death associated with ferroptosis. Ferrostatin-1, on the other hand, is a potent inhibitor of ferroptosis, which can upregulate the level of ferroportin to prevent lipid peroxide formation and protect against cell death. In an in vitro model of sepsis-induced ALI, ferrostatin-1 effectively inhibited lipid peroxidation and damage in THP-1 macrophages induced by LPS [53]. Shimizu et al. suggested that intraperitoneal injection of extracellular cold-inducible RNA-binding protein (eCIRP) reduced the expression of GPX4 in lung tissue and increased lipid ROS, while ferrostatin-1 treatment significantly reduced this increase [68].

GPX4 plays a central role in inhibiting ferroptosis by reducing lipid ROS [50, 69]. It achieves this by catalyzing the oxidation of GSH to oxidized glutathione (GSSG), effectively eliminating lipid peroxides and shielding cell membranes from the harmful effects of polyunsaturated fatty acid peroxidation [70]. Hence, GPX4 is a vital negative regulator of oxidative damage that inhibits ferroptosis, with its downregulation being a common method for identifying ferroptosis [71, 72]. In a sepsis-induced ALI animal model using cecal ligation and puncture (CLP), GPX4 expression was significantly reduced, coinciding with increased MDA levels, iron levels, and lung tissue injury scores [68]. Cao et al. demonstrated that in a sepsis-induced ALI mouse model, increased iron content and decreased GPX4 expression correlated with lung tissue damage and lipid peroxidation, while mitochondrial aldehyde dehydrogenase 2 (ALDH2) exerted a protective role by reducing ferroptosis and increasing GPX4 levels [73].

The function of GPX4 in ferroptosis is intrinsically connected to SLC7A11, a critical component of the xCT transporter system that facilitates the uptake of cystine required for GSH synthesis. SLC7A11's role in sustaining GSH production is vital for GPX4's activity, as GPX4 utilizes GSH to detoxify lipid peroxides, thereby preventing ferroptosis. In sepsis-induced ALI, both GPX4 and SLC7A11 levels decrease with ferroptosis activation 60. Zhang et al. confirmed that in an ALI model, lung alveolar epithelial cells showed increased levels of Fe^{2+} and MDA, decreased levels of GSH, downregulated expression of GPX4 and SLC7A11 and upregulated expression of ACSL4, while YAP1 could function with an endogenous protective mechanism against ALI [74]. Additionally, inhibiting STEAP family member 1 (STEAP1) in a sepsis-induced ALI model reduced inflammatory responses and ROS generation, increased NRF2 and GSH levels by activating the SLC7A11/GPX4 axis, and suppressed ferroptosis, thereby protecting pulmonary endothelium [75]. Recent research found that in a CLP-induced ALI model, hydrogen sulfide (H2S) attenuated sepsis-induced ALI ferroptosis by increasing GPX4 and SLC7A11 expression in lung tissues, blocking mTOR signaling to inhibit autophagy activation, improving histopathological changes, alleviating lung tissue damage, and reducing lung injury severity [76]. All these results implied that inhibiting ferroptosis by activation of SLC7A11/GPX4 may be a potential therapeutic target for sepsis-induced ALI.

3.3 The role of ferroptosis in other organ damage caused by sepsis and its association with lung injury

Emerging evidence highlights the substantial involvement of cellular ferroptosis in organ-specific injuries during sepsis. In the context of sepsis-induced liver injury, ferroptosis plays a crucial role in the development of liver damage. Consequently, inhibiting ferroptosis has emerged as a novel therapeutic approach for mitigating septic liver injury. For example, the traditional Chinese medicine Wenqingyin (WQY) attenuates sepsis-mediated liver injury by targeting and inhibiting iron toxicity in hepatocytes [77]. It has been found that YAP1 prevents ferritin degradation, reducing ROS generation and ferroptosis-mediated iron toxicity in hepatocytes in septic liver injury [78]. In sepsis-induced kidney injury, in vitro studies have shown that ginsenoside Rg1 increases HK-2 cell viability and reduces iron accumulation and lipid peroxidation, thereby alleviating septic kidney injury [79]. Melatonin treatment in vivo has been shown to attenuate septic kidney injury by upregulating the NRF2/HO-1 pathway, inhibiting ferroptosis [80]. In cardiac injury, suppressing tumor protein 53 (p53) and ferritin levels enhances GPX4 and SLC7A11, protecting against sepsis-induced cardiac injury by inhibiting ferroptosis in mouse cardiomyocytes [81, 82].

While ferroptosis plays a direct role in organ-specific injuries, the interconnection between organ injuries lies in the systemic inflammatory response and the release of inflammatory mediators. In sepsis, the activated inflammatory response can promote iron accumulation and cellular iron death, which further exacerbate inflammation and tissue damage. This interconnectedness creates a complex web of organ injury, where lung injury can influence the progression of liver, kidney, and heart injury, and vice versa [83, 84]. However, research in this field remains relatively limited, and further investigations, both in basic science and clinical studies, are necessary to fully understand the impact of sepsis-induced lung injury on organ damage in other organ systems.

3.4 Ferroptosis as a potential target for the treatment of sepsis-induced ALI and its challenges

In recent years, an increasing number of cellular and animal studies have highlighted the potential of targeting ferroptosis as a therapeutic approach for sepsis-induced ALI. However, the majority of these investigations have been limited to cellular and animal models.

Some promising developments include the identification of itaconate as a candidate drug for treating ALI by inhibiting ferroptosis [53]. Additionally, the QiShengYiQi pill (QSYQ), a traditional Chinese medicinal formulation, has shown the ability to preserve the integrity of the pulmonary vascular barrier by suppressing ferroptosis in CLP mice. This provides a scientific basis for considering QSYQ as a treatment for sepsis-induced ALI [85]. In sepsis-induced ALI, Ferulic acid has demonstrated the potential to improve alveolar epithelial barrier function by activating the NRF2/HO-1 pathway, thereby inhibiting ferroptosis in alveolar epithelial cells. This offers a protective effect against sepsis-induced ALI, adding new evidence to the field of sepsis treatment [86]. Furthermore, F-box and WD repeat domain-containing 7 (FBXW7) have been found to mediate the ubiquitination and degradation of AUF1 in ferroptosis, counteracting the ferroptotic response through its regulation of NRF2 and the AU-rich element (ARE)-binding factor 1 (AUF1). Activation of the AUF1 pathway may hold promise for the treatment of sepsis-induced ALI [87].

Collectively, these studies suggest that targeting iron metabolism and lipid peroxidation has the potential to mitigate lung injury by preventing ferroptosis in sepsis-induced ALI. However, there is currently a paucity of clinical studies focused on the application of ferroptosis as a therapeutic target in sepsis-induced ALI. Therefore, further clinical research is needed to validate the findings from these cellular and animal experiments in the future. Moreover, several challenges, including issues related to selectivity, timing, potential off-target effects, and the complex interplay with other biological processes, must be addressed. Further research and development efforts are necessary to optimize therapeutic approaches targeting cellular iron death and translate these findings into effective treatments for sepsis-induced lung injury.

4. Challenges and future directions for ferroptosis as a therapeutic target of sepsis-induced ALI

Despite the promising insights into ferroptosis and its role in sepsis-induced ALI, numerous challenges and avenues for future research persist. The current understanding of ferroptosis in the context of sepsis-induced ALI remains in its early stages, demanding further investigation to unravel the intricate mechanisms and pathways involved. To translate these findings into effective clinical interventions, several challenges must be addressed:

1. Comprehensive exploration of the interplay between various ferroptosis mediators such as GPX4, SLC7A11, and ferroportin, and their impact on cellular iron metabolism and lipid peroxidation in sepsis-induced ALI is warranted.

2. Sepsis-induced ALI exhibits substantial heterogeneity in clinical manifestations and responses to treatment. Understanding how individual variability influences ferroptosis pathways can provide insights into personalized therapeutic approaches.

3. A significant challenge lies in translating preclinical findings into clinical practice. Many therapeutic approaches targeting ferroptosis are still in experimental stages and require rigorous evaluation through clinical trials. While inhibitors, such as ferrostatin-1, exhibit potential, their safety and efficacy in human subjects, particularly in the complex clinical context of sepsis, necessitate thorough assessment. The development and testing of combination therapies that synergistically target ferroptosis, inflammation, and other relevant mechanisms represent an important future direction.

Furthermore, future research should focus on a more comprehensive elucidation of the molecular mechanisms underlying ferroptosis in sepsis-induced ALI. The exploration and validation of specific biomarkers associated with cellular ferroptosis and organ damage are crucial endeavors. Additionally, the development of personalized treatment strategies tailored to individual patient characteristics should be pursued and subjected to rigorous clinical investigation.

5. Conclusion

Ferroptosis has emerged as a promising therapeutic target for sepsis-induced lung injury and other organ injuries. This review has emphasized the growing significance of ferroptosis in the pathophysiology of sepsis-induced ALI. The intricate interplay among various cellular mechanisms, including inflammation, oxidative stress, iron metabolism, and lipid peroxidation, along with the involvement of key proteins such as ACSL4, GPX4, SLC7A11, and ALOX15, as well as regulators like ferroportin and ferrostatin-1, underscores the multifaceted role of ferroptosis in the progression of sepsis-induced ALI. While these findings open new avenues for therapeutic interventions, they also present challenges, particularly in fully comprehending the underlying mechanisms and translating these insights into clinical practice. The potential for targeting ferroptosis in the treatment of sepsis-induced ALI is substantial, yet it necessitates a cautious and well-informed approach due to the complexity and variability of the disease. In conclusion, ferroptosis represents a promising but challenging frontier in the endeavor to mitigate the impact of sepsis-induced ALI. Future research should strive to unravel the intricacies of ferroptosis pathways and work toward the development of safe, effective, and personalized therapeutic strategies that have the potential to revolutionize the management of sepsis-induced ALI.

Acknowledgements

We thank the Natural Science Foundation of Guangdong Province and the Guangzhou Science and Technology Bureau for the financial support.

This work was supported by the National Natural Science Foundation of China (82472180), the Guangdong Basic and Applied Basic Research Foundation (2024A1515010969), and the characteristic innovation project of general universities in Guangdong province (2023KTSCX108).

Conflict of interest

The authors declare no conflict of interest.

Author details

Yuanhang Fan[1], Wanrong Wu[1], Jiao Liu[2], Daolin Tang[3], Zhenhui Zhang[1*] and Yichun Wang[1*]

1 Department of Critical Care Medicine, Guangdong Provincial Key Laboratory of Major Obstetric Diseases, Guangdong Provincial Clinical Research Center for Obstetrics and Gynnecology, The Third Affiliated Hospital, Guangzhou Medical University, Guangzhou, China

2 DAMP Laboratory, Guangdong Provincial Key Laboratory of Major Obstetric Diseases, Guangdong Provincial Clinical Research Center for Obstetrics and Gynecology, The Third Affiliated Hospital, Guangzhou Medical University, Guangzhou, China

3 Department of Surgery, UT Southwestern Medical Center, Dallas, TX, USA

*Address all correspondence to: zzhmed@126.com and wangyichun2005@163.com

References

[1] Ladhani HA, Yowler CJ, Claridge JA. Burn wound colonization, infection, and sepsis. Surgical Infections. 2021;**22**(1):44-48. DOI: 10.1089/sur.2020.346

[2] Gotts JE, Matthay MA. Sepsis: Pathophysiology and clinical management. British Medical Journal. 2016;**353**:i1585. DOI: 10.1136/bmj.i1585

[3] Salomão R, Ferreira BL, Salomão MC, Santos SS, Azevedo LCP, Brunialti MKC. Sepsis: Evolving concepts and challenges. Brazilian Journal of Medical and Biological Research. 2019;**52**(4):e8595. DOI: 10.1590/1414-431X20198595

[4] Chen L, Huang Q, Zhao T, Sui L, Wang S, Xiao Z, et al. Nanotherapies for sepsis by regulating inflammatory signals and reactive oxygen and nitrogen species: New insight for treating COVID-19. Redox Biology. 2021;**45**:102046. DOI: 10.1016/j.redox.2021.102046

[5] Rimmelé T, Payen D, Cantaluppi V, Marshall J, Gomez H, Gomez A, et al. Immune cell phenotype and function IN SEPSIS. Shock. 2016;**45**(3):282-291. DOI: 10.1097/SHK.0000000000000495

[6] Stoller J, Halpin L, Weis M, Aplin B, Qu W, Georgescu C, et al. Epidemiology of severe sepsis: 2008-2012. Journal of Critical Care. 2016;**31**(1):58-62. DOI: 10.1016/j.jcrc.2015.09.034

[7] Xie J, Wang H, Kang Y, Zhou L, Liu Z, Qin B, et al. The epidemiology of sepsis in Chinese ICUs: A national cross-sectional survey. Critical Care Medicine. 2020;**48**(3):e209-e218. DOI: 10.1097/CCM.0000000000004155

[8] Kumar V. Pulmonary innate immune response determines the outcome of inflammation during pneumonia and sepsis-associated acute lung injury. Frontiers in Immunology. 2020;**11**:1722. DOI: 10.3389/fimmu.2020.01722

[9] Hwang J-S, Kim K-H, Park J, Kim SM, Cho H, Lee Y, et al. Glucosamine improves survival in a mouse model of sepsis and attenuates sepsis-induced lung injury and inflammation. The Journal of Biological Chemistry. 2019;**294**(2):608-622. DOI: 10.1074/jbc.RA118.004638

[10] Sevransky JE, Martin GS, Shanholtz C, Mendez-Tellez PA, Pronovost P, Brower R, et al. Mortality in sepsis versus non-sepsis induced acute lung injury. Critical Care. 2009;**13**(5):1-6. DOI: 10.1186/cc8048

[11] Blank R, Napolitano LM. Epidemiology of ARDS and ALI. Critical Care Clinics. 2011;**27**(3):439-458. DOI: 10.1016/j.ccc.2011.05.005

[12] Sevransky JE, Levy MM, Marini JJ. Mechanical ventilation in sepsis-induced acute lung injury/acute respiratory distress syndrome: An evidence-based review. Critical Care Medicine. 2004;**32**(11):S548-S553. DOI: 10.1097/01.ccm.0000145947.19077.25

[13] Polidoro RB, Hagan RS, de Santis Santiago R, Schmidt NW. Overview: Systemic inflammatory response derived from lung injury caused by SARS-CoV-2 infection explains severe outcomes in COVID-19. Frontiers in Immunology. 2020;**11**:1626. DOI: 10.3389/fimmu.2020.01626

[14] Chen G, Hou Y, Li X, Pan R, Zhao D. Sepsis-induced acute lung injury in young rats is relieved by calycosin through inactivating the HMGB1/MyD88/NF-κB pathway and

NLRP3 inflammasome. International Immunopharmacology. 2021;**96**:107623. DOI: 10.1016/j.intimp.2021.107623

[15] Xia W, Pan Z, Zhang H, Zhou Q, Liu Y. Inhibition of ERRα aggravates sepsis-induced acute lung injury in rats via provoking inflammation and oxidative stress. Oxidative Medicine and Cellular Longevity. 2020;**2020**:2048632. DOI: 10.1155/2020/2048632

[16] Sikora JP, Karawani J, Sobczak J. Neutrophils and the systemic inflammatory response syndrome (SIRS). International Journal of Molecular Sciences. 2023;**24**(17):13469. DOI: 10.3390/ijms241713469

[17] Prauchner CA. Oxidative stress in sepsis: Pathophysiological implications justifying antioxidant co-therapy. Burns. 2017;**43**(3):471-485. DOI: 10.1016/j.burns.2016.09.023

[18] Kumar S, Saxena J, Srivastava VK, Kaushik S, Singh H, Abo-El-Sooud K, et al. The interplay of oxidative stress and ROS scavenging: Antioxidants as a therapeutic potential in sepsis. Vaccines (Basel). 2022;**10**(10):1575. DOI: 10.3390/vaccines10101575

[19] Unar A, Bertolino L, Patauner F, Gallo R, Durante-Mangoni E. Pathophysiology of disseminated intravascular coagulation in sepsis: A clinically focused overview. Cells. 2023;**12**(17):2120. DOI: 10.3390/cells12172120

[20] Iba T, Umemura Y, Wada H, Levy JH. Roles of coagulation abnormalities and microthrombosis in sepsis: Pathophysiology, diagnosis, and treatment. Archives of Medical Research. 2021;**52**(8):788-797. DOI: 10.1016/j.arcmed.2021.07.003

[21] van der Poll T, van de Veerdonk FL, Scicluna BP, Netea MG. The immunopathology of sepsis and potential therapeutic targets. Nature Reviews Immunology. 2017;**17**(7):407-420. DOI: 10.1038/nri.2017.3623

[22] Nedeva C, Menassa J, Puthalakath H. Sepsis: Inflammation is a necessary evil. Frontiers in Cell and Developmental Biology. 2019;**7**:108. DOI: 10.3389/fcell.2019.00108

[23] Chen X, Liu Y, Gao Y, Shou S, Chai Y. The roles of macrophage polarization in the host immune response to sepsis. International Immunopharmacology. 2021;**96**:107791. DOI: 10.1016/j.intimp.2021.107791

[24] Souza-Fonseca-Guimaraes F, Parlato M, Philippart F, Misset B, Cavaillon JM, Adib-Conquy M, et al. Toll-like receptors expression and interferon-γ production by NK cells in human sepsis. Critical Care. 2012;**16**(5):R206. DOI: 10.1186/cc11838

[25] Hirano Y, Ode Y, Ochani M, Wang P, Aziz M. Targeting junctional adhesion molecule-C ameliorates sepsis-induced acute lung injury by decreasing CXCR4+ aged neutrophils. Journal of Leukocyte Biology. 2018;**104**(6):1159-1171. DOI: 10.1002/JLB.3A0218-050R

[26] Derwall M, Martin L, Rossaint R. The acute respiratory distress syndrome: Pathophysiology, current clinical practice, and emerging therapies. Expert Review of Respiratory Medicine. 2018;**12**(12):1021-1029. DOI: 10.1080/17476348.2018.1548280

[27] Park I, Kim M, Choe K, Song E, Seo H, Hwang Y, et al. Neutrophils disturb pulmonary microcirculation in sepsis-induced acute lung injury. The European Respiratory Journal. 2019;**53**(3):1800786. DOI: 10.1183/13993003.00786-2018

[28] Wang Q-L, Yang L, Peng Y, Gao M, Yang MS, Xing W, et al. Ginsenoside Rg1 regulates SIRT1 to ameliorate sepsis-induced lung inflammation and injury via inhibiting endoplasmic reticulum stress and inflammation. Mediators of Inflammation. 2019;**2019**:6453296. DOI: 10.1155/2019/6453296

[29] Wang Y, Deng F, Zhong X, Du Y, Fan X, Su H, et al. Dulaglutide provides protection against sepsis-induced lung injury in mice by inhibiting inflammation and apoptosis. European Journal of Pharmacology. 2023;**949**:175730. DOI: 10.1016/j.ejphar.2023.175730

[30] Chen X, Cai X, Le R, Zhang M, Gu X, Shen F, et al. Isoliquiritigenin protects against sepsis-induced lung and liver injury by reducing inflammatory responses. Biochemical and Biophysical Research Communications. 2018;**496**(2):245-252. DOI: 10.1016/j.bbrc.2017.11.159

[31] Lu J, Liu J, Li A. Roles of neutrophil reactive oxygen species (ROS) generation in organ function impairment in sepsis. Journal of Zhejiang University. Science. B. 2022;**23**(6):437-450. DOI: 10.1631/jzus.B2101075

[32] Wang H, Sun X, Lu Q, Zemskov EA, Yegambaram M, Wu X, et al. The mitochondrial redistribution of eNOS is involved in lipopolysaccharide induced inflammasome activation during acute lung injury. Redox Biology. 2021;**41**:101878. DOI: 10.1016/j.redox.2021.101878

[33] Hu Q, Wang Q, Han C, Yang Y. Sufentanil attenuates inflammation and oxidative stress in sepsis-induced acute lung injury by downregulating KNG1 expression. Molecular Medicine Reports. 2020;**22**(5):4298-4306. DOI: 10.3892/mmr.2020.11526

[34] Chen J, Li C, Liang Z, Li C, Li Y, Zhao Z, et al. Human mesenchymal stromal cells small extracellular vesicles attenuate sepsis-induced acute lung injury in a mouse model: The role of oxidative stress and the mitogen-activated protein kinase/nuclear factor kappa B pathway. Cytotherapy. 2021;**23**(10):918-930. DOI: 10.1016/j.jcyt.2021.05.009

[35] Li Z, Yin M, Zhang H, Ni W, Pierce RW, Zhou HJ, et al. BMX represses thrombin-PAR1–mediated endothelial permeability and vascular leakage during early sepsis. Circulation Research. 2020;**126**(4):471-485. DOI: 10.1161/CIRCRESAHA.119.315769

[36] Seo J, Do Yoo J, Kim M, Shim G, Oh YK, Park RW, et al. Fibrinolytic nanocages dissolve clots in the tumor microenvironment, improving the distribution and therapeutic efficacy of anticancer drugs. Experimental and Molecular Medicine. 2021;**53**(10):1592-1601. DOI: 10.1038/s12276-021-00688-7

[37] Lauw FN, Dekkers PEP, te Velde AA, Speelman P, Levi M, Kurimoto M, et al. Interleukin-12 induces sustained activation of multiple host inflammatory mediator systems in chimpanzees. The Journal of Infectious Diseases. 1999;**179**(3):646-652. DOI: 10.1086/314636

[38] López-Zambrano M, Rodriguez-Montesinos J, Crespo-Avilan GE, Muñoz-Vega M, Preissner KT. Thrombin promotes macrophage polarization into M1-like phenotype to induce inflammatory responses. Thrombosis and Haemostasis. 2020;**120**(04):658-670. DOI: 10.1055/s-0040-1703007

[39] Iba T, Levy JH. Inflammation and thrombosis: Roles of neutrophils, platelets and endothelial cells and their interactions in thrombus formation

during sepsis. Journal of Thrombosis and Haemostasis. 2018;**16**(2):231-241. DOI: 10.1111/jth.13911

[40] Lv J, Guo X, Zhao H, Zhou G, An Y. Xuebijing administration alleviates pulmonary endothelial inflammation and coagulation dysregulation in the early phase of Sepsis in rats. Journal of Clinical Medicine. 2022;**11**(22):6696. DOI: 10.3390/jcm11226696

[41] Robinson N, Ganesan R, Hegedűs C, Kovács K, Kufer TA, Virág L. Programmed necrotic cell death of macrophages: Focus on pyroptosis, necroptosis, and parthanatos. Redox Biology. 2019;**26**:101239. DOI: 10.1016/j.redox.2019.101239

[42] Kopeina GS, Zhivotovsky B. Programmed cell death: Past, present and future. Biochemical and Biophysical Research Communications. 2022;**633**:55-58. DOI: 10.1016/j.bbrc.2022.09.022

[43] Dixon SJ, Lemberg KM, Lamprecht MR, Skouta R, Zaitsev EM, Gleason CE, et al. Ferroptosis: An iron-dependent form of nonapoptotic cell death. Cell. 2012;**149**(5):1060-1072. DOI: 10.1016/j.cell.2012.03.042

[44] Xie Y, Hou W, Song X, Yu Y, Huang J, Sun X, et al. Ferroptosis: Process and function. Cell Death and Differentiation. 2016;**23**(3):369-379. DOI: 10.1038/cdd.2015.158

[45] Tang D, Kroemer G. Ferroptosis. Current Biology. 2020;**30**(21):R1292-R1297. DOI: 10.1016/j.cub.2020.09.068

[46] Cheung JCT, Deng G, Wong N, Dong Y, Ng SSM. More than a duologue: In-depth insights into epitranscriptomics and ferroptosis. Frontiers in Cell and Developmental Biology. 2022;**10**:982606. DOI: 10.3389/fcell.2022.982606

[47] Moreira AC, Mesquita G, Gomes MS. Ferritin: An inflammatory player keeping iron at the core of pathogen-host interactions. Microorganisms. 2020;**8**(4):589. DOI: 10.3390/microorganisms8040589

[48] Lee J-Y, Kim WK, Bae K-H, Lee SC, Lee E-W. Lipid metabolism and ferroptosis. Biology. 2021;**10**(3):184. DOI: 10.3390/biology10030184

[49] Hirschhorn T, Stockwell BR. The development of the concept of ferroptosis. Free Radical Biology and Medicine. 2019;**133**:130-143. DOI: 10.1016/j.freeradbiomed.2018.09.043

[50] Ursini F, Maiorino M. Lipid peroxidation and ferroptosis: The role of GSH and GPx4. Free Radical Biology and Medicine. 2020;**152**:175-185. DOI: 10.1016/j.freeradbiomed.2020.02.027

[51] Gong Y, Wang N, Liu N, Dong H. Lipid peroxidation and GPX4 inhibition are common causes for myofibroblast differentiation and ferroptosis. DNA and Cell Biology. 2019;**38**(7):725-733. DOI: 10.1089/dna.2018.4541

[52] Li N, Wang W, Zhou H, Wu Q, Duan M, Liu C, et al. Ferritinophagy-mediated ferroptosis is involved in sepsis-induced cardiac injury. Free Radical Biology and Medicine. 2020;**160**:303-318. DOI: 10.1016/j.freeradbiomed.2020.08.009

[53] He R, Liu B, Xiong R, Geng B, Meng H, Lin W, et al. Itaconate inhibits ferroptosis of macrophage via Nrf2 pathways against sepsis-induced acute lung injury. Cell Death Discovery. 2022;**8**(1):43. DOI: 10.1038/s41420-021-00807-3

[54] Lv Y, Chen D, Tian X, Xiao J, Xu C, Du L, et al. Protectin conjugates in

tissue regeneration 1 alleviates sepsis-induced acute lung injury by inhibiting ferroptosis. Journal of Translational Medicine. 2023;**21**(1):293. DOI: 10.1186/s12967-023-04111-9

[55] Zhang C, Liu Z, Zhang Y, Ma L, Song E, Song Y. "Iron free" zinc oxide nanoparticles with ion-leaking properties disrupt intracellular ROS and iron homeostasis to induce ferroptosis. Cell Death and Disease. 2020;**11**(3):183. DOI: 10.1038/s41419-020-2384-5

[56] Burke MJ, Salzer WL, Devidas M, Dai Y, Gore L, Hilden JM, et al. Replacing cyclophosphamide/cytarabine/mercaptopurine with cyclophosphamide/etoposide during consolidation/delayed intensification does not improve outcome for pediatric B-cell acute lymphoblastic leukemia: A report from the COG. Haematologica. 2019;**104**(5):986. DOI: 10.3324/haematol.2018.204545

[57] Kleist SA, Knoop KA. Understanding the elements of maternal protection from systemic bacterial infections during early life. Nutrients. 2020;**12**(4):1045. DOI: 10.3390/nu12041045

[58] Huang Q, Ding Y, Fang C, Wang H, Kong L. The emerging role of ferroptosis in sepsis, opportunity or challenge? Infection and Drug Resistance. 2023;**16**:5551-5562. DOI: 10.2147/IDR.S419993

[59] Wang Y-M, Gong F-C, Qi X, et al. Mucin 1 inhibits ferroptosis and sensitizes vitamin E to alleviate sepsis-induced acute lung injury through GSK3β/Keap1-Nrf2-GPX4 pathway. Oxidative Medicine and Cellular Longevity. 2022;**2022**:2405943. DOI: 10.1155/2022/2405943

[60] Zhang J, Zheng Y, Wang Y, Wang J, Sang A, Song X, et al. YAP1 alleviates sepsis-induced acute lung injury via inhibiting ferritinophagy-mediated ferroptosis. Frontiers in Immunology. 2022;**13**:884362. DOI: 10.3389/fimmu.2022.884362

[61] Zarjou A, Black LM, McCullough KR, Hull TD, Esman SK, Boddu R, et al. Ferritin light chain confers protection against sepsis-induced inflammation and organ injury. Frontiers in Immunology. 2019;**10**:131. DOI: 10.3389/fimmu.2019.00131

[62] Yuan H, Li X, Zhang X, Kang R, Tang D. Identification of ACSL4 as a biomarker and contributor of ferroptosis. Biochemical and Biophysical Research Communications. 2016;**478**(3):1338-1343. DOI: 10.1016/j.bbrc.2016.08.124

[63] Liao P, Wang W, Wang W, Kryczek I, Li X, Bian Y, et al. CD8(+) T cells and fatty acids orchestrate tumor ferroptosis and immunity via ACSL4. Cancer Cell. 2022;**40**(4):365-378.e6. DOI: 10.1016/j.ccell.2022.02.003

[64] Wang W, Xu R, Zhao H, Xiong Y, He P. CircEXOC5 promotes ferroptosis by enhancing ACSL4 mRNA stability via binding to PTBP1 in sepsis-induced acute lung injury. Immunobiology. 2022;**227**(4):152219. DOI: 10.1016/j.imbio.2022.152219

[65] Lai K, Song C, Gao M, Deng Y, Lu Z, Li N, et al. Uridine alleviates sepsis-induced acute lung injury by inhibiting ferroptosis of macrophage. International Journal of Molecular Sciences. 2023;**24**(6):5093. DOI: 10.3390/ijms24065093

[66] Cheng PL, Chen HH, Jiang YH, Deng Y, Lu Z, Li N, et al. Using RNA-Seq to investigate immune-metabolism features in immunocompromised patients with sepsis. Frontiers in Medicine (Lausanne). 2021;**8**:747263. DOI: 10.3389/fmed.2021.747263

[67] Evans CE, Zhang X, Machireddy N, Zhao YY. The unexpected protective role of thrombosis in sepsis-induced inflammatory lung injury via endothelial Alox15. medRxiv. 2023. 2023.03.29.23287934. DOI: 10.1101/2023.03.29.23287934

[68] Shimizu J, Murao A, Nofi C, Wang P, Aziz M. Extracellular CIRP promotes GPX4-mediated ferroptosis in sepsis. Frontiers in Immunology. 2022;**13**:903859. DOI: 10.3389/fimmu.2022.903859

[69] Imai H, Matsuoka M, Kumagai T, Sakamoto T, Koumura T. Lipid peroxidation-dependent cell death regulated by GPx4 and ferroptosis. Apoptotic and Non-Apoptotic Cell Death. 2017;**403**:143-170. DOI: 10.1007/82_2016_508

[70] Chen X, Li J, Kang R, Klionsky DJ, Tang D. Ferroptosis: Machinery and regulation. Autophagy. 2021;**17**(9):2054-2081. DOI: 10.1080/15548627.2020.1810918

[71] Gao M, Monian P, Pan Q, Zhang W, Xiang J, Jiang X. Ferroptosis is an autophagic cell death process. Cell Research. 2016;**26**(9):1021-1032. DOI: 10.1038/cr.2016.95

[72] Seibt TM, Proneth B, Conrad M. Role of GPX4 in ferroptosis and its pharmacological implication. Free Radical Biology and Medicine. 2019;**133**:144-152. DOI: 10.1016/j.freeradbiomed.2018.09.014

[73] Cao Z, Qin H, Huang Y, Zhao Y, Chen Z, Hu J, et al. Crosstalk of pyroptosis, ferroptosis, and mitochondrial aldehyde dehydrogenase 2-related mechanisms in sepsis-induced lung injury in a mouse model. Bioengineered. 2022;**13**(3):4810-4820. DOI: 10.1080/21655979.2022.2033381

[74] Zhang J, Qingyuan W, Xinyi LI, Yanlin W. Role of Yes-associated protein 1 in acute lung injury in septic mice: The relationship with ferroptosis. Chinese Journal of Anesthesiology. 2022;**42**(8):970-973. DOI: 10.3760/cma.j.cn131073.20220412.00817

[75] Zou X, Liu C, Huang Z, Xiang S, Li K, Yuan Y, et al. Inhibition of STEAP1 ameliorates inflammation and ferroptosis of acute lung injury caused by sepsis in LPS-induced human pulmonary microvascular endothelial cells. Molecular Biology Reports. 2023;**50**(7):5667-5674. DOI: 10.1007/s11033-023-08403-7

[76] Li J, Li M, Li L, Ma J, Yao C, Yao S. Hydrogen sulfide attenuates ferroptosis and stimulates autophagy by blocking mTOR signaling in sepsis-induced acute lung injury. Molecular Immunology. 2022;**141**:318-327. DOI: 10.1016/j.molimm.2021.12.003

[77] Xie L, Zhou C, Wu Y, Fu X, Zhang G, Han X, et al. Wenqingyin suppresses ferroptosis in the pathogenesis of sepsis-induced liver injury by activating the Nrf2-mediated signaling pathway. Phytomedicine. 2023;**114**:154748. DOI: 10.1016/j.phymed.2023.154748

[78] Wang J, Zhu Q, Li R, Zhang J, Ye X, Li X. YAP1 protects against septic liver injury via ferroptosis resistance. Cell & Bioscience. 2022;**12**(1):163. DOI: 10.1186/s13578-022-00902-7

[79] Guo J, Wang R, Min F. Ginsenoside Rg1 ameliorates sepsis-induced acute kidney injury by inhibiting ferroptosis in renal tubular epithelial cells. Journal of Leukocyte Biology. 2022;**112**(5):1065-1077. DOI: 10.1002/JLB.1A0422-211R

[80] Qiu W, An S, Wang T, Li J, Yu B, Zeng Z, et al. Melatonin suppresses ferroptosis via activation of the

Nrf2/HO-1 signaling pathway in the mouse model of sepsis-induced acute kidney injury. International Immunopharmacology. 2022;**112**:109162. DOI: 10.1016/j.intimp.2022.109162

[81] Chen Z, Cao Z, Gui F, Zhang M, Wu X, Peng H, et al. TMEM43 protects against sepsis-induced cardiac injury via inhibiting ferroptosis in mice. Cells. 2022;**11**(19):2992. DOI: 10.3390/cells11192992

[82] Zhou B, Zhang J, Chen Y, Liu Y, Tang X, Xia P, et al. Puerarin protects against sepsis-induced myocardial injury through AMPK-mediated ferroptosis signaling. Aging (Albany NY). 2022;**14**(8):3617. DOI: 10.18632/aging.204033

[83] Herrero R, Sánchez G, Asensio I, López E, Ferruelo A, Vaquero J, et al. Liver–lung interactions in acute respiratory distress syndrome. Intensive Care Medicine Experimental. 2020;**8**(Suppl 1):48. DOI: 10.1186/s40635-020-00337-9

[84] Doi K, Ishizu T, Fujita T, Noiri E. Lung injury following acute kidney injury: Kidney–lung crosstalk. Clinical and Experimental Nephrology. 2011;**15**:464-470. DOI: 10.1007/s10157-011-0459-4

[85] Li Z, Yu Y, Bu Y, Liu C, Jin J, Li W, et al. QiShenYiQi pills preserve endothelial barrier integrity to mitigate sepsis-induced acute lung injury by inhibiting ferroptosis. Journal of Ethnopharmacology. 2023:117610. DOI: 10.1016/j.jep.2023.117610

[86] Tang X, Liu J, Yao S, Zheng J, Gong X, Xiao B. Ferulic acid alleviates alveolar epithelial barrier dysfunction in sepsis-induced acute lung injury by activating the Nrf2/HO-1 pathway and inhibiting ferroptosis. Pharmaceutical Biology. 2022;**60**(1):2286-2294. DOI: 10.1080/13880209.2022.2147549

[87] Wang Y, Chen D, Xie H, Jia M, Sun X, Peng F, et al. AUF1 protects against ferroptosis to alleviate sepsis-induced acute lung injury by regulating NRF2 and ATF3. Cellular and Molecular Life Sciences. 2022;**79**(5):228. DOI: 10.1007/s00018-022-04248-8

Chapter 4

Challenges in Critical Care Lung Ultrasound

Pedro Yasfir González-Noris

Abstract

Nowadays, lung ultrasonography is routinely used in critical care medicine during bedside rounds in several intensive care units across the world. Despite its increasing popularity, some hurdles persist in the efficient deployment of lung ultrasonography. This chapter focuses on challenges like limited training opportunities, difficulty in interpretation, and how other techniques like transesophageal lung ultrasonography (TELUS) might be advantageous in some situations. Certain devices equipped with advanced software can significantly aid in the learning process by providing appropriate feedback, and in low-income settings, the use of lung ultrasonography has been shown to be beneficial. Furthermore, in comparison with other modalities such as chest radiography, the diagnostic accuracy may be equivalent or superior using lung ultrasound.

Keywords: lung ultrasound, TELUS, training, protocols, diagnostic accuracy

1. Introduction

Some of the challenges of lung ultrasound are essentially patient-dependent. Obese patients are frequently difficult to examine because of the thickness of their ribcage and soft tissues. Furthermore, subcutaneous emphysema can alter the propagation of ultrasound beams. Lung ultrasonography (LUS) is recognized for its utility in assessing diuretic responsiveness in acute heart failure and cardiogenic pulmonary illness. Conversely, when the analysis of natriuretic peptide B lines is unfeasible, it may serve as an excellent alternative [1]. LUS presents several advantages over chest radiography: it is devoid of radiation, economically viable, permits follow-up examinations, aids in treatment assessment, is easily accessible in diverse environments, is straightforward to master, and can be employed immediately as a point-of-care instrument [2].

In certain situations, such as heart failure and cardiogenic pulmonary edema accompanying acute exacerbation of chronic obstructive pulmonary disease, differentiation may pose challenges; however, Lajili et al. demonstrated that the diagnostic efficacy of lung ultrasound and LUS score for heart failure in the context of acute exacerbation of chronic pulmonary disease is satisfactory, with a cutoff of 5 indicating good sensitivity and a cutoff of 30 indicating good specificity. An LUS score below 5 can effectively exclude heart failure, whereas a value beyond 30 indicates a higher likelihood of heart failure [3].

The evaluation of pleural anomalies is crucial for differentiating between ARDS and cardiogenic edema; however, it may pose difficulties for inexperienced practitioners. In certain cases, the integration of LUS with targeted cardiac ultrasound may be warranted [4]. Pleural effusion is readily identifiable; however, discerning the origin and assessing the volume can prove more difficult. B-lines are readily identifiable; however, their genesis and clinical interpretation may provide challenges for assessment. Lung consolidation is readily identifiable; nevertheless, differentiating between atelectasis and pneumonia necessitates that the sonographer possess the ability to recognize dynamic air bronchograms and interpret color Doppler, which likely represents at least intermediate proficiency [5].

The diagnostic accuracy of lung ultrasound has been characterized in various respiratory pathologies. Pneumonia has a sensitivity of 89% and a specificity of 94%. The positive predictive value for pneumonia is 88%, while the negative predictive value is 95%. Pneumothorax has a sensitivity of 88% and a specificity of 100%. The positive predictive value for pneumothorax is 100%, while the negative predictive value is 99%. This illustrates why the lung point serves as a pathognomonic marker for pneumothorax. Meanwhile, chronic obstructive pulmonary disease and asthma exacerbation have a sensitivity of 89%, a specificity of 97%, a positive predictive value of 93%, and a negative predictive value of 95%. Acute pulmonary edema has a sensitivity of 97%, specificity of 95%, positive predictive value of 87%, and negative predictive value of 99% [6]. Additionally, the accuracy of the diagnosis of pneumonia in the intensive care unit is significantly higher compared to the accuracy of chest X-rays [7]. The evidence presented may be a significant factor in advocating for the integration of this impact into all residency programs for critical care medicine globally.

2. Training

The application of lung ultrasonography is increasingly gaining popularity globally in critical care medicine; nevertheless, a standardized training model is needed. Moreover, in several residency programs, the utilization of ultrasonography is optional rather than mandatory.

There are different programs regarding lung ultrasound. Four levels of expertise have been described: The fundamental level consists of a straightforward identification of A-lines, B-lines, and consolidations [8]. An intermediate level may encompass pleural movement analysis (sliding, lung pulse, lung point) and supplementary skills such as pleural effusion quantification, air-bronchogram analysis, and a systematic diagnostic approach to acute respiratory failure; advanced knowledge may involve quantitative lung ultrasound as a monitoring instrument (calculation of lung ultrasound score and ventilator-associated pneumonia lung ultrasound score); and the expert level incorporates both qualitative and quantitative lung ultrasound in the clinical management of acute respiratory failure patients and as a guide for mechanical ventilation strategy. Clinical investigation must validate this hypothesis. Achieving sufficient training, which is now lacking, is also a topic of uncertainty [9].

3. Protocols

There are different protocols to approach the lung systematically in critical care medicine, and the scale most used is the lung ultrasonography scale (LUS). COVID-19

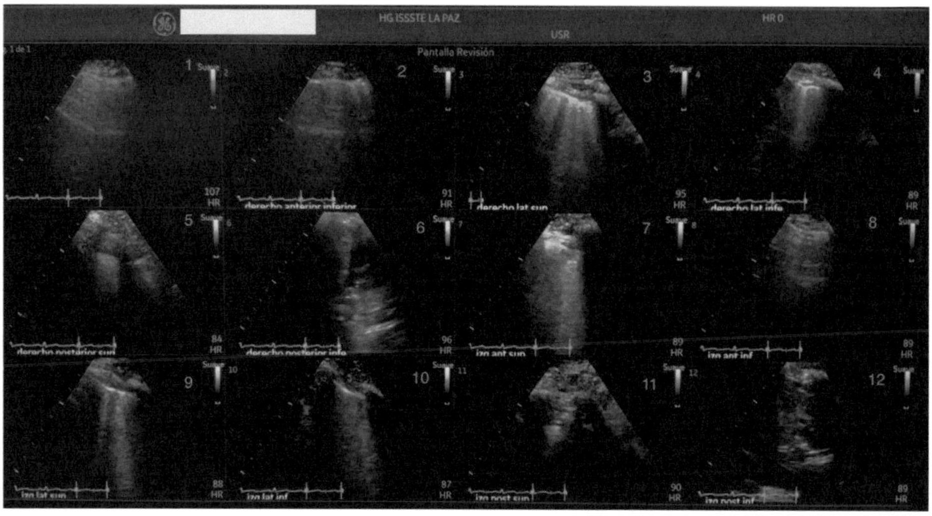

Figure 1.
Depicts a 12-point LUS in a patient with ARDS and pneumonia. Heterogeneous findings. Numbers: 1, 2, 8 A lines. Numbers: 3, 5, 9, and 10 B lines. Number: 4 A-B lines. Number: 7 subpleural consolidation and B lines. Numbers: 6, 11, 12 air bronchogram—consolidated lung. Image created by the author.

was involved in many publications of lung ultrasound; certainly, one of the protocols, like 12-zone ultrasound scanning, appears to be the ideal protocol for identifying disease severity [10]. Some of the challenges are to demonstrate a reduction in mortality using personalized mechanical ventilation guided by ultrasound in patients with acute respiratory distress syndrome, using a 12-point LUS exam [11]. Conceivably, the protocol using 12 points might be the standard of lung approach systematically in the intensive care unit at the bedside, to know daily changes. The following series of images, which show heterogeneous findings in a patient with COVID-19 pneumonia, illustrates how our institution routinely follows this protocol (**Figure 1**). However, this protocol uses transthoracic probes.

4. Transesophageal lung ultrasound (TELUS)

Transesophageal lung ultrasonography is mostly used in critical care medicine when transthoracic lung ultrasound does not provide enough image quality to resolve a clinical question. In this case, without contraindications, TELUS often produces satisfactory image quality. TELUS is often used when patient-related concerns, like obesity, significant edema, substantial musculature, chest wall considerations, or the difficulties in positioning the patient for sufficient transtoracic lung imaging, occur.

One advantage of TELUS is its capacity to properly scan the posterior lungs of a supine patient with severe sickness; hence, accessing places is usually difficult to see by transthoracic ultrasonography. Often, during a typical transthoracic exam in the supine patient with severe illness, the dependent areas of the lungs (inferoposterior) and the blind spots produced by the scapulae (superoposterior) are inaccessible with transthoracic ultrasound. Advanced applications of TELUS encompass real-time imaging to facilitate interventions, including drainage catheter placement and ventilator recruitment maneuvers. Concerning the latter, TELUS can facilitate the detection of lung recruitment through the application of positive end-expiratory pressure in acute respiratory distress syndrome while simultaneously evaluating right and left ventricular function as part of heart-lung interactions, such as cor pulmonale [12]. The use of TELUS has been described in hypoxemic patients with COVID-19 in an emergency scenario, approaching diagnosis and guiding mechanical ventilation [13].

TELUS provides a complimentary lung imaging method, transthoracic lung ultrasound, for the point-of-care evaluation of respiratory failure. The short effort and time required to get significant information, particularly about the lung bases, renders TELUS easily integrable for the bedside physician during critical care transesophageal echocardiography (TEE). As other centers implement critical care TEE, it will be crucial to investigate its incremental effects on a larger scale. The indications for TELUS are patient-dependent. The most common indications include differential diagnosis of acute hypoxemia, differential diagnosis of reduced respiratory system compliance, qualitative and quantitative evaluation of suspected pleural effusion, monitoring the impact of ventilator settings and prone positioning in ARDS, and assessing extravascular lung water to inform fluid and diuretic therapy. Contraindications to TELUS, include esophageal pathologic features, recent upper gastrointestinal surgery, and bleeding tendency [12, 14].

4.1 Lung examination

It is necessary to separate each lung along the craniocaudal axis into apical, middle, and basal regions. The origin of the left subclavian artery is used as a landmark to identify the apical regions. The superior pulmonary veins are used to mark the middle regions. Finally, the inferior vena cava is right atrial. From a cardiocentric starting position at 12:00, the TEE probe is rotated counterclockwise to examine the left lung, with continued rotation to examine the right lung until a full rotation is completed [12].

Our institution uses TELUS alongside TEE, particularly in challenging scenarios, as illustrated in the following figures, which depict a patient with cardiogenic shock who subsequently develops pneumonia and pleural effusion. As mentioned, the left lung is easier to acquire images of because the aorta offers a better beam view. **Figure 2** shows the posterior base, **Figure 3** shows the posterior medium, and **Figure 4** shows the posterior apical region.

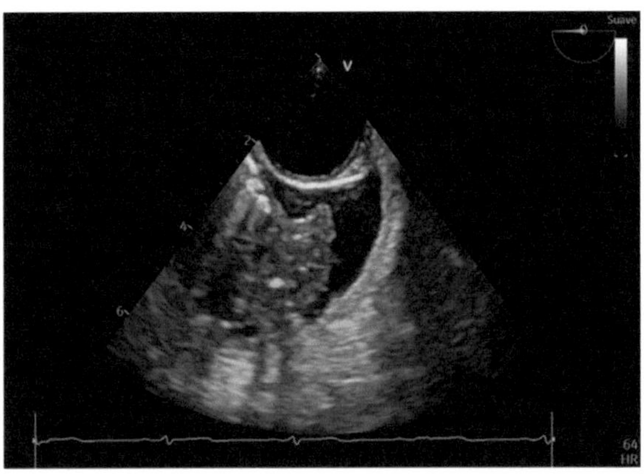

Figure 2.
Aortic view. Air bronchogram. Hyperechoic air bubbles trapped in bronchi are seen surrounded by lung consolidation and pleural effusion. Image created by the author.

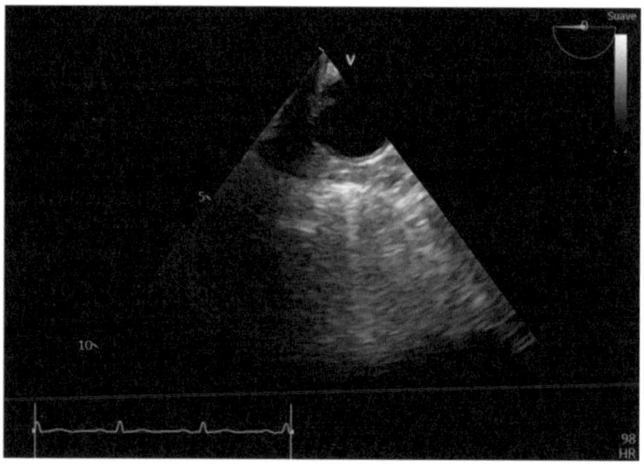

Figure 3.
B line and thickened pleural line. Image created by the author.

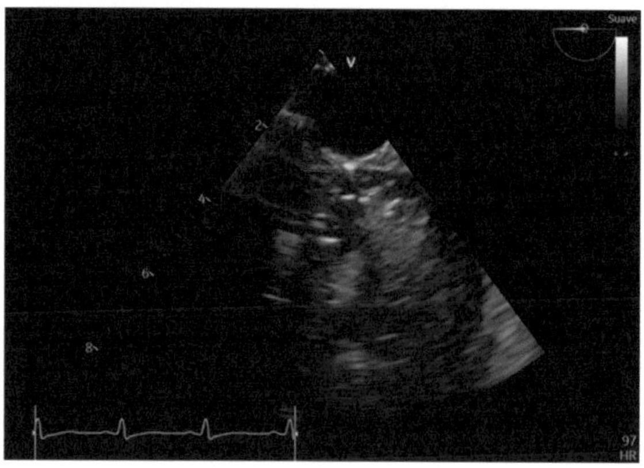

Figure 4.
Air bronchogram and consolidation. Image created by the author.

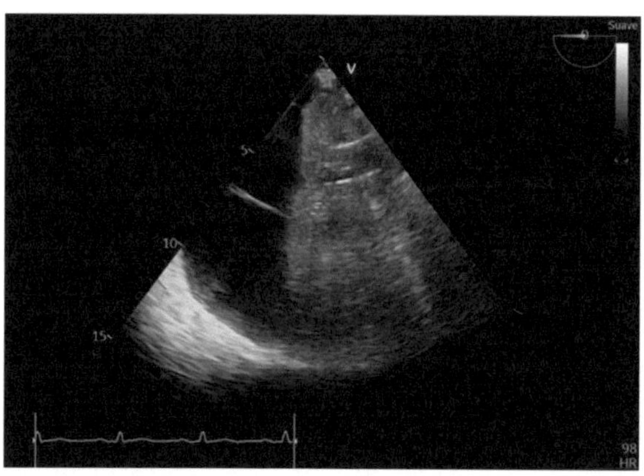

Figure 5.
Consolidation and pleural effusion. Image created by the author.

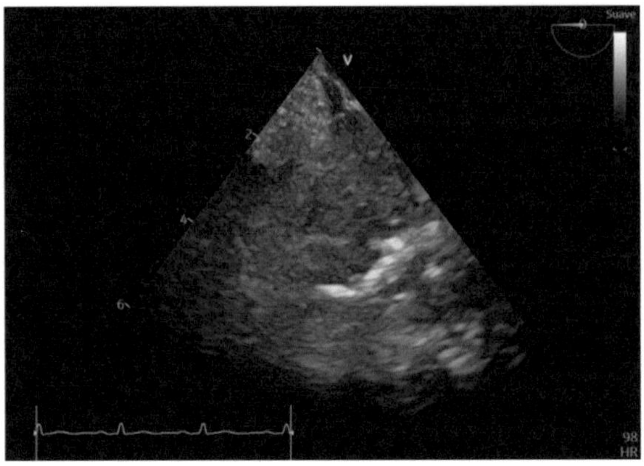

Figure 6.
Air bronchogram and consolidated lung. Image created by the author.

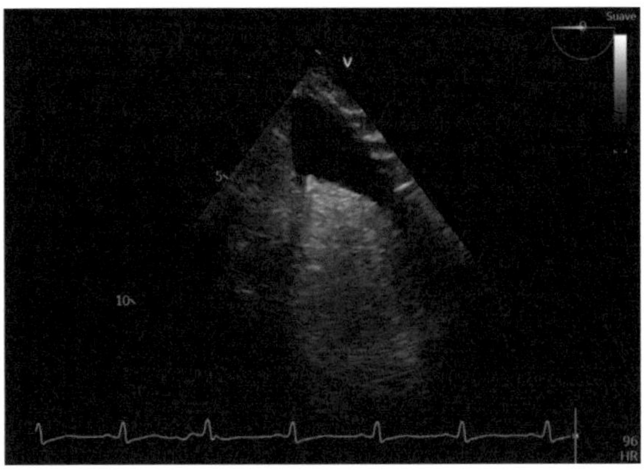

Figure 7.
Pleural effusion and atelectasis. Image created by the author.

Nonetheless, the right lung may present greater challenges due to the proximity of the esophagus to the dorsal vertebrae. Otherwise, it can be seen in certain respiratory diseases. **Figure 5** shows the posterior base, **Figure 6** shows the posterior medium, and **Figure 7** shows the posterior apical.

5. Future directions

5.1 ARDS and mechanical ventilation

Since the relevance of lung ultrasound in the diagnosis of respiratory diseases [15] was the cornerstone for advancing the use of lung ultrasound. LUS is also helpful in conditions most prevalent in low-income settings; for instance, one of the causes of death in malaria is ARDS. Furthermore, the Kigali modifications of the Berlin criteria have helped to diagnose ARDS by allowing ultrasound to identify bilateral pulmonary edema instead of chest radiography or tomography [16]. For this reason, LUS will be more available in the future in these settings around the world. The LUS score may be used effectively to assess the need for surfactant replacement therapy or mechanical ventilation in newborns experiencing respiratory distress [17]. Likewise in adults needs to be validated the use of lung ultrasound-guided mechanical ventilation in ARDS [11].

5.2 Artificial intelligence

Some of the challenges in LUS are identifying B-lines; for this reason, there are different software programs that can be helpful. The use of artificial intelligence introduces objectivity, improves inter-rater reliability, and enhances quality assurance with good sensibility and specificity in the context of A and B lines; however, it is necessary to add tools to identify lung sliding and consolidations [18]. Deep learning models applied to analysis have shown that deep learning algorithms are able to perform at a high level of accuracy [19]. Innovative artificial intelligence methodologies must be established to deliver real-time feedback to users during imaging sessions. Artificial intelligence possesses significant potential to enhance the quality of LUS images and to assist the operator during the acquisition process [20]. For instance, it has been demonstrated that trained healthcare professionals aided by artificial intelligence achieved comparable performance to expert LUS users in acquiring images meeting diagnostic standards following brief software-focused training [21]. Moreover, in pleural effusion, deep learning models are accurate compared to the algorithm and experts [22]. Nevertheless, the pleural line automatic recognition algorithm automatically finds the pleural line and works just as well as bedside chest X-ray for diagnosing pneumothorax and is more convenient and quicker [23].

6. Conclusions

Every intensive care unit around the world should consider using lung ultrasound due to its low cost, benefits in low-income settings, and superior diagnostic capabilities compared to other options. Furthermore, different approaches like TELUS need to be a mandatory part of the academic residency program of critical care medicine. Meanwhile, the use of artificial intelligence in lung ultrasound enhances the inter-rater reliability of the observer.

Acknowledgements

Thank you to all of the critical care attending staff and critical care nurses of the intensive care unit in the General Hospital ISSSTE La Paz.

This is for everyone who believes in lung ultrasound.

Conflict of interest

The author declares no conflict of interest.

Notes

The images used in this chapter were developed by the author.

Author details

Pedro Yasfir González-Noris
Intensive Care Unit, General Hospital ISSSTE, La Paz, Mexico

*Address all correspondence to: drpedroygonzalez@gmail.com

References

[1] Gargani L. Lung ultrasound: A new tool for the cardiologist. Cardiovascular Ultrasound. 2011;**9**:6

[2] Buonsenso D, De Rose C. Implementation of lung ultrasound in-to middle -income countries: A new challenge global health? European Journal of Pediatrics. 2022;**181**(1):1-8

[3] Lajili F, Toumia M, Sekma A, Bel Haj Ali K, Sassi S, Zorgati A, et al. Value of lung ultrasound sonography B-lines quantification as a marker of heart failure in COPD exacerbation. International Journal of Chronic Obstructive Pulmonary Disease. 2024;**19**:1767-1774. DOI: 10.2147/COPD.S447819

[4] Smit MR, Mayo PH, Mongodi S. Lung ultrasound for diagnosis and management of ARDS. Intensive Care Medicine. 2024;**50**:1143-1145. DOI: 10.1007/s00134-024-07422-7

[5] Kraaijenbrink BVC, Mousa A, Bos LD, Paulus F, Tuinman PR. Defining basic (lung) ultrasound skills: Not so basic after all? Intensive Care Medicine. 2022;**48**:628-629

[6] Northern T, Broyles MG, Nooli NP, Peirce A, Tuck BC, Coker BJ. Applications of perioperative lung ultrasound: From the clinic to the ICU. International Anesthesiology Clinics. 2022;**60**(3):41-44. DOI: 10.1097/AIA.0000000000000370

[7] Dhawan J, Singh G. Bedside lung ultrasound as an independent tool to diagnose pneumonia in comparison to chest X-ray: An observational prospective study from intensive care units. Indian Journal of Critical Care Medicine. 2022;**26**(8):920-929. DOI: 10.5005/jp-journals-10071-24283

[8] Arbelot C, Dexheimer Neto FL, Gao Y, Brisson H, Chunyao W, Lv J, et al. Lung ultrasound in emergency and critically ill patients number of supervised exams to reach basic competence. Anesthesiology. 2020;**132**:899-907

[9] Mongodi S, Bonomi F, Vaschetto R, Robba C, Salve G, Volta CA, et al. Point-of-care ultrasound training for residents in anaesthesia and critical care: Results of a national survey comparing residents and training program directors' perspectives. BMC Medical Education. 2022;**22**:647

[10] Rinaldi L, Lugarà M, Simeon V, Perrotta F, Romano C, Iadevaia C, et al. Application and internal validation of lung ultrasound score in COVID-19 setting: The ECOVITA observational study. Pulmonology. 2025;**31**(1):2416842. DOI: 10.1016/j.pulmoe.2024.04.012. Epub 2024 Oct 25

[11] Sinnige JS, Smit MR, Ghose A, de Grooth H-J, Itenov TS, Ischaki E, et al. Personalized mechanical ventilation guided by ultrasound in patients with acute respiratory distress syndrome (PEGASUS): Study protocol for an international randomized clinical trial. Trials. 2024;**25**:308

[12] Weber AG, Mastroianni F, Koenig S, Mayo PH. Transesophageal lung ultrasonography as part of the critical care transesophageal echocardiography examination. Chest. 2022;**161**(6):e335-e336. DOI: 10.1016/j.chest.2022.01.025. Epub 2022 Jan 23

[13] Cavayas YA, Girard M, Desjardins G, et al. Transesophageal lung ultrasonography: A novel technique for investigating hypoxemia. Canadian Journal of Anesthesia/Journal canadien

d'anesthésie. 2016;**63**:1266-1276. DOI: 10.1007/s12630-016-0702-2

[14] Hilberath JN, Oakes DA, Shernan SK, Bulwer BE, D'Ambra MN, Eltzschig HK. Safety of transesophageal echocardiography. Journal of the American Society of Echocardiography. 2010;**23**(11):1115-1127; quiz 1220-1. DOI: 10.1016/j.echo.2010.08.013

[15] Lichtenstein DA, Mezière GA. Relevance of lung ultrasound in the diagnosis of acute respiratory failure: The BLUE protocol. Chest. 2008;**134**(1):117-125. DOI: 10.1378/chest.07-2800. Epub 2008 Apr 10. Erratum in: Chest. 2013 Aug;144(2):721

[16] Tran TT, Hlaing M, Krause M. Point-of-care ultrasound: Applications in low- and middle-income countries. Current Anesthesiology Reports. 2021;**11**(1):69-75. DOI: 10.1007/s40140-020-00429-y. Epub 2021 Jan 6

[17] Razak A, Faden M. Neonatal lung ultrasonography to evaluate need for surfactant or mechanical ventilation: A systematic review and meta-analysis. Archives of Disease in Childhood. Fetal and Neonatal Edition. 2020;**105**:164-171

[18] Nekoui M, Seyed Bolouri SE, Forouzandeh A, Dehghan M, Zonoobi D, Jaremko JL, et al. Enhancing lung ultrasound diagnostics: A clinical study on an artificial intelligence tool for the detection and quantification of A-lines and B-lines. Diagnostics. 2024;**14**(22):2526. DOI: 10.3390/diagnostics14222525

[19] Baloescu C, Toporek G, Kim S, McNamara K, Liu R, Shaw MM, et al. Automated lung ultrasound B-line assessment using a deep learning algorithm. IEEE Transactions on Ultrasonics, Ferroelectrics, and Frequency Control. 2020;**67**:2312-2320

[20] Demi L, Wolfram F, Klersy C, De Silvestri A, Ferretti VV, Muller M, et al. New international guidelines and consensus on the use of lung ultrasound. Journal of Ultrasound in Medicine. 2023;**42**(2):309-344. DOI: 10.1002/jum.16088. Epub 2022 Aug 22

[21] Baloescu C, Bailitz J, Cheema B, Agarwala R, Jankowski M, Eke O, et al. Artificial intelligence-guided lung ultrasound by nonexperts. JAMA Cardiology. 2025;**10**(3):245-253. DOI: 10.1001/jamacardio.2024.4991

[22] Vukovic D, Wang A, Antico M, Steffens M, Ruvinov I, van Sloun RJ, et al. Automatic deep learning-based pleural effusion segmentation in lung ultrasound images. BMC Medical Informatics and Decision Making. 2023;**23**(1):274. DOI: 10.1186/s12911-023-02362-6

[23] Yang C, Zhao H, Wang A, Li J, Gao J. Comparison of lung ultrasound assisted by artificial intelligence to radiology examination in pneumothorax. Journal of Clinical Ultrasound. 2024;**52**(8):1051-1055. DOI: 10.1002/jcu.23756. Epub 2024 Jun 29

Chapter 5

Intensive Care Management of Stroke

Hussain Ayyaz and Saskin Vitaly Alexandrovich

Abstract

Stroke is a leading cause of disability and mortality worldwide. The management of stroke involves several important stages, including prehospital, hospital, and outpatient care. The hospital phase of stroke management begins with critical care in many countries. Recent advances in clinical research and critical care have led to significant improvements in stroke management. In this chapter, we will discuss the current definition, classification, pathogenesis, and management of different types of stroke in the critical care setting. We will discuss the algorithm for the management of different types of stroke. The current practice of intravenous thrombolysis, mechanical thrombectomy in ischemic stroke and subarachnoid hemorrhage will be discussed.

Keywords: ischemic stroke, intracerebral hemorrhage, subarachnoid hemorrhage, intracranial aneurysm, intravenous thrombolysis

1. Introduction

Cerebrovascular diseases constitute a significant public health concern, constituting a worldwide epidemic that poses substantial threats to the life and well-being of the global population [1–4].

According to the World Health Organization, stroke is characterized as the sudden onset of clinical symptoms indicative of focal or diffuse brain dysfunction, which persist for more than 24 hours or result in death, provided that no alternative causes, other than those of cerebrovascular origin, can be identified [5].

This definition encompasses all types of strokes, including ischemic, hemorrhagic stroke (subarachnoid hemorrhage and intracerebral hemorrhage), and strokes not classified as either hemorrhagic or ischemic.

Stroke outcomes are affected by various factors, and many patients require critical care both in the early and late stages of stroke [6–8]. The primary objectives of admission to specialized intensive care for stroke patients include treatment, as well as diagnosis, prophylaxis, and treatment of specific complications. Stroke patients require a personalized therapeutic strategy considering various factors such as the size and location of hemorrhage and ischemic lesions, the hemodynamic status, and severity of neurological impairment using the National Institute of Health Stroke Scale (NIHSS).

Core principles of intensive care of stroke patients are:

1. Management of acute revascularization period of ischemic stroke

2. Hemodynamic optimization

3. Airway management and ventilatory support

4. Management of cerebral edema and intracranial hypertension

5. Supportive care

2. Management of acute revascularization period ischemic stroke

The acute vascularization of ischemic stroke can be achieved through intravenous thrombolysis or mechanical thrombectomy, or a combination of both methods.

Commonly used intravenous thrombolytic drugs include recombinant tissue plasminogen activator (rt-PA) (such as alteplase and tenecteplase) and recombinant non-immunogenic Staphylokinase [9–11].

According to current American Heart Association (AHA)/ASA guidelines, intravenous thrombolysis (IVT) is recommended for eligible patients within 4.5 hours of symptom onset of ischemic stroke [12–14]. Mechanical thrombectomy (MT) alone is recommended if IVT is contraindicated. MT + IVT is standard for large vessel occlusion (LVO) patients within 6 hours. MT ≤24 h is indicated in select patients with imaging mismatch (e.g., WAKE-UP Stroke, DWI/FLAIR mismatch, and DAWN/DEFUSE-3 criteria) [15–21].

The primary method for objectively monitoring intravenous thrombolysis (IVT) is through repeated CT scans or high-field MRI. This should be conducted 24 hours after the thrombolytic procedure in all patients, or immediately if clinical signs of deterioration are observed. Evaluate neurological status during IVT and for 24 hours after its completion. Recommended NIHSS assessment frequency: every 15 minutes during thrombolytic administration (1 hour); every 30 minutes for the next 6 hours; every 60 minutes until 24 hours post-procedure [22–24].

In the context of IVT, a reduction of at least 4 points or more on the NIHSS scale within 24 hours is considered a "successful recanalization" or modified Thrombolysis In Cerebral Infarction (mTICI) 2b or 3. This parameter serves as a primary criterion of the effectiveness of IVT [14, 25, 26].

2.1 Blood pressure management during acute revascularization period

During IVT and the first 24 hours, continuous monitoring blood pressure is recommended. If systolic BP exceeds 185 mmHg and/or diastolic BP exceeds 110 mmHg during IVT, the procedure should be paused, and efforts should be made to reduce the blood pressure below these limits. If successful, IVT can be continued once the BP is within the acceptable range [14, 27].

The use of oral and sublingual dosage forms is not preferred for managing hypertension due to their inability to provide a controlled and rapid hypotensive effect [14, 27]. Intravenous antihypertensive drugs are recommended in such cases (**Table 1**).

Drug	Stroke Context	Dosing Protocol	Max Dose	Key Considerations
First-Line Agents				
Urapidil	Ischemic hemorrhagic	Bolus: 12.5–25 mg IV Infusion: start 5 mg/h	40 mg/h	α_1-blocker with central 5-HT_1A agonism; used in Europe/Asia [28].
Labetalol	Ischemic (thrombolysis)	Bolus: 10–20 mg IV over 1–2 min; repeat every 10 min	300 mg total	α/β-blocker; first-line for IVT candidates [14, 27, 29]. Avoid in asthma, heart failure patients.
	Hemorrhagic	Infusion: 2–8 mg/min	300 mg/ day	
Nicardipine	Hemorrhagic	Start at 5 mg/h; titrate by 2.5 mg/h every 15 min	15 mg/h	Dilute to reduce phlebitis risk; preferred for titratability.
	Ischemic (thrombolysis)	Start at 5 mg/h	15 mg/h	
Clevidipine	General hypertensive emergency	Start at 1–2 mg/h IV; titrate by 1–2 mg/h every 5–10 min	32 mg/h	Rapid onset; preferred for labile BP.
Nimodipine	Hemorrhagic (Prophylaxis of vasospasm after aneurysmal subarachnoid hemorrhage) [30];	1 mg/hour (5 mL/h) first 2 hours, after 2 hours 2 mg/ hour (10 mL/h) (Alternative for patients who cannot tolerate oral medications)		Must be administered through a central line.
Alternatives and second Line				
Enalaprilat	Ischemic and hemorrhagic	1.25 mg IV over 5 min, repeat every 6 hrs.	5 mg total	ACE inhibitor; prevent hypovolemia to reduce the risk of a significant hypotension.
Esmolol	Tachycardia-associated	Bolus: 500 μg/kg IV over 1 min; Infusion: 50–300 μg/kg/min	N/A	Ultra-short acting; avoid in heart block.
Nitroprusside	Refractory hypertension	Start at 0.25 μg/kg/ min; titrate every 5 min	10 μg/kg/ min	Monitor for cyanide toxicity (max 4-hour use)
Azamethonium bromide	Ischemic and hemorrhagic	0–150 mg IV infusion, titrate to effect	450 mg/ day	Rarely used; historical interest (ganglionic blocker).
Hydralazine	Ischemic and hemorrhagic	10–20 mg IV, repeat every 15 min (max 3 doses)	60 mg total	Direct vasodilator; may cause reflex tachycardia.

Table 1.
Intravenous antihypertensive drugs in acute period of stroke.

There are additional potential complications associated with thrombolytic therapy, including anaphylactoid reactions and arterial hypotension. Anaphylactoid reactions during intravenous thrombolysis are often related to the concurrent use of ACE inhibitors or prior administration of drugs from this group. The occurrence of anaphylaxis requires immediate discontinuation of thrombolytic therapy. Management includes the use of H1-antihistamines, and glucocorticosteroids may be indicated in severe cases. Adrenaline is recommended for anaphylactic shock; however, its use should be minimized in other situations due to the increased risk of intracerebral hemorrhages associated with hypertension [14, 27].

2.2 Hemorrhagic complications of IVT

Monitoring indirect signs of cerebral hemorrhagic complications is essential. These signs include a significant deterioration in the patient's neurological status (an increase in the total NIHSS score ≥ 4 points or an increase of >2 points from baseline) occurring during or within 24–36 hours after IVT, as well as the onset of meningeal signs (neck muscle stiffness, Bekhterev's zygomatic syndrome, Kernig's symptom, Brudzinsky, Mondonesi, Mendel, etc.). Signs of intracranial hemorrhage are criteria for stopping thrombolytic therapy immediately and conducting an urgent CT scan [14, 26, 27, 31, 32].

Sites of extracranial bleeding are:

- Damaged Skin: Includes any cuts, abrasions, wounds, surgical sites, IV-line insertion sites, sites of recent blood draws, intramuscular injection sites) – these are common points for oozing or hematoma formation under thrombolysis [33–35].

- Genitourinary Tract (Bladder/Kidneys): Hematuria, bleeding from urinary catheter insertion sites [33–35].

- Gastrointestinal Tract: Hematemesis, blood in stool, can be melena or hematochezia, blood *via* nasogastric/orogastric tube: aspiration of blood or coffee-ground material from the stomach.

- Hidden hematomas: particularly those resulting from falls or trauma in the prehospital stage, should be monitored for signs such as unexplained pain, swelling, or bruising at potential trauma sites (e.g., flank, thigh, back, and abdomen). Also, watch for indicators of compartment syndrome (severe pain, pallor, paresthesia, paralysis, pulselessness) in an extremity, unexplained decreases in hemoglobin/hematocrit, and tachycardia or hypotension that may suggest internal blood loss [36–38].

The occurrence of life-threatening bleeding is an indication for the immediate cessation of thrombolytic therapy [10, 14, 27, 37, 39].

3. Hemodynamic optimization

3.1 Maintaining cerebral perfusion

Maintaining adequate cerebral perfusion is a key goal of intensive care management for patients with ischemic stroke. However, identifying the optimal blood pressure range during intensive care for these patients is still an unresolved issue. Increasing blood pressure through infusion therapy and the use of vasopressors can improve cerebral blood flow, brain oxygenation, and metabolic processes. On the other hand, this intervention may be associated with various potential complications, including acute respiratory distress syndrome and myocardial injury.

Maintaining blood pressure within MAP of >70 mmHg is essential to balance improved cerebral perfusion and the risk of cardiovascular and pulmonary complications in patients with ischemic stroke without reperfusion therapies. This strategy aims to enhance patient outcomes and ensure safer intensive care for ischemic stroke patients. Patients with long-term hypertension may require a different blood pressure target.

3.2 Hypertension management

Elevated blood pressure is frequently observed in the early stages of ischemic stroke, as it helps to sustain cerebral perfusion, particularly in the affected areas of the brain [29, 40–43].

Evidence suggests that a decrease in blood pressure during the initial hours following ischemic stroke is correlated with poor neurological outcome. Conversely, excessively elevated blood pressure levels are also considered potentially hazardous [29, 44].

Current guidelines recommend that the patient who is not undergoing intravenous thrombolysis have their arterial blood pressure reduced to below 220/120 mmHg within the first 24 hours following the onset of ischemic stroke [14, 44].

3.3 Blood pressure management in intracerebral hemorrhage (ICH)

Optimal blood pressure levels in patients with acute hemorrhagic stroke are undetermined due to conflicting views. While high blood pressure can worsen outcomes by increasing hematoma size, it may also help maintain cerebral perfusion. Lowering blood pressure has shown mixed results; some studies suggest it reduces hematoma growth, but larger studies have not confirmed significant benefits from aggressive reduction [42, 43, 45, 46].

However, the Expert consensus statement the European Stroke Organization in the 2025 guidelines recommends targeting systolic blood pressure below 140 mmHg within 6 hours for minor to moderate ICH patients (hematoma volume < 30 ml). For patients with a large volume of ICH (over 30 ml) and high initial systolic blood pressure (>220 mmHg), or if surgery is planned, blood pressure reduction should be approached with caution. The blood pressure-lowering treatment should ideally start within the first 2 hours of symptom onset [43, 44].

3.4 Antihypertensive drugs used in stroke

Intravenous short-acting antihypertensive medications are recommended in the acute phase of stroke, due to their ability to rapidly and effectively control blood pressure [14, 29, 41–43].

Oral antihypertensives are generally avoided in the initial hours of acute stroke management when significant blood pressure reduction is required, due to their slow and unpredictable effects as well as challenges with titration. These medications become more relevant later for transitioning to maintenance therapy once the patient's condition has stabilized [29, 41–43, 46].

The selection of antihypertensive medications and the appropriate duration of treatment remain unclear and under investigation. To achieve a rapid and sustained antihypertensive effect while mitigating the risk of excessive hypotension, it is advisable to administer drugs with rapid onset of action and shorter duration of action. Some of these drugs and their doses are summarized in **Table 1**.

3.5 Management of cerebral vasospasm and cerebral ischemia in subarachnoid hemorrhage

- The administration of calcium channel blockers, specifically nimodipine, is advised prophylactically prior to the onset of instrumental or clinical indications of vasospasm, as its efficacy is limited to prevention and it is ineffective once vasospasm has developed. Nimodipine may be prescribed orally at a dosage of 60 mg every 4 hours or *via* continuous intravenous infusion. Contraindications include known hypersensitivity to the drug and a predisposition to persistent arterial hypotension.

- Maintenance of normovolemia should be achieved through the controlled administration of colloid and crystalloid solutions, with monitoring of central venous pressure (CVP) and urine output.

- Currently, there are no proven therapies for established vasopasm. Management should focus on supporting cerebral perfusion, including the prevention of hypotension and hypovolemia, maintenance of appropriate electrolyte balance, and reduction of intracranial pressure (ICP).

- Triple-H therapy (hypervolemia, hemodilution, hypertension) is not recommended during the preoperative period. Furthermore, the efficacy of antioxidants and anti-inflammatory agents, including hormonal drugs, has not been substantiated.

3.6 Fluid infusion

The choice of fluid infusion depends on a detailed assessment of the patient's intravascular volume status. Both colloid and crystalloid solutions are used for fluid infusion therapy. Crystalloids (e.g., 0.9% saline, lactated Ringer's) are first line for most cases due to lower cost and wider availability. Colloids (e.g., albumin and hydroxyethyl starch) may be considered in specific scenarios (e.g., severe hypoalbuminemia and capillary leak), but their use is limited by cost, potential renal/hepatic effects, and lack of proven mortality benefit [30, 42–44, 47].

The typical maintenance fluid requirement is 30–40 mL/kg/day (adjusted for age, weight, comorbidities). Additionally, insensible losses (respiration, perspiration ~500 mL/day), fever (+10–15% per °C above 38°C), drains, polyuria, diarrhea, or vomiting should be considered. Subtract enteral intake from total fluid requirements to avoid overhydration [14, 30, 43].

The main goals of fluid therapy are to maintain euvolemia and achieve zero water balance. These are assessed using clinical indicators like blood pressure, capillary refill time, urine output, lactate levels, and central venous pressure if possible. Daily fluid intake should match fluid output, monitored by intake/output records and daily weight changes [14, 30, 42–44].

4. Airway management and ventilatory support

The primary goals of respiratory support in patients with stroke are to achieve adequate arterial oxygenation ($SpO_2 \geq 94\%$, PaO_2 70–100 mmHg) and maintain normocapnia (PaCO2 35–45 mmHg) under conditions of minimal intrathoracic pressure [14, 30, 31, 42–44, 48].

Indications for endotracheal intubation and mechanical ventilation in patients with stroke include: [14, 30, 31, 42, 47, 48].

- Reduced level of consciousness and coma (Glasgow Coma Scale score ≤ 8);
- Apnea;
- Irregular breathing patterns, or agonal respiration;
- Tachypnea exceeding 30 breaths per minute, not attributable to hyperthermia or severe unresolved hypovolemia;
- Clinical signs of hypoxemia and/or hypercapnia ($PaO_2 < 60$ mmHg, SpO2 < 90%, $PaCO_2 > 55$ mmHg);
- Uncontrolled status epilepticus.

Indications for Tracheostomy

- Consider if mechanical ventilation is expected to exceed 48 hours.
- Benefits: Reduced sedation needs, improved comfort, lower risk of ventilator-associated pneumonia (VAP).

4.1 Mechanical ventilation in stroke patients

Ventilator Settings for Optimal Gas Exchange.

Tidal volume (VT): 7–8 mL/kg ideal body weight [43, 44, 48].
Respiratory rate: Adjusted to maintain normocapnia ($PaCO_2$ 35–45 mmHg).
PEEP: ≥5 cmH_2O (prevents atelectasis).
FiO_2: 30–50% (titrated to $SpO_2 \geq 92\%$).
Humidification: Essential to avoid airway drying (use heat-moisture exchangers filters or heated humidifiers).

4.2 Acute lung injury (ALI) or ARDS management

Lung-protective ventilation:

Tidal volume > 4–6 mL/kg IBW [48, 49].
Peak airway pressure < 35 cm H_2O; mean pressure < 27 cm H_2O.
Flow pattern: Decelerating waveform (peak flow 40–70 L/min).

Rescue therapies for refractory hypoxemia:

- Prone positioning (improves V/Q matching).
- Alveolar recruitment maneuvers (transiently increase PEEP).
- High MAP (individualized hemodynamic monitoring).

Non-Invasive Ventilation (NIV).

Respiratory failure without absolute intubation criteria is the main indication of NIV [14, 30, 43, 44].

Advantages:

- No sedation required.
- Preserves cough/swallowing.
- Reduces VAP risk.

Contraindications:

- Coma/stupor, bulbar dysfunction (aspiration risk).
- Absent cough reflex, facial trauma/sinusitis.

Weaning and Extubation Criteria.

Prerequisites:

- Stable hemodynamics.
- Adequate spontaneous breathing (e.g., passed spontaneous breathing trial).
- Normal cough/gag reflex (assessed *via* endoscopic vocal cord exam or dye swallow test).

5. Management of cerebral edema and intracranial hypertension

5.1 Intracranial hypertension/cerebral edema

Ischemic cytotoxic injury can trigger cellular swelling *via* excitotoxicity, free radicals, and calcium influx. Raised intracranial pressure (ICP) worsens ischemia and edema, accelerating secondary injury [50–53].

Malignant cerebral edema is characterized by life-threatening ICP elevation and herniation risk which has Incidence 2–8% and mortality is 40–80% [14, 43, 54, 55].

Key predictors of malignant cerebral edema are ≥50% middle cerebral artery territory involvement on brain imaging, infarct volume > 82 cm^3 within 6 hours of onset of the symptom onset and large hemispheric infarct (supratentorial) [14, 43, 54, 55].

Medical Management of Raised ICP.

Optimize Physiology: [14, 30, 42–44].

- Head elevation 30°, midline position.

- Minimize PEEP (ventilated patients).
- Avoid hypo-osmolar fluids.
- Maintain sedation/analgesia (prevent coughing/bucking).
- Aggressive fever control.

Hyperosmolar Therapy (Individualized):

Hypertonic normal saline or mannitol is usually used for the medical treatment of edema and high ICP. However, insufficient evidence for the routine use of mannitol or hypertonic normal saline in AIS-related malignant edema [14, 30, 42, 43].

Use tailored to the patient profile.

ICP Monitoring:

- Consider as part of multimodal monitoring in ICU.
- Limited evidence for routine use in acute ischemic stroke; not standard [14].

5.2 Hyperosmolar therapy in intracranial hypertension

Hyperosmolar therapy is commonly used to treat brain edema and intracranial hypertension in patients with conditions such as traumatic brain injury, ischemic stroke, intracranial hemorrhages, and hepatic encephalopathy. The primary mechanism of action involves creating an osmolar gradient between brain tissues and the vascular bed, which facilitates the removal of fluid from the cranial cavity and results in a reduction in ICP [30, 42–44, 53].

Hyperosmolar therapy involves the use of hypertonic sodium chloride solutions, with different concentrations, such as 3.0, 7.5, and 23.4%, as well as mannitol with concentrations between 5 and 25%. The effects of hypertonic sodium chloride typically begin within 5 minutes and can last up to 12 hours. Mannitol's effects start within 10–20 minutes after administration and last for 4–6 hours [30, 42–44, 53].

5.3 Surgical management (decompressive hemicraniectomy - DHC)

The primary goal of DHC is to reduce mortality by relieving ICP and preventing herniation.

DHC reduces mortality and poor outcomes if performed within 48 hours. And no benefit if delayed to 96 hours [14, 30, 43, 55].

DHC consistently reduces mortality by ~50% but survivors often have major disability. Benefits are time-dependent and age-dependent [14, 30, 43, 55].

6. General supportive care

6.1 Blood glucose control

Both hypoglycemia and hyperglycemia have weak correlations with neurological outcomes in stroke. The SHINE trial showed that an intensive intravenous insulin protocol aimed at maintaining glucose levels between 80 and 130 mg/dL

(4.44–7.21 mmol/L) resulted in less favorable 90-day outcomes than a sliding scale insulin regimen, which targeted 80–179 mg/dL (4.44–9.93 mmol/L). Current guidelines recommend keeping blood glucose levels between 8 and 10 mmol/L [14, 30, 42, 43, 56].

6.2 Seizures

Early seizures can occur within 7 days of ischemic stroke, often due to acute metabolic or ischemic changes. Late seizures can be observed in some patients after 7 days and are more likely due to structural changes, gliosis, or epileptogenesis [14, 30, 42, 43].

Risk factors for post-stroke seizures include:

- Higher severity of stroke (large infarcts, higher NIHSS score)
- Cortical localization (frontal, parietal, or temporal lobes involvement)
- Hemorrhagic transformation (increases brain tissue irritability)
- Younger age (higher risk compared to older adults, possibly due to increased neuronal excitability)

Recommended Antiepileptic Drugs (AEDs):

- Levetiracetam, lamotrigine, and lacosamide are preferred for their favorable safety profiles, fewer drug interactions, and minimal sedation. They also have a lower risk of exacerbating post-stroke cognitive deficits compared to older AEDs like phenytoin or valproate [14, 43].
- It is advisable to avoid enzyme-inducing AEDs (e.g., phenytoin and carbamazepine) in elderly patients or those on multiple medications.

The American Heart Association (AHA) advises against the use of prophylactic antiepileptic drugs due to the lack of proven benefit in preventing late seizures and the potential for increased side effects [14].

Author details

Hussain Ayyaz[1*] and Saskin Vitaly Alexandrovich[2]

1 Department of Anaesthesiology and Intensive Care Medicine, Northern State Medical University, Arkhangelsk, Russian Federation

2 Regional Vascular Center, First City Hospital, Northern State Medical University, Arkhangelsk, Russian Federation

*Address all correspondence to: ayyaz@mail.ru

References

[1] GBD 2015 Neurological Disorders Collaborator Group. Global, regional, and national burden of neurological disorders during 1990-2015: A systematic analysis for the Global Burden of Disease Study 2015. Lancet Neurology. 2017;**16**(11):877-897. DOI: 10.1016/S1474-4422(17)30299-5

[2] WHO. The Top 10 Causes of Death. Switzerland: World Health Organization; 2024. Available from: https://www.who.int/news-room/fact-sheets/detail/the-top-10-causes-of-death [Accessed: July 9, 2025]

[3] Feigin VL, Brainin M, Norrving B, et al. World stroke organization: Global stroke fact sheet 2025. Int J Stroke Off J Int Stroke Soc. 2025;**20**(2):132-144. DOI: 10.1177/17474930241308142

[4] Feigin VL, Brainin M, Norrving B, et al. World stroke organization (WSO): Global stroke fact sheet 2022. International Journal of Stroke: Official Journal of the International Stroke Society. 2022;**17**(1):18-29. DOI: 10.1177/17474930211065917

[5] Feigin V, Norrving B, Sudlow CLM, Sacco RL. Updated criteria for population-based stroke and transient ischemic attack incidence studies for the 21st century. Stroke. 2018;**49**:2248-2255. DOI: 10.1161/STROKEAHA.118.022161

[6] Kasemsap N, Vorasoot N, Kongbunkiat K, Tiamkao S, Boonsawat W, Sawanyawisuth K. Factors associated with favorable outcomes in acute severe stroke patients: A real-world, national database study. Biomedical Reports. 2022;**17**(3):74. DOI: 10.3892/br.2022.1557

[7] Fan R, Gu J, Zhang J, et al. Risk factors for stroke outcomes in adults: Stroke in China. Medicine (Baltimore). 2023;**102**(49):e36606. DOI: 10.1097/MD.0000000000036606

[8] Asgedom SG, Gebrewahd DT, Abdi MG, Wondie YA, Mekonnen BA, Belete KT. Treatment outcome and risk factors of ischemic stroke among adult patients in two selected hospital in Addis Ababa, Ethiopia. Brain Disorders. 2025;**19**:100242. DOI: 10.1016/j.dscb.2025.100242

[9] Xiong Y, Wakhloo AK, Fisher M. Advances in acute ischemic stroke therapy. Circulation Research. 2022;**130**(8):1230-1251. DOI: 10.1161/CIRCRESAHA.121.319948

[10] Miller SE, Warach SJ. Evolving thrombolytics: From alteplase to tenecteplase. Neurotherapeutics : The Journal of the American Society for Experimental NeuroTherapeutics. 2023;**20**(3):664-678. DOI: 10.1007/s13311-023-01391-3

[11] Gusev EI, Martynov MY, Nikonov AA, et al. Non-immunogenic recombinant staphylokinase versus alteplase for patients with acute ischaemic stroke 4·5 h after symptom onset in Russia (FRIDA): A randomised, open label, multicentre, parallel-group, non-inferiority trial. Lancet Neurology. 2021;**20**(9):721-728. DOI: 10.1016/S1474-4422(21)00210-6

[12] Kleindorfer DO, Towfighi A, Chaturvedi S, et al. 2021 guideline for the prevention of stroke in patients with stroke and transient ischemic attack: A guideline from the American Heart Association/American Stroke Association. Stroke. 2021;**52**(7):e364-e467. DOI: 10.1161/STR.0000000000000375

[13] Warner JJ, Harrington RA, Sacco RL, Elkind MSV. Guidelines for the early Management of Patients with Acute Ischemic Stroke: 2019 update to the 2018 guidelines for the early Management of Acute Ischemic Stroke. Stroke. 2019;**50**(12):3331-3332. DOI: 10.1161/STROKEAHA.119.027708

[14] Powers WJ, Rabinstein AA, Ackerson T, et al. Guidelines for the early Management of Patients with Acute Ischemic Stroke: 2019 update to the 2018 guidelines for the early Management of Acute Ischemic Stroke: A guideline for healthcare professionals from the American Heart Association/American Stroke Association. Stroke. 2019;**50**(12):e344-e418. DOI: 10.1161/STR.0000000000000211

[15] Li Y, Ma CH. Advancements in imaging for the diagnosis of wake-up stroke. The Neurologist. 2025;**30**(1):55-59. DOI: 10.1097/NRL.0000000000000585

[16] Nguyen TN, Abdalkader M, Fischer U, et al. Endovascular management of acute stroke. Lancet (London, England). 2024;**404**(10459):1265-1278. DOI: 10.1016/S0140-6736(24)01410-7

[17] Chen H, Lee JS, Michel P, Yan B, Chaturvedi S. Endovascular stroke thrombectomy for patients with large ischemic core: A review. JAMA Neurology. 2024;**81**(10):1085-1093. DOI: 10.1001/jamaneurol.2024.2500

[18] Goyal M, Menon BK, van Zwam WH, et al. Endovascular thrombectomy after large-vessel ischaemic stroke: A meta-analysis of individual patient data from five randomised trials. Lancet (London, England). 2016;**387**(10029):1723-1731. DOI: 10.1016/S0140-6736(16)00163-X

[19] Morsi S, Ghozy S, Elfil M, et al. Endovascular thrombectomy for DAWN- and DEFUSE-3 ineligible acute ischemic stroke patients: A systematic review and meta-analysis. Journal of Neurology. 2024;**271**(5):2230-2237. DOI: 10.1007/s00415-024-12198-3

[20] Ryan D, Chang V, Ouf A. Utilization of DWI-FLAIR mismatch for intravenous thrombolysis in an elderly patient with stroke. The Neurohospitalist. 2025:19418744251343999. DOI: 10.1177/19418744251343999

[21] Nogueira RG, Jadhav AP, Haussen DC, et al. Thrombectomy 6 to 24 hours after stroke with a mismatch between deficit and infarct. The New England Journal of Medicine. 2018;**378**(1):11-21. DOI: 10.1056/NEJMoa1706442

[22] Seners P, Turc G, Tisserand M, et al. Unexplained early neurological deterioration after intravenous thrombolysis. Stroke. 2014;**45**(7):2004-2009. DOI: 10.1161/STROKEAHA.114.005426

[23] Faigle R, Marsh EB, Llinas RH, Urrutia VC, Gottesman RF. ICAT: A simple score predicting critical care needs after thrombolysis in stroke patients. Critical Care. 2016;**20**(1):26. DOI: 10.1186/s13054-016-1195-7

[24] Seners P, Turc G, Oppenheim C, Baron JC. Incidence, causes and predictors of neurological deterioration occurring within 24 h following acute ischaemic stroke: A systematic review with pathophysiological implications. Journal of Neurology, Neurosurgery, and Psychiatry. 2015;**86**(1):87-94. DOI: 10.1136/jnnp-2014-308327

[25] Hacke W, Kaste M, Bluhmki E, et al. Thrombolysis with alteplase 3 to 4.5 hours after acute ischemic stroke. The New England Journal of Medicine.

2008;**359**(13):1317-1329. DOI: 10.1056/NEJMoa0804656

[26] Saqqur M, Molina CA, Salam A, et al. Clinical deterioration after intravenous recombinant tissue plasminogen activator treatment: A multicenter transcranial Doppler study. Stroke. 2007;**38**(1):69-74. DOI: 10.1161/01.STR.0000251800.01964.f6

[27] Berge E, Whiteley W, Audebert H, et al. European stroke organisation (ESO) guidelines on intravenous thrombolysis for acute ischaemic stroke. European Stroke Journal. 2021;**6**(1):I-LXII. DOI: 10.1177/2396987321989865

[28] Chen C, Song L, Yang J, et al. Regional differences in early BP management after acute ischemic stroke in the ENCHANTED international randomized controlled trials. Frontiers in Neurology. 2021;**12**:687862. DOI: 10.3389/fneur.2021.687862

[29] Bath PM, Song L, Silva GS, et al. Blood pressure management for ischemic stroke in the first 24 hours. Stroke. 2022;**53**(4):1074-1084. DOI: 10.1161/STROKEAHA.121.036143

[30] Hoh BL, Ko NU, Amin-Hanjani S, et al. 2023 Guideline for the Management of Patients with Aneurysmal Subarachnoid Hemorrhage: A guideline from the American Heart Association/American Stroke Association. Stroke. 2023;**54**(7):e314-e370. DOI: 10.1161/STR.0000000000000436

[31] Unnithan AKA, Das JM, Mehta P. Hemorrhagic stroke. In: StatPearls. USA: StatPearls Publishing; 2025 [Accessed: July 10, 2025]. Available from: http://www.ncbi.nlm.nih.gov/books/NBK559173/

[32] Hussein AM, Bayoumy IM, Abdulghani KO, Eissa MA, Ahmed EM, Abou Elmaaty AA. Predictors of clinical outcome in post-thrombolysis among sample of Egyptian patients with acute ischemic stroke. The Egyptian Journal of Neurology, Psychiatry and Neurosurgery. 2025;**61**(1):1. DOI: 10.1186/s41983-024-00931-8

[33] Morawo A. Intravenous thrombolysis in acute ischemic stroke. In: Stroke - Management Pearls. London, UK: IntechOpen; 2023. DOI: 10.5772/intechopen.111731

[34] Han TS, Gulli G, Fry CH, et al. Adverse consequences of immediate thrombolysis-related complications: A multi-Centre registry-based cohort study of acute stroke. Journal of Thrombosis and Thrombolysis. 2022;**53**(1):218-227. DOI: 10.1007/s11239-021-02523-2

[35] Miller DJ, Simpson JR, Silver B. Safety of thrombolysis in acute ischemic stroke: A review of complications, risk factors, and newer technologies. The Neurohospitalist. 2011;**1**(3):138-147. DOI: 10.1177/1941875211408731

[36] An SA, Kim J, Kim SH, Kim WC. Abdominal wall hemorrhage after intravenous thrombolysis for acute ischemic stroke. BMC Neurology. 2013;**13**:6. DOI: 10.1186/1471-2377-13-6

[37] Charbonnier G, Bonnet L, Biondi A, Moulin T. Intracranial bleeding after reperfusion therapy in acute ischemic stroke. Frontiers in Neurology. 2021;**11**:11. DOI: 10.3389/fneur.2020.629920

[38] Fonseca AC, Geraldes R, Reimão S, Pinho e Melo T, Ferro JM. Neck hematoma after intravenous thrombolysis for stroke treatment. Cerebrovasc Dis Basel Switz. Cerebrovascular Diseases. 2010;**30**(1):101-102. DOI: 10.1159/000314712

[39] Baig MU, Bodle J. Thrombolytic therapy. In: StatPearls. USA: StatPearls Publishing; 2025. Available from: http://www.ncbi.nlm.nih.gov/books/NBK557411/ [Accessed: July 10, 2025]

[40] De Georgia M, Bowen T, Duncan KR, Chebl AB. Blood pressure management in ischemic stroke patients undergoing mechanical thrombectomy. Neurological Research and Practice. 2023;**5**(1):12. DOI: 10.1186/s42466-023-00238-8

[41] Gąsecki D, Kwarciany M, Kowalczyk K, Narkiewicz K, Karaszewski B. Blood pressure Management in Acute Ischemic Stroke. Current Hypertension Reports. 2020;**23**(1):3. DOI: 10.1007/s11906-020-01120-7

[42] Greenberg SM, Ziai WC, Cordonnier C, et al. Guideline for the Management of Patients with Spontaneous Intracerebral Hemorrhage: A guideline from the American Heart Association/American Stroke Association. Stroke. 2022;**2022**:e282-e361. DOI: 10.1161/STR.0000000000000407

[43] Steiner T, Purrucker JC, de Sousa DA, et al. European Stroke Organisation (ESO) and European Association of Neurosurgical Societies (EANS) guideline on stroke due to spontaneous intracerebral haemorrhage. European Stroke Journal. 2025;**0**(0):I-80. DOI: 10.1177/23969873251340815

[44] Sandset EC, Anderson CS, Bath PM, et al. European Stroke Organisation (ESO) guidelines on blood pressure management in acute ischaemic stroke and intracerebral haemorrhage. European Stroke Journal. 2021;**6**(2):X48-L89. DOI: 10.1177/23969873211012133

[45] Ma L, Hu X, Song L, et al. The third intensive care bundle with blood pressure reduction in acute cerebral haemorrhage trial (INTERACT3): An international, stepped wedge cluster randomised controlled trial. The Lancet. 2023;**402**(10395):27-40. DOI: 10.1016/S0140-6736(23)00806-1

[46] Qureshi AI, Palesch YY, Foster LD, et al. Blood pressure-attained analysis of ATACH 2 trial. Stroke. 2018;**49**(6):1412-1418. DOI: 10.1161/STROKEAHA.117.019845

[47] Ganti L. Management of acute ischemic stroke in the emergency department: Optimizing the brain. International Journal of Emergency Medicine. 2025;**18**:7. DOI: 10.1186/s12245-024-00780-5

[48] Robba C, Poole D, McNett M, et al. Mechanical ventilation in patients with acute brain injury: Recommendations of the European Society of Intensive Care Medicine consensus. Intensive Care Medicine. 2020;**46**(12):2397-2410. DOI: 10.1007/s00134-020-06283-0

[49] The Acute Respiratory Distress Syndrome Network. Ventilation with lower tidal volumes as compared with traditional tidal volumes for acute lung injury and the acute respiratory distress syndrome. The New England Journal of Medicine. 2000;**342**(18):1301-1308. DOI: 10.1056/NEJM200005043421801

[50] Dirnagl U, Iadecola C, Moskowitz MA. Pathobiology of ischaemic stroke: An integrated view. Trends in Neurosciences. 1999;**22**(9):391-397. DOI: 10.1016/s0166-2236(99)01401-0

[51] Chamorro Á, Meisel A, Planas AM, Urra X, van de Beek D, Veltkamp R. The immunology of acute stroke. Nature Reviews. Neurology. 2012;**8**(7):401-410. DOI: 10.1038/nrneurol.2012.98

[52] Simard JM, Kent TA, Chen M, Tarasov KV, Gerzanich V. Brain oedema in focal ischaemia: Molecular pathophysiology and theoretical implications. Lancet Neurology. 2007;**6**(3):258-268. DOI: 10.1016/S1474-4422(07)70055-8

[53] Cook AM, Morgan Jones G, Hawryluk GWJ, et al. Guidelines for the acute treatment of cerebral edema in neurocritical care patients. Neurocritical Care. 2020;**32**(3):647-666. DOI: 10.1007/s12028-020-00959-7

[54] Oppenheim C, Samson Y, Manaï R, et al. Prediction of malignant middle cerebral artery infarction by diffusion-weighted imaging. Stroke. 2000;**31**(9):2175-2181. DOI: 10.1161/01.str.31.9.2175

[55] Zerna C, Thomalla G, Campbell BCV, Rha JH, Hill MD. Current practice and future directions in the diagnosis and acute treatment of ischaemic stroke. The Lancet. 2018;**392**(10154):1247-1256. DOI: 10.1016/S0140-6736(18)31874-9

[56] Johnston KC, Bruno A, Pauls Q, et al. Intensive vs standard treatment of Hyperglycemia and functional outcome in patients with acute ischemic stroke: The SHINE randomized clinical trial. Journal of the American Medical Association. 2019;**322**(4):326-335. DOI: 10.1001/jama.2019.9346

Chapter 6

Eye Care in the Intensive Care Unit

Negin Sanadgol, Daniel Pethers, David Merle and Mertcan Sevgi

Abstract

Critically ill patients in the intensive care unit (ICU) are especially at high risk of ocular surface damage due to sedation, mechanical ventilation, and impairment of protective eye mechanisms (e.g., reduced blink reflex and tear production). Inadequate eye care can lead to exposure keratopathy, a corneal surface drying and epithelial breakdown from incomplete eyelid closure, which can affect over half of mechanically ventilated ICU patients in the UK and may progress to corneal ulceration (microbial keratitis) with corneal scarring or even permanent vision loss. Although largely preventable with simple measures, eye care is often overlooked in ICU settings amid the focus on acute life-threatening conditions. Recognising this risk, clinical guidelines (e.g., from the Royal College of Ophthalmologists and Intensive Care Society) advocate routine eye assessments and prophylactic interventions (such as frequent lubricating ointment application and eyelid taping) to maintain corneal moisture and integrity and prevent ICU-related ocular complications. Evidence-based protocols and staff education have demonstrated substantial benefits, dramatically reducing the incidence of exposure keratopathy to less than 5%. Vigilant eye care is therefore a simple yet critical preventive intervention in the ICU that mitigates the risk of exposure keratopathy and corneal ulcers, thereby safeguarding vision and improving patient outcomes.

Keywords: eye care, ophthalmology, ICU, intensive care, exposure keratopathy, vision, eye care protocol

1. Introduction

Ophthalmic complications frequently occur in critically ill patients yet often receive less attention than other organ-system issues. In the ICU setting, where the priority is maintaining vital functions and preventing life-threatening events, the eyes can be inadvertently overlooked. Exposure keratopathy, the most common ICU-related ocular surface disorder, occurs when the tear film and eyelids fail to fully protect the cornea, leading to surface drying and small breaks in the epithelium (punctate erosions). It affects 20–42% of ICU patients and may reach 60% in those sedated for more than 48 hours [1]. Without preventive care, impaired tear production, lagophthalmos (incomplete eyelid closure), and reduced blinking rate can lead to discomfort, infection, scarring, and, in severe cases, permanent vision loss.

Most of these complications are avoidable with straightforward, cost-effective interventions [2, 3]. This chapter reviews the anatomy and physiology of the ocular surface, highlights ICU-specific risk factors, and presents a practical, protocol-based framework for assessment, monitoring, and prevention. Aimed at non-ophthalmic clinicians, it emphasises the integration of "eye checks" into existing nursing routines, a simple grading system for eyelid closure, evidence-based lubrication and lid-closure techniques, and clear criteria for ophthalmology referral. By adopting these strategies, ICU teams can reduce ocular morbidity and help preserve patients' vision.

2. Understanding the ocular surface unit: From normal function to ICU-related pathophysiology

To effectively prevent and manage eye disease in critically ill patients, it's important to understand the eye's normal protective mechanisms. This understanding clarifies how critical illness and ICU interventions can disrupt this delicate balance, leading to the ocular surface complications frequently seen in this setting.

Under normal conditions, several coordinated mechanisms safeguard ocular health [4]:

1. Continuous tear production lubricates the ocular surface and provides antimicrobial defence.

2. Blinking spreads tears evenly and clears debris.

3. Eyelid closure protects the cornea from mechanical injury and prevents evaporation during rest.

4. Bell's phenomenon (upward rotation of the eyeballs during eyelid closure) offers an additional layer of protection.

5. Intact corneal sensation triggers reflex tearing and blinking in response to irritation.

These functions are not isolated but reflect the integrated operation of the Ocular Surface Unit—a complex, functional system essential for maintaining clear vision and defending the eye from external insults. This unit is not merely a collection of separate structures but a complex, integrated set of anatomical and functional components. It includes the cornea, conjunctiva, eyelids, eyelashes, tear film, and both the main and accessory lacrimal glands, as well as the meibomian glands (**Figure 1**). The lacrimal glands produce the aqueous layer of the tear film, while the meibomian glands contribute its lipid layer, and the tear film itself acts as a protective barrier and nutrient medium. Together, these structures work in concert to maintain surface integrity, lubrication, optical clarity, and immunological defence.

Disruption to any part of this delicate system can compromise the entire unit, predisposing patients to ocular surface disease (OSD), exposure keratopathy, chemosis (conjunctival swelling), and Microbial conjunctivitis and keratitis [6]. In the ICU, critical illness and its management can significantly disturb this balance. Understanding the structure and function of the Ocular Surface Unit is therefore essential for effective prevention and management of eye disease in critically ill patients [7].

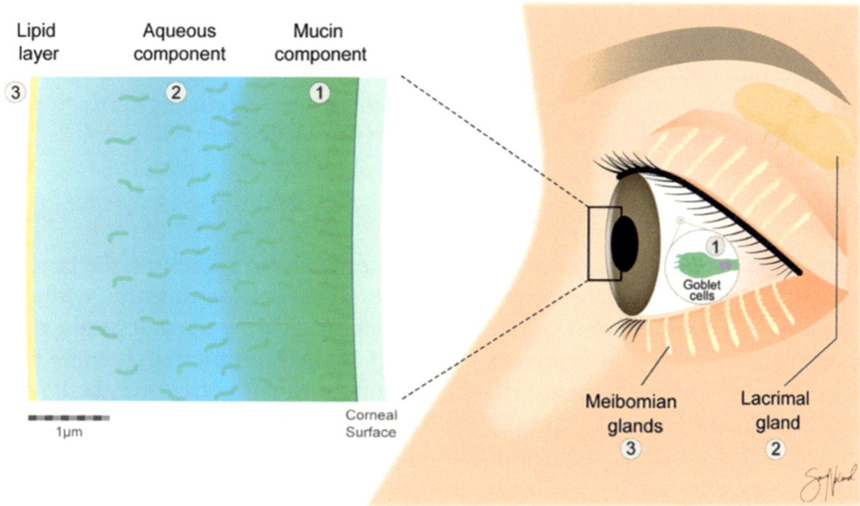

Figure 1.
This cross-sectional depiction of the precorneal tear film illustrates its three principal layers. (1) The mucin layer, located closest to the corneal surface and secreted by goblet cells in the conjunctiva, supports tear film stability by promoting water retention and increasing viscosity. (2) The aqueous layer, which makes up the majority of the tear film volume, is mainly produced by the lacrimal glands with contributions from the conjunctival epithelium. (3) The outer lipid layer, synthesised primarily by the meibomian glands, lowers surface tension and limits evaporation. Image credit: Sara Tellefsen Nøland [5].

2.1 Tear film

The tear film as a key component of the ocular surface unit is a trilaminar fluid layer that covers the cornea and conjunctiva. It consists of:

- An outer lipid layer that reduces evaporation and stabilises the tear film.
- A middle aqueous layer that provides moisture, oxygen, nutrients, and antimicrobial proteins.
- An inner mucin layer that enables even spreading of the tear film across the hydrophobic corneal surface.

The tear film is essential for ocular surface health. It lubricates the eye, provides a smooth optical surface, nourishes the avascular cornea, and serves as a primary defence against infection [11].

2.2 Cornea

The cornea is a transparent, avascular structure that forms the anterior surface of the eye, overlying the anterior chamber iris and pupil. Functioning as the eye's principal refractive component, its smooth curvature is essential for directing incoming light onto the retina. The outermost layer, the corneal epithelium, serves as a primary barrier against microbial invasion and environmental insults. As the cornea lacks its own vasculature, the epithelium relies entirely on the tear film for hydration, oxygenation, and nutrient delivery, and on the eyelids for mechanical protection and tear distribution [14, 15].

In the ICU, the cornea is highly vulnerable. Lagophthalmos and reduced blinking promotes tear film evaporation, causing dryness of the epithelial surface, which can lead to exposure keratopathy if left untreated. Damaged epithelial cells lose viability leading to increased susceptibility to microbial invasion. The cornea is also prone to direct mechanical injury, potentially resulting in superficial corneal abrasions.

2.3 Conjunctiva

The conjunctiva is a thin, transparent mucous membrane that lines the inner surface of the eyelids (palpebral conjunctiva) and folds back to cover the white part of the eye, the sclera (bulbar conjunctiva). It contains goblet cells that produce mucin, a key component of the tear film, and contributes to tear production, helping to lubricate the eye. It also plays a role in ocular immune defence. In critically ill patients, the conjunctiva is particularly prone to swelling or oedema, known as chemosis. This swelling can be dramatic, causing the conjunctiva to appear boggy and protrude between the eyelids, further hindering complete lid closure and exacerbating corneal exposure (**Figure 2**) [17].

2.4 Eyelids

The eyelids' primary functions are to protect the globe from injury and excessive light, and crucially, to distribute the tear film evenly across the ocular surface through blinking. Complete closure during sleep or periods of rest is vital for preventing corneal drying. In the ICU, eyelid function is frequently compromised. Reduced level of consciousness, sedation, and neuromuscular blockade significantly reduce or eliminate the blink reflex and diminish the tone of the orbicularis oculi muscle, leading to lagophthalmos. Facial oedema, often associated with fluid resuscitation or prone positioning, can also mechanically prevent full closure. Lagophthalmos is a major risk factor for the development of exposure to keratopathy and subsequent complications.

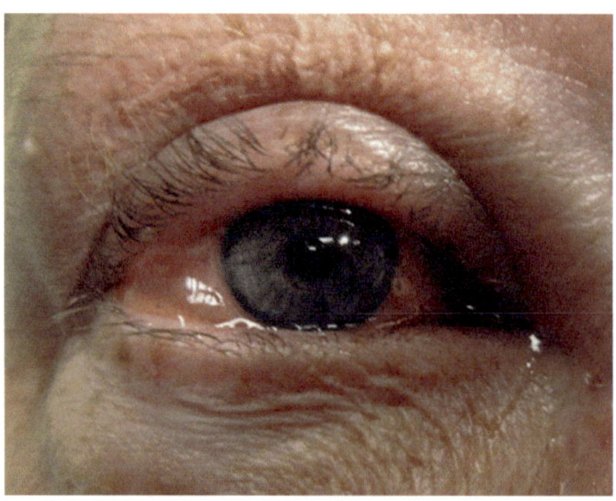

Figure 2.
Clinical image of a patient presenting with conjunctival chemosis [16].

3. Risk factors for ocular complications in ICU

Inability to fully close the eyelids, whether due to lagophthalmos or conjunctival chemosis, and a reduced blink rate are key contributors to ocular complications in ICU patients. Several factors compound this risk, including mechanical ventilation, particularly with high oxygen flow or elevated positive end expiratory pressure (PEEP), prone positioning to manage acute respiratory distress syndrome (ARDS), generalised oedema, and prolonged ICU stays. Recognising these risk factors is essential for identifying patients who require proactive ocular protection. For example, *a deeply sedated, mechanically ventilated patient with eyelid swelling and exposed corneas is at significantly elevated risk and necessitates aggressive prophylactic eye care*. In contrast, an alert, interactive patient is far less susceptible. Notably, the duration of sedation and ICU stay directly correlates with ocular risk, one study reported lagophthalmos in 17–75% of ICU patients and corneal epithelial defects in over half of those sedated for more than 48 hours. A clear understanding of these underlying pathophysiological mechanisms is critical for implementing effective, targeted prevention strategies (**Table 1**) [18].

Categories	Risk factors for ocular complications
Patient-related factors	**Fluid maldistribution**
	Positive fluid balance, fluid overload states, and conditions causing low oncotic pressure can cause facial oedema, lid swelling and chemosis (a pronounced conjunctival oedema that prevents the lids from closing fully).
	Altered level of consciousness (Low GCS)
	Reduces blink rate and eye safety reflexes.
	Systemic issues or Nerve dysfunction
	Facial nerve dysfunction (e.g. from stroke or trauma) can impair eyelid function.
Treatment-related factors	**Neuromuscular blocking agents or Sedatives**
	Reduces blink rate, impairs blink reflex and is precursor to lagophthalmos.
	Diminishes the tonic contraction of the orbicularis oculi muscle necessary for complete closure.
	Continuous positive airway pressure (CPAP) and oxygen masks
	Air leaks around endotracheal tubes, CPAP/BiPAP masks, or high-flow nasal cannula can directly accelerate tear evaporation and dry the ocular surface.
	Mechanical Positive Pressure Ventilation
	Increased jugular pressure causes conjunctival oedema (chemosis) increasing risk of lagophthalmos.
	Ventilating patients in prone position (face-down)
	Direct injury during positioning
	Gravitational force causing conjunctival oedema (chemosis) increasing risk of lagophthalmos. Rare complications of Ischemic optic neuropathy (ION) and acute angle-closure glaucoma (AACG).

Categories	Risk factors for ocular complications
ICU Environment-related factors	**Duration of ICU Stay**
	Increased length of stay associated with increased risk of OSD.
	Challenging environmental conditions
	Exposure to bright lights, low humidity, and frequent nursing interventions.
	Adhesive tapes used to secure tubes or to tape eyelids may also injure the skin or cornea if improperly applied.
	Critical care transfers are high-risk situations in which eye care can be overlooked, increasing the risk of ocular injury during transport.
	Other Medications/Procedures
	Unintentional contact of Topical medications like aerosolized bronchodilators (e.g. nebulized ipratropium bromide).
	Cardiological drugs (e.g., Amiodarone, Beta-blockers) and antibiotics (e.g., Penicillin, Rifampicin, Metronidazole) can affect perfusion and lead to oedema and chemosis.
	Anticholinergics reduce tear production.
	Procedures such as endotracheal suctioning if unsecured can cause inadvertent trauma to the eye in the form of corneal scratches or Increased exposure to microorganisms.

Table 1.
Key risk factors for ocular complications in critically ill patients involve disrupted protective mechanisms and are categorised into three interrelated groups: patient-related, treatment-related, and ICU environment-related contributing to ocular surface disease (OSD) [8, 9].

4. Assessment and monitoring of eye health in the ICU

Routine assessment of the eyes should be part of daily ICU care, just like tracking vital signs or skin integrity. The challenge is that many ICU patients cannot report eye symptoms, so clinicians must rely on regular examinations. As a general guideline, inspect the patient's eyes at least once every shift (i.e. at least every 8–12 hours) using a good light source. Detailed key components of ocular assessment in ICU include:

Alternate: Routine eye assessment is a standard of care in the ICU, much like vital signs or skin integrity checks. Many of these patients cannot report symptoms, clinicians are responsible for regular eye examinations, ensuring inspection with a good light source at least every 8–12 hours (once per shift). The key components of this ICU ocular assessment are as follows:

4.1 Inspect eyelid closure

The Royal College of Ophthalmologists and Intensive Care Society recommend documenting eyelid closure and eye appearance once per shift throughout the ICU stay [19]. Nurses or physicians should note whether the eyelids are fully closed, partially open, or fully open at rest. If lids are open, estimate the exposed extent (for example, "approximately 3 mm of cornea exposed").

4.1.1 Grade lagophthalmos severity

If the patient cannot fully close their eyes, assess the severity of lagophthalmos. A simple grading system is used:

- *Grade 0:* Complete eyelid closure at rest.
- *Grade 1:* Incomplete closure with exposure of the conjunctiva (sclera) only.
- *Grade 2:* Incomplete closure with any degree of corneal exposure (even if minimal).

This grading system directly guides preventive measures, with grades 1 and 2 indicating a high risk of corneal drying and the need for appropriate intervention, as outlined in **Table 2**.

4.2 Observe for redness, swelling, discharge

Check for the presence of tearing, redness of the conjunctiva, cloudiness of the cornea, or any discharge. A penlight or flashlight held close can illuminate subtle corneal changes even if the patient's eyes are only slightly open; additionally, gently lifting the upper eyelid can allow inspection of the cornea if needed, but this must be done carefully to avoid causing an abrasion. Documentation of findings is important, e.g. "Eyes closed and moist" or "Right eye partially open, cornea clear, lubricating ointment applied."

4.2.1 Recognising ocular redness and corneal abnormalities

Ocular redness may signal irritation or infection. Diffuse conjunctival hyperaemia often indicates dryness or non-specific irritation (**Figure 3A**); however, marked redness accompanied by purulent discharge, such as crusting of the eyelashes or yellow secretions, arises strong suspicion for infectious conjunctivitis until ruled out as shown in **Figure 3B**. Chemosis, a gelatinous swelling of the conjunctiva, should be documented if present, as it increases the risk of exposure-related complications. Corneal clarity is a critical marker of ocular health with the normal cornea being transparent, any loss of clarity, including haze, dullness, or visible opacities, is abnormal and may reflect oedema, epithelial breakdown, or early infection. In sedated or unresponsive patients, corneal haze may be the only external sign of a developing corneal ulcer. *Any persistent corneal opacity should be treated as an ophthalmic emergency and escalated promptly for specialist review.*

4.3 Use of fluorescein dye

Nursing protocols in some ICUs allow fluorescein screening for corneal abrasions. For instance, if a patient has new conjunctival redness or evidence of exposed cornea, a fluorescein check can confirm an epithelial defect. Fluorescein strips (which are touched to a drop of saline then to the lower conjunctiva) are inexpensive and could be part of ICU supply. The dye will stain areas of missing epithelium bright green under cobalt blue light. However, care must be taken to moisten the strip adequately and avoid scratching the cornea during the test. In practice, many ICU teams will defer fluorescein exams to ophthalmology consultants unless they have specific training. At minimum, if an eye is red or suspicious, an order for an ophthalmology evaluation or at least fluorescein check is warranted. *Some bedside exam tips: using a blue light, a corneal abrasion will glow bright yellow-green, whereas an intact cornea remains dark* (as in **Figure 4**).

Grade of Exposure/ Lagophthalmos Grading	Preventive Strategy	Available Options	Detailed Instruction	Application Illustration
Grade 0 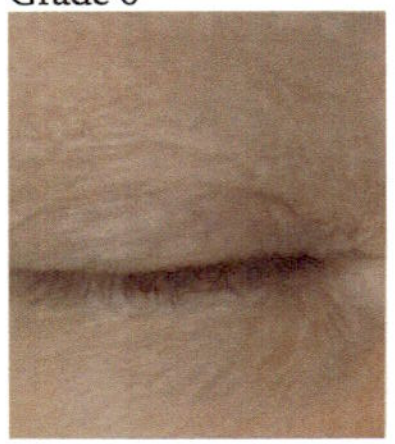	No prevention procedure is needed.			
Grade 1 Conjunctival exposure with no corneal exposure 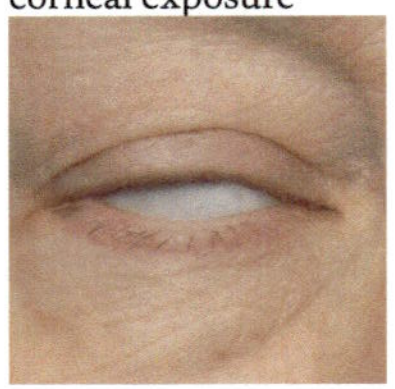	Lubrication of the Ocular Surface + Monitor corneal clarity each shift	• Artificial Tear Drops Short duration due to evaporation within minutes. Thus, drops alone must be applied very frequently (every 1–2 hours) to be protective.	In conscious patients, provide education on hand hygiene, correct eye drop application, and the schedule of applying drops every two hours with ointment before bedtime if required.	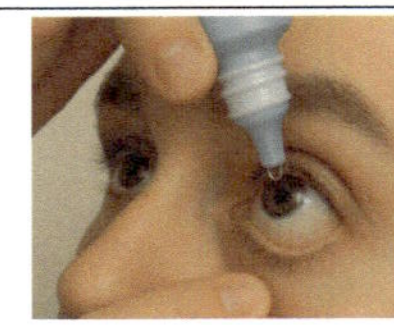
		• Lubricating Gels • Ophthalmic Ointments Liberal use of ointment lubricants into the eye four times daily e.g. simple eye ointment.	1. Clean the previous dried ointment and examine the eye abnormalities. 2. Liberal use of ointment by pulling the lower eyelid down with a finger and inserting the ointment over the top of the lower lid into the gap between the lid and the conjunctiva.	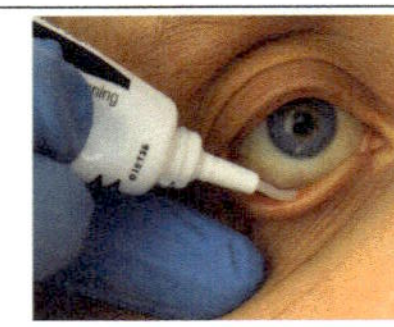

Grade of Exposure/ Lagophthalmos Grading	Preventive Strategy	Available Options	Detailed Instruction	Application Illustration
Grade 2 Conjunctival + Some Corneal exposure. 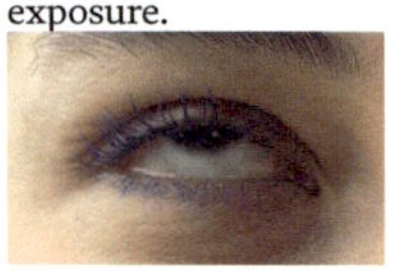	Lubrication of the Ocular Surface + Eyelid closure	• Manual closure	A temporary measure done by Nursing Staff for a moment to re-spread tears or ointment.	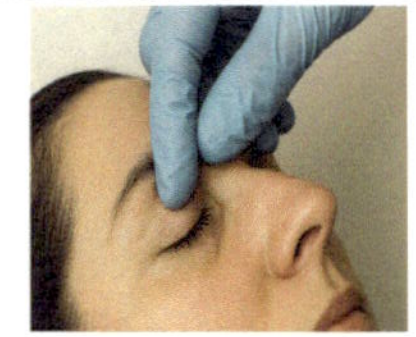
		• Eyelid Taping	Using medical tape to secure the lids in a closed position, Fully close lids via horizontally tape avoiding gaps and pressure	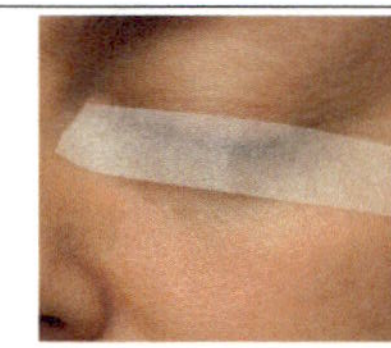
		• Hydrogel/Silicone Pads or Dressings These are preferred when periorbital oedema or severe chemosis prevents effective application of adhesive tape or cling film.	They should be kept moist and changed every shift and fully cover the closed lids and be monitored. Care must be taken that the pad does not inadvertently shift and scratch the eye.	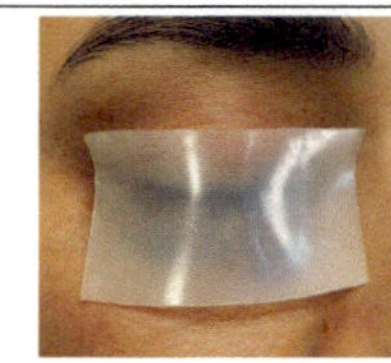

Table 2.
This table outlines the clinical grading of lagophthalmos and the recommended interventions for each grade. The classification is intended to guide the intensity of ocular care required, with higher grades indicating increased risk of exposure-related complications and the need for more intensive protective strategies. Clinical judgement should always guide individual patient management, especially in the context of sedation level, facial anatomy, and overall clinical status (Images are generated by ChatGPT, May 2025 except for image A which is from Royal college of ophthalmology handbook [10] and image B from one of our colleagues. Images are generated by ChatGPT, May and July 2025 (except for image B, which is provided by one of our colleagues).

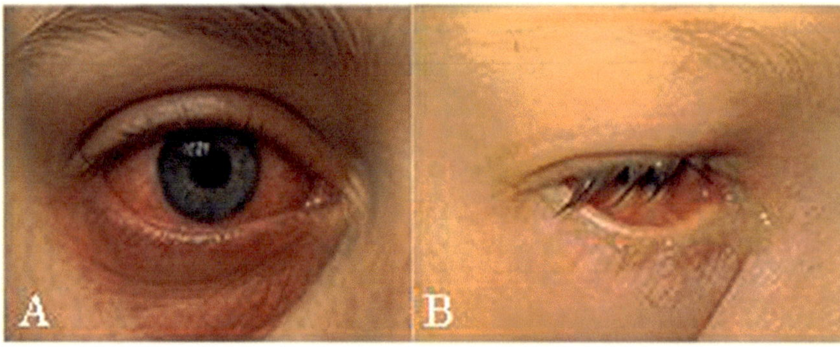

Figure 3.
Conjunctival involvement in ICU patients with: (A) diffuse redness with no discharge, (B) Purulent sticky discharge and redness [10, 19]. Image A: Generated by ChatGPT, July 2025. Image B: From reference [10].

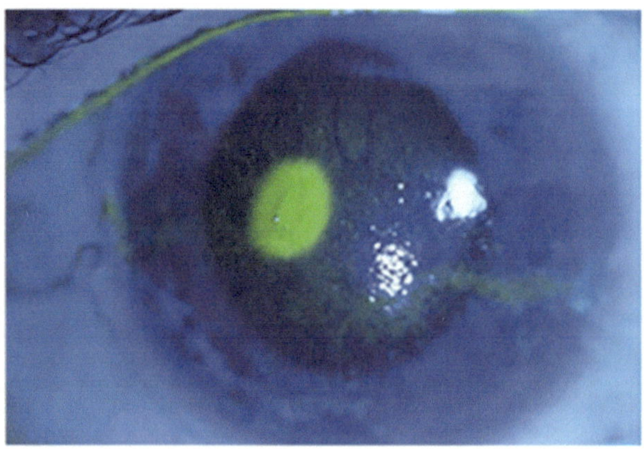

Figure 4.
Corneal ulcer illumination under blue light with fluorescein dye [20]. Used with permission from Dr. David Merle.

4.3.1 Frequency of exams

Regular eye examination in low-risk patients (awake, blinking normally) should be performed daily, often aligning with routine care activities such as turning or oral care. During these intervals, the care provider can check the cornea and refresh lubrication as needed. However, in high-risk patients (such as those on mechanical ventilation with sedation and/or presence of lagophthalmos), eye inspections should occur at least every 4 hours, not just once per shift. Incorporating eye checks into existing ICU checklists can be helpful, for example, adding an "Eye care, [DONE]" item to the ventilator bundle [21] or sedation vacation checklist ensures that this critical task is not overlooked.

4.4 When to escalate

In general, if the eye does not appear normal despite routine preventive care, early ophthalmology input is advisable to prevent irreversible complications. ICU clinicians should have well-defined criteria for involving ophthalmology, based on expert consensus and clinical guidelines. Key referral triggers include:

a. *Persistent red, sticky eye not improving within 24 hours,* which may represent infectious conjunctivitis requiring microbiological investigation and targeted treatment.

b. *Any corneal opacity or white spot,* suggestive of a corneal ulcer, which warrants urgent ophthalmology consultation.

c. *A cloudy pupil or presence of hypopyon,* raising concern for intraocular infection (e.g. endophthalmitis), which constitutes an emergency referral.

d. *Uncertainty about ocular findings,* particularly when examination is limited but clinical suspicion remains high.

In summary, regular and proactive monitoring is the key. Eyes should be checked during each shift, their condition documented, and any concerns acted on early. ICU nurses are often the first to notice changes, and thorough assessments can identify problems while they are still reversible. Eye checks should be as routine and prioritised as pressure area assessments. With consistent monitoring in place, we can now turn to the interventions that help prevent these complications.

5. Prevention strategies for ocular complications

Preventive eye care in the ICU is simple, low-cost, and highly effective, when applied diligently. The goal is to maintain corneal moisture, integrity, and cleanliness. Evidence-based protocols emphasise a combination of lubrication and eye closure techniques as the cornerstone, with adjustments based on individual risk. Below, we detail the key preventive measures and current evidence for each [22].

5.1 Lubrication of the ocular surface

5.1.1 Lubrication: A core strategy for ocular protection in the ICU

Regular ocular lubrication plays a central role in preventing corneal dryness, abrasion, and infection in critically ill patients. For high-risk individuals, such as those who are comatose or intubated, lubrication should be initiated at the time of ICU admission, rather than delayed until clinical signs of dryness emerge. Prevention is considerably more effective than managing established epithelial breakdown. A fixed schedule, for example ointment every 4 hours, should be followed and adjusted as needed. If signs of dryness appear, additional drops can be added between ointment applications. Reapplication is also necessary after any activity that exposes the eyes, such as repositioning, suctioning, or personal care. If redness or surface dryness develops, increase lubrication to every 2 hours until reviewed by ophthalmology. Lubricants replace or supplement the tear film and help maintain corneal hydration when blink reflexes or eyelid closure are impaired. The main types used in ICU care are outlined below:

5.1.1.1 Artificial tear drops

Saline-based and easy to apply, but evaporate rapidly (within minutes), requiring frequent reapplication (every 2 hours). This is often impractical in sedated or ventilated patients.

5.1.1.2 Lubricating gels

being more viscous than drops, gels offer longer protection (2–4 hours) and are suitable for moderate-frequency use. Temporary visual blurring is not a concern in unconscious patients.

5.1.1.3 Ophthalmic ointments

Petroleum-based or antibiotic ointments provide the longest coverage (4–6 hours or more). Though they blur vision and leave residue, they are preferred for high-risk patients due to their prolonged effect and ease of use. A typical regimen involves a 1 cm ribbon applied every 4 hours.

5.1.1.4 Evidence-based practice

A 2024 meta-analysis of 959 ICU patients demonstrated that lubricating gels or ointments were significantly more effective than artificial tear drops alone in preventing ocular surface disease. Polyethylene film covers used alongside gel or ointment had comparable efficacy. Drops or eyelid taping alone were consistently less protective [23].

Application Tips:

- Apply lubricating drops before ointments to ensure absorption.
- For incomplete lid closure, place ointment in the lower fornix and gently close the eyelids.
- Avoid touching the eye with the applicator.
- Use preservative-free drops to reduce irritation.

5.2 Ensuring complete eye closure

Keeping the eyelids gently closed over the eye is a fundamental protective strategy. This can be achieved in several ways:

Manual Lid Closure: Close the patient's eyes by gently shutting the lids with a finger can be done during routine care. However, the lids will usually reopen due to loss of tone, so this is at best a temporary measure (e.g. periodically throughout the day a nurse might close the lids for a moment to re-spread tears or ointment). Manual closure alone is not sufficient long-term.

Eyelid Taping: Taping the eyelids closed is a simple and effective method to protect the eyes in ICU patients with incomplete lid closure, particularly those with Grade 2 exposure. Ointment should be applied first to maintain corneal moisture, followed by hypoallergenic paper tape placed horizontally across the closed lids, avoiding pressure on the eye or trapping the eyelashes. *Tape should adhere to the skin, not the globe, and be replaced at least once per shift to allow for inspection and prevent skin irritation*. Incorrect taping, such as over an open eye or with lashes caught on the cornea, can cause abrasions, so proper technique and staff training are essential. In awake or lightly sedated patients, taping may cause distress, and alternative approaches or periodic breaks may be needed. Taping should only be used when clinically indicated, if the eyelids close fully, it is not necessary.

Moisture Chambers (Eye Covers): A moisture chamber protects the eyes by trapping humidity over the ocular surface. The simplest method uses a 10 × 10 cm piece of clear polyethylene film (e.g. cling film) placed over closed eyelids and secured with tape. It forms a loose seal, conforming to facial contours without touching the cornea. This approach is low-cost, easy to apply, and has been shown to be as effective as ointment alone in preventing corneal drying. Combined use of film and lubricant provides added protection. In one RCT, polyethylene covers significantly reduced corneal damage compared to taping, even with both groups receiving lubrication. The film should be replaced every shift and not reused between patients [23].

Commercial moisture goggles or domes are also available. They form a sealed chamber around the orbit and are helpful when tape is poorly tolerated. However, poor fit, pressure on the orbit, or dried-out foam seals can cause harm if not monitored and adjusted regularly. Overall, cling film offers a simple, effective alternative to taping, especially in sedated or unconscious patients, and is now commonly used as a first-line option in many ICUs.

Hydrogel Pads or Dressings: Another option for patients with significant periorbital oedema is to use a moist hydrogel dressing (e.g. a piece of water-gel pad) over the eyes. These pads both keep the eye moist and apply gentle pressure to keep lids closed. They are useful when standard tape is unable to be used due to oedema or if the conjunctiva is so swollen that cling film is hard to apply. They should be kept moist and changed every shift. Care must be taken that the pad does not inadvertently shift and scratch the eye, it must fully cover the closed lids and be monitored.

Tarsorrhaphy (Suturing the Eyelids): Tarsorrhaphy is a minor surgical procedure performed by an ophthalmologist in which the eyelids are partially sutured together to protect the cornea. It is rarely required as a preventive measure and is typically reserved for severe cases, such as marked chemosis or facial nerve paralysis that cannot be managed with standard methods. In ICU settings, temporary tarsorrhaphy may be considered when the cornea remains at risk despite maximal lubrication and taping, for example, in patients with eyelid burns or persistent chemosis during prone ventilation. While effective in ensuring eyelid closure, tarsorrhaphy limits the ability to perform ongoing eye examinations, and is therefore considered a last resort.

5.3 Practical considerations beyond lubrication and taping

5.3.1 Eyelid hygiene

- Clean eyelids once or twice daily using sterile water or saline on gauze to remove dried ointment or mucus and reduce bacterial load.

- Perform cleansing before lubrication to ensure optimal corneal contact and minimise infection risk.

5.3.2 Avoiding harmful practices

- Routine saline irrigation is discouraged, as it can disrupt the tear film and increase dryness.

- Avoid using cotton balls or wipes on the cornea to prevent micro abrasions and contamination.

- Do not tape eyes open or apply tape directly over the globe—these are common but avoidable sources of iatrogenic injury.

5.3.3 Positioning and humidification

- Adjust ventilator tubing and oxygen masks to prevent direct airflow across the eyes.
- Maintain adequate room humidity or use humidified ventilation to reduce ocular drying.
- Where appropriate, sedation breaks may allow voluntary blinking, which helps redistribute tears.

5.3.4 Protection during procedures

- Ensure eyes are closed and protected before any procedure under sedation or anaesthesia (e.g., bronchoscopy, CT, central line placement).
- Incorporate eye protection into pre-procedure safety checklists, as routinely done in the operating theatre.

5.3.5 Prone positioning eye care

- Prone patients, particularly those with ARDS, are at increased risk of ocular compression, facial oedema, and chemosis, and require careful eye protection [12].
- Apply lubricating ointment to both eyes at least every 4 hours, and ensure eyelids are fully closed using tape or cling film prior to prone positioning.
- Use foam cushions or head holders to suspend the face and relieve orbital pressure. If these are unavailable, alternate head positions and confirm that no tubing or pillows are exerting pressure on the eyes.
- During each prone session, perform at least one eye check by gently lifting the head to assess for swelling or pressure-related injury. Persistent chemosis or conjunctival prolapse despite taping may require ophthalmology referral for temporary tarsorrhaphy or canthotomy.
- Eye protection should be embedded in positioning protocols and checklists, particularly considering COVID-19 experiences where optic nerve complications were reported.

6. Common ocular complications in critically ill patients

Several distinct ocular pathologies can develop in ICU patients, most involving the ocular surface (cornea and conjunctiva) as shown in **Table 3**. These often occur in combination or sequentially, for instance, exposure-related dryness can lead to corneal abrasions, which in turn predispose to infection. The following are the most frequently encountered problems:

Grade	Ocular surface complication	Schematic ocular appearance
Grade 0	No ocular surface disease	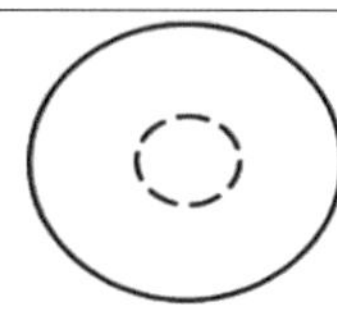
Grade 1	Punctate epithelial erosions (PEEs) involving the inferior third of the cornea	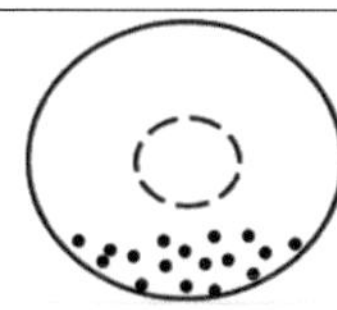
Grade 2	PEEs involving more than the inferior third of the corneal surface	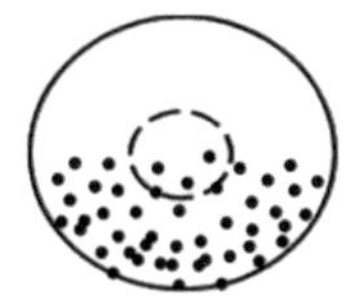
Grade 3	Macro Epithelial defect (MED)	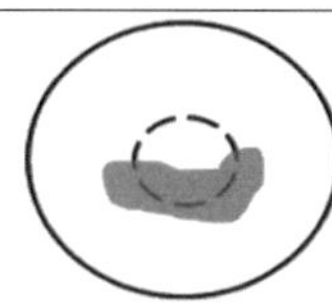
Grade 4	Stromal whitening in the presence of epithelial defect (SWED)	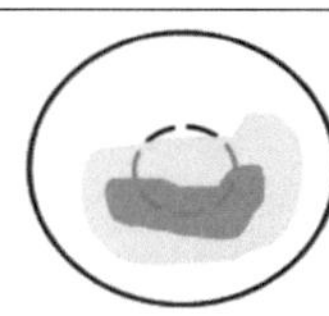
Grade 5	Stromal scar	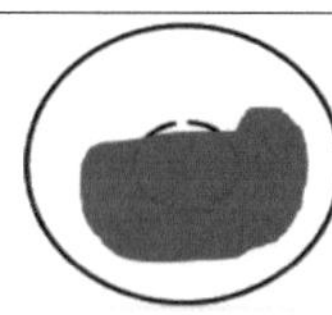
Grade 6	Microbial keratitis	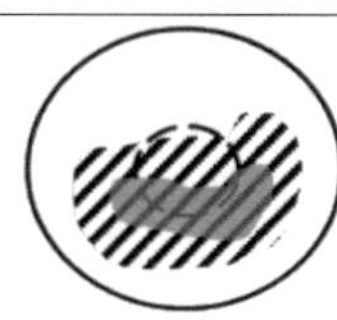

Table 3.
The classification and grading of ocular surface disease [12, 13].

6.1 Exposure keratopathy (exposure keratitis)

6.1.1 Definition

Exposure keratopathy (EK) refers to corneal injury caused by prolonged exposure of the ocular surface to the environment, typically resulting from lagophthalmos and/or insufficient blinking compromising the tear film protection (**Figure 5**). The exposed cornea experiences excessive tear film evaporation, leading to desiccation, epithelial breakdown, and inflammation, which, if untreated, can progress to

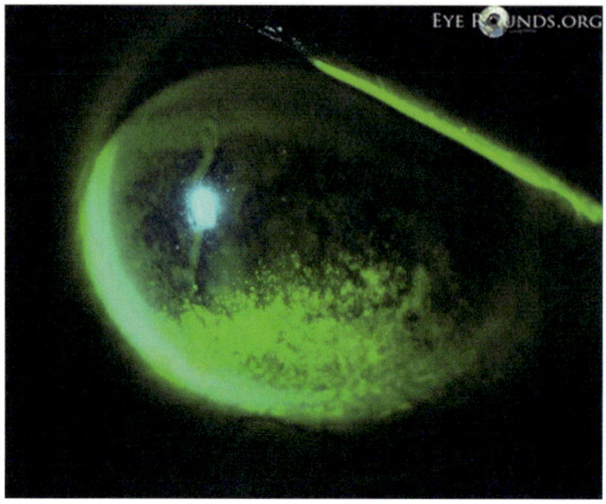

Figure 5.
Punctate epithelial erosions (PEE) [24].

secondary infection. EK can be regarded as a severe form of dry eye disease, commonly affecting critically ill patients, particularly those in the ICU.

EK is the most common ocular complication observed in ICU patients. Reported prevalence rates vary considerably, typically ranging from roughly 20–42% depending on patient factors, with higher rates seen in those who are sedated, mechanically ventilated, or unconscious [25, 26]. A systematic review of 3484 records reported a pooled prevalence of EK at 34% (34.1% in adults and 40.9% in children) and an incidence of 23% (26.0% in adults and 12.0% in children) [8]. Prevalence can also vary depending on the ICU environment and the nature of the patient population. Higher rates have been reported among the patients receiving deep sedation or neuromuscular blockade such as those in general medical, neurological and surgical ICUs, while slightly lower rates are seen in paediatric units such as PICUs where sedation practices and ventilation techniques are non-invasive most of the time [27].

6.1.2 Course of onset

Even short-term exposure, lasting only a few hours, can induce significant corneal changes, including epithelial dehydration, initial thinning, and aggregation of inflammatory cells within the stroma. However, in ICU patients, exposure keratopathy typically develops within the first 2–7 days of admission and may become evident as early as 48 hours in high-risk individuals. Clinically, exposure keratopathy first appears as areas of dry, dull corneal surface and conjunctival injection. The patient's conjunctiva may look red, and the cornea loses its normal lustrous reflection. In an awake patient, this causes irritation, foreign-body sensation, and blurry vision; however, in an unconscious patient, there are no subjective symptoms, so early examinations are critical. If not promptly recognised and managed, EK can rapidly progress from minor surface dryness to serious ocular damage. Initial punctate epithelial erosions can evolve into corneal ulcers, microbial keratitis, stromal melting, and even corneal perforation. Severe cases can result in permanent vision loss, with devastating consequences for survivors.

6.1.3 Diagnosis

Diagnosis of EK in the ICU setting relies heavily on clinical examination, as patients are frequently sedated, intubated, or otherwise unable to communicate visual symptoms. Evaluation begins with inspection for lagophthalmos, conjunctival injection, and chemosis, followed by assessment of the corneal surface using a penlight or ophthalmoscope for signs of dryness, dullness, or haziness suggestive of epithelial damage. The hallmark diagnostic sign is the presence of corneal epithelial defects, best visualised with fluorescein dye testing. After instilling preservative-free fluorescein, examination under cobalt blue light reveals epithelial defects ranging from fine, scattered dots (punctate epithelial erosions, PEE), typically seen in the inferior cornea where exposure (**Figure 5**) is greatest, to larger, confluent areas of epithelial loss (macro-epithelial defects or corneal abrasions), or even frank corneal ulcers. Additional findings may include mucous filaments adhering to the corneal surface or severe chemosis preventing eyelid closure. Given the rapid risk of progression, daily bedside examinations with a low threshold for fluorescein testing are crucial for early detection and timely intervention in these vulnerable patients.

6.2 Corneal abrasions and superficial injuries

A corneal abrasion is a superficial injury involving the loss of the corneal epithelium. In ICU patients, abrasions may result from various causes, including direct trauma (e.g. unintentional contact with a suction catheter, endotracheal tube, or the edge of a mask during repositioning), poorly applied adhesive tape that touches the cornea, or severe exposure keratopathy where areas of dry epithelium detach. In many cases, the clinical appearance of a corneal abrasion reflects spontaneous breakdown and detachment of desiccated epithelium, rather than a scratch caused by an external object. Regardless of the cause, the clinical features are similar: a well-demarcated epithelial defect that stains with fluorescein and is often associated with redness and irritation. Corneal abrasions in critically ill patients have a high propensity to progress to infectious keratitis if not managed aggressively. The normal corneal epithelium serves as a barrier to microbes; when that barrier is breached, bacteria can invade the cornea.

6.3 Microbial keratitis (MK)

Microbial keratitis is an ophthalmic emergency that requires immediate ophthalmology consultation and aggressive treatment to prevent corneal perforation and permanent vision loss. It occurs when microorganisms, bacteria, fungi, or parasites, invade the corneal stroma, almost always following an initial breach in the protective epithelial barrier. In the ICU, the most significant predisposing factor is untreated or progressive exposure keratopathy, where devitalised epithelium provides a portal of entry for pathogens. The progression from tear film instability and dryness to exposure keratopathy, and subsequently to microbial keratitis, represents a common and well-recognised trajectory of ocular surface deterioration in critically ill patients. The presence of chemosis can further exacerbate this risk by impairing eyelid closure and promoting retention of debris or organisms on the corneal surface. The risk is heightened in ventilated patients, where the ocular surface is more prone to colonisation, and procedures such as open tracheal suctioning may directly inoculate the eye with respiratory pathogens. These factors underscore the importance of early preventative strategies, including regular lubrication and ensuring adequate eyelid closure from the outset of ICU admission, particularly in patients at elevated risk. Warning signs of corneal infection in an ICU patient include increasing cloudiness or opacity in the cornea, persistent redness, a "sticky" eye with discharge, or failure of an epithelial defect to improve over 24–48 hours despite treatment. ICU staff should suspect a corneal ulcer in such cases and obtain prompt ophthalmology consultation.

While contact lens wear is the leading cause of MK in the general population [28], the profile in the ICU may differ. Studies have found that sedated ICU patients often have the ocular surface colonised by organisms such as *Staphylococcus aureus* and *Pseudomonas aeruginosa*. Pseudomonas is a virulent Gram-negative bacteria known to cause rapidly progressive corneal ulcers. In the ICU, any corneal defect can act as an entry point for such bacteria, leading to a corneal ulcer with stromal infiltrate (white opacity) and sometimes a hypopyon (inflammatory pus layer inside the eye) Notably, Pseudomonas keratitis carries a risk of corneal perforation in under 72 hours if untreated [29]. If not treated accordingly, microbial keratitis can result in corneal perforation within just 24–48 hours, a true ophthalmic emergency [29]. Gram-positive organisms like *Staphylococcus aureus* (including MRSA) and coagulase-negative staphylococci, which can be part of the normal ocular or skin flora, are also common, especially when the ocular surface is compromised. Other Gram-negative bacteria such as Klebsiella and Acinetobacter species are also relevant in the hospital environment. Fungal keratitis, caused by yeasts (Candida spp.) or moulds (Aspergillus, Fusarium spp.), should be considered, especially in immunocompromised patients, those on long-term antibiotics or steroids, or following trauma involving vegetative matter (though less common in typical ICU settings) (**Figure 6**) [32, 33].

Diagnosis requires a high index of suspicion in any ICU patient with a red eye or corneal changes, particularly when exposure keratopathy is present. While slit lamp examination provides the best view, careful inspection with a bright penlight and fluorescein staining can often identify suspicious lesions at the bedside. Definitive diagnosis and targeted treatment rely on obtaining corneal scrapings for Gram stain, bacterial and fungal cultures, and sensitivity testing. This procedure is typically performed by an ophthalmologist.

Treatment for microbial keratitis should begin immediately after obtaining cultures, without waiting for results. Empiric therapy typically involves hourly broad-spectrum topical antibiotics. Options include fortified combination therapy

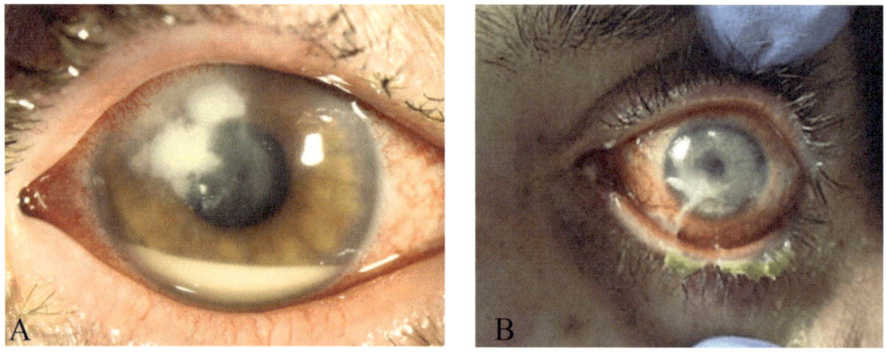

Figure 6.
Microbial keratitis with: (A) Hypopyon, fungal infections keratitis and conjunctivitis, (B) Bacterial keratitis with conjunctival injection most prominent inferiorly, mucopurulent conjunctival discharge, large inferior corneal epithelial defects [30, 31].

(e.g., vancomycin plus tobramycin) or fluoroquinolone monotherapy (e.g., moxifloxacin), with the choice guided by infection severity, likely pathogens, resistance patterns, and specialist preference. Once culture and sensitivity results are available (usually within 24–72 hours), antibiotic therapy should be adjusted accordingly.

6.4 Conjunctival chemosis (ventilator eye)

Chemosis is the swelling of the conjunctiva due to fluid accumulation. In an ICU patient, it often presents as a gelatinous, translucent bulging of the conjunctival tissue, sometimes so pronounced that it protrudes between the eyelids. Chemosis is common in critically ill patients, with reported incidences of 80% in up ventilated ICU patients and 92% of those with lagophthalmos [13].

Multiple factors contribute to periocular oedema in critically ill patients. Positive pressure ventilation may impair orbital venous return, a process further exacerbated by tightly secured endotracheal tube taping, which can increase local pressure. Additional contributors include fluid overload, hypoalbuminemia, venous congestion from elevated intrathoracic pressure or prolonged prone positioning, and systemic inflammation, all of which promote fluid extravasation into the periorbital tissues. Conditions such as congestive heart failure, renal failure, or capillary leak syndromes (e.g. sepsis) commonly cause facial oedema and chemosis. Additionally, tight taping of endotracheal tubes or nasal cannulas can further impede venous and lymphatic drainage around the eyes, worsening periocular oedema [1].

While chemosis itself is not directly vision-threatening, it is a marker of underlying issues and predisposes to exposure injury. The swollen conjunctiva can physically push the eyelids apart or prevent them from sealing, causing lagophthalmos even in an unconscious patient. The oedematous conjunctiva also impairs tear film distribution and oxygenation of the cornea. In effect, severe chemosis can cause or exacerbate exposure keratopathy. Moreover, the stagnant fluid in a chemotic conjunctiva may serve as a culture media for bacteria, increasing infection risk. ICU staff should pay attention to conjunctival oedema during eye exams. Management involves addressing the root cause (e.g. improving volume status, reducing PEEP if possible) and vigilant eye protection (frequent lubrication and ensuring eyelids are closed). In extreme cases where chemosis prevents lid closure despite these measures, an ophthalmologist may need to intervene (for instance, by temporary tarsorrhaphy, suturing the corners of the eyelids partially, to protect the cornea until swelling resolves). The presence of chemosis signals that the eyes are at major risk and should be lubricated at least every 2 hours and taped or covered, as recommended by protocols for high-risk patients.

6.5 Other common ocular surface issues

Additional ocular findings in ICU patients include subconjunctival haemorrhages (small bleeding under the conjunctiva, often from coughing or coagulopathy are benign and self-resolving) and exposure-related keratoconjunctivitis sicca (severe dry eye with keratinization in very prolonged ICU stays, rarely). Crust formation on lashes and eyelid margins is common due to evaporated tears and ointments; while not harmful per se, it underscores the need for regular eye cleaning. ICU patients may also have pupillary abnormalities (e.g. dilated or unequal pupils) usually due to neurological injury or medications, rather than primary eye pathology, these are monitored as part of neuro exams but can confuse the ocular picture if, for instance, a dilated nonreactive pupil is from nebulized atropine in the eye versus a sign of intracranial pathology. Clinicians should be aware of any ophthalmic drugs given (such as atropine drops during eye exams or nebuliser exposure) that could affect pupil exam findings [34].

In summary, the bulk of ICU eye complications involve the anterior segment (cornea and conjunctiva) and stem from drying, exposure, and secondary infection. These problems are often interrelated, and spiral exposure leads to abrasion, which invites infection, which worsens inflammation and can culminate in permanent damage. Thankfully, with diligent preventive care, most of these complications are avoidable or readily treatable if caught early. The next sections will discuss how to assess the eyes of ICU patients and implement protective strategies to minimise these issues.

7. Uncommon but serious ocular complications in ICU

While ocular surface disorders are the most common issues, ICU patients can also experience less frequent ophthalmologic emergencies that require specialised management [35]. These tend to be related to severe systemic conditions or specific interventions. Recognising these scenarios is important, as they can lead to permanent blindness if not promptly addressed.

7.1 Endogenous endophthalmitis (intraocular infection)

It is a serious intraocular infection resulting from haematogenous spread of pathogens into the eye, typically affecting patients with fungemia or persistent bacteraemia. In ICU settings, *Candida Albicans* is the most common cause, particularly in patients with central venous catheters, parenteral nutrition, or prolonged antibiotic use [36]. Less commonly, *Staphylococcus aureus* or Streptococcus species can cause endophthalmitis in the context of high-grade bacteraemia or endocarditis. Clinical signs may be subtle in sedated patients, check for a white pupillary reflex, hypopyon, or hazy fundus view. While older guidelines recommended routine screening in all patients with candidemia, a 2019 systematic review of over 7000 patients found that only ~1% required ophthalmic intervention [37]. Current practice supports a targeted approach: eye examination is indicated if symptoms are present, if the patient cannot report symptoms but is at high risk, or if any concerning signs are seen. For suspected fungal endophthalmitis, ophthalmology consultation is essential, and systemic antifungal selection should account for intraocular penetration e.g. intravenous voriconazole and echinocandins (**Figure** 7) [38].

7.2 Ischemic optic neuropathy and cortical blindness

Ischaemic Optic Neuropathy (ION) is a rare but devastating complication in critically ill patients, caused by infarction of the optic nerve due to prolonged hypotension, anaemia, or low-flow states. Posterior ION, more common in the ICU, may occur following cardiac arrest, massive haemorrhage, ECMO cannulation, or septic shock. Prone positioning, frequently used in ARDS management, has also been implicated, particularly in COVID-19 patients, likely due to increased venous pressure and reduced arterial inflow to the optic nerve. Case reports have described bilateral ION and irreversible vision loss following prolonged prone positioning [39]. Diagnosis is often delayed, as fundus findings may appear normal initially, and vision

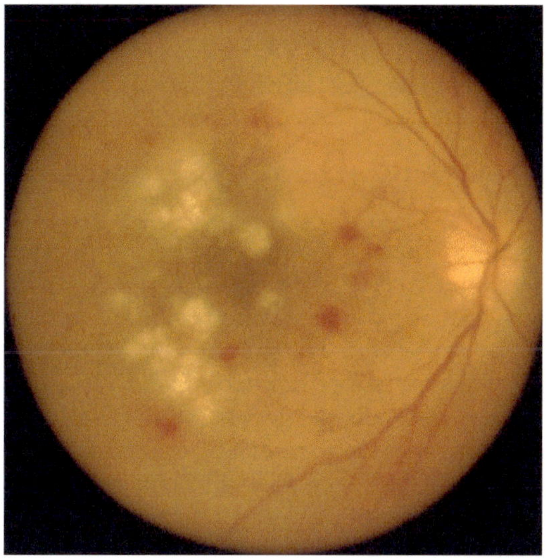

Figure 7.
Fundus-style retinal image illustrating creamy-white, fluffy intraretinal lesions with surrounding haemorrhages consistent with Candida retinitis. (Image generated by ChatGPT, May 2025).

loss is usually recognised only after sedation is lifted. ICU teams can reduce risk by maintaining adequate mean arterial pressure and haemoglobin, especially in patients with cardiovascular disease or borderline perfusion. In selected high-risk cases (e.g. major haemorrhage or prolonged hypotension), some centres consider periodic optic nerve sheath diameter monitoring or structured eye checks, though this is difficult in practice. If a patient reports new vision loss or fails to respond to visual stimuli upon awakening, urgent ophthalmology and neurology assessment is essential to distinguish ION from cortical blindness. Unfortunately, once vision loss occurs, it is almost always permanent, making prevention through early haemodynamic optimisation the only effective intervention.

7.3 Acute glaucoma (angle-closure glaucoma)

s a sight-threatening emergency that can occur in ICU patients, particularly when nebulised anticholinergics or adrenergic, such as ipratropium bromide, reach the eyes, triggering pupillary dilation in anatomically predisposed individuals with narrow iridocorneal angles. This leads to a rapid rise in intraocular pressure (IOP), often presenting in awake patients with severe eye pain, a red eye, blurred vision with halos, a fixed mid-dilated pupil, and systemic symptoms like headache, nausea, or vomiting. In sedated patients, pain and visual complaints may be absent, but clues include a hazy cornea from corneal oedema, a mid-dilated non-reactive pupil, or one eye that feels rock-hard on gentle palpation through the eyelid, this firm globe is a key bedside finding [40]. Sustained IOP >40–50 mmHg can cause permanent optic nerve damage within hours, making this an ophthalmologic emergency. Immediate treatment includes IV acetazolamide, topical agents (e.g. beta-blockers, pilocarpine), osmotic therapy (e.g. mannitol), and urgent laser iridotomy. Prevention is equally critical: shield the eyes during aerosol treatments, use closed ventilator circuits when possible, or apply moist gauze over the eyes if using nebuliser masks. Scopolamine patches may also provoke pupil dilation and should be used with caution. In prone patients, especially with head-down tilt, increased orbital venous pressure may contribute to angle closure in at-risk eyes; therefore, avoiding excessive head dependency and ensuring orbital pressure is minimised is advised.

7.4 Orbital compartment syndrome (orbital apex syndrome)

Orbital Compartment Syndrome is a vision-threatening emergency caused by a rapid rise in intraocular pressure, most commonly due to retrobulbar haemorrhage following trauma, but also possible from prolonged external compression during prone positioning or spontaneous bleeding in coagulopathic ICU patients. It presents with acute proptosis, a tense, rock-hard globe, tight eyelids (often difficult to manually open), severe conjunctival chemosis, and rapidly declining vision or pupillary responses. If suspected, action must be immediate, lateral canthotomy and cantholysis should ideally be performed within minutes to decompress the orbit and restore perfusion [41]. While performing a canthotomy is not within the typical scope of practice for ICU physicians, the expertise of emergency physicians or ophthalmologists is crucial in cases requiring this procedure. If no specialist is immediately available and vision is at risk, documented cases support canthotomy being performed by critical care or trauma teams under remote guidance. Prevention hinges on avoiding direct orbital pressure, particularly during prone ventilation, and on early identification of bleeding risk in coagulopathic patients (e.g. those on ECMO or with severe thrombocytopenia). In certain high-risk surgical patients, prophylactic canthotomy or partially open eyelid closures may be left intentionally by surgeons to reduce risk. There is no routine orbital pressure monitoring, so awareness and rapid response are crucial.

8. Consultation and multidisciplinary management

The value of a standardised ICU eye-care protocol cannot be overstated. In the UK, practice varied widely, but once a universal guideline was rolled out, documentation rates climbed, and ocular complications fell [42]. Embedding eye care into routine patient checks, especially since pupils are already examined regularly in critical care, offers a natural "hook" for assessing corneal integrity, tear film status, and eyelid closure. One quality-improvement project even wove an eye-care checklist into the standard nursing documentation, not only ensuring every shift included eye assessment but also enabling meaningful audit of care delivery [43].

Despite these advancements, gaps in consistent eye care persist. In most ICUs, nurses already perform routine high-risk checks: pressure-area assessments, vascular line inspections, and ventilator circuit reviews for patients who cannot mobilise. Eye care for those at elevated risk (e.g., intubated, sedated, or with lagophthalmos) should be embedded in the same checklist framework. Staffing pressures, heavy workloads, and the specialised nature of ophthalmic assessment can still undermine consistency. Many nurses report feeling under-prepared to recognise early corneal changes or manage lubrication protocols. Targeted education, formal teaching on ICU-relevant eye diseases, hands-on skills sessions with fluorescein staining, and case-based discussions helps bridge this niche knowledge gap. When eye-care responsibilities are clearly assigned and reinforced through both documentation and ongoing training, protocol adherence improves, and more patients receive reliable, high-quality ocular protection [44, 45].

9. Conclusion

Ocular complications are common in critically ill patients but are largely preventable when addressed through a structured, multidisciplinary approach. *By identifying high-risk individuals* at admission and applying a simple eyelid-closure grading system, ICU teams can tailor interventions, ranging from routine lubrication to moisture chambers and lid-taping, according to a patient's needs. Integrating an "eye check" into existing care bundles (pressure-area, line inspections, ventilator circuits) ensures that ocular assessment is performed alongside other standard safety measures each shift.

Education and audit are essential for sustaining protocol adherence. Targeted training in basic ophthalmic examination, fluorescein staining, and documentation reinforces nursing competence and highlights early signs of exposure keratopathy, conjunctivitis, or corneal ulceration. When advanced pathology is suspected, clear referral criteria expedite ophthalmology involvement and reduce the risk of permanent visual sequelae.

Incorporating these evidence-based practices into routine ICU workflows not only reduces the incidence of corneal drying, abrasions, and infections but also preserves visual function—as an integral aspect of comprehensive critical-care outcomes.

Acknowledgements

The authors would like to acknowledge the use of AI-assisted tools, specifically ChatGPT-4o and Google Gemini, in supporting the writing of this document. We also acknowledge ChatGPT-4o for its assistance in generating some synthetic imaging.

Author contributions

- Negin Sanadgol: Conceptualization, Writing – original draft.
- Mertcan Sevgi: Conceptualization, Writing – review and editing.
- Daniel Pethers: Writing – review and editing, Validation.
- David Merle: Writing – review and editing, Validation.

Funding

[DRAFT: UCL funding contribution once approved].

Ethical statement

Not applicable.

Data availability statement

Source data not available for this article.

Conflict of interest

The authors declare no conflict of interest.

Author details

Negin Sanadgol[1*], Daniel Pethers[2], David Merle[1,3] and Mertcan Sevgi[1,3]

1 Institute of Ophthalmology, University College London, London, United Kingdom

2 NHS Greater Glasgow and Clyde, Major Trauma/Critical Care, Glasgow, Scotland

3 Moorfields Eye Hospital NHS Foundation Trust, London, United Kingdom

*Address all correspondence to: negin.sanadgol.24@ucl.ac.uk

References

[1] Hearne BJ, Hearne EG, Montgomery H, Lightman SL. Eye care in the intensive care unit. Journal of the Intensive Care Society. 2018;**19**(4):345-350. DOI: 10.1177/1751143718764529

[2] Kousha O, Kousha Z, Paddle J. Incidence, risk factors and impact of protocolised care on exposure keratopathy in critically ill adults: A two-phase prospective cohort study. Critical Care (London, England). 2018;**22**(1):5. DOI: 10.1186/s13054-017-1925-5

[3] Nikseresht T et al. Lubratex eye ointment with polyethylene cover significantly reduces corneal abrasion in ICU patients: A randomized controlled trial. Scientific Reports. 2024;**14**(1):20443. DOI: 10.1038/s41598-024-71601-1

[4] Kaye AD et al. Postoperative management of corneal abrasions and clinical implications: A comprehensive review. Current Pain and Headache Reports. 2019;**23**(7):48. DOI: 10.1007/s11916-019-0784-y

[5] Magno MS et al. Chambered warm moist air eyelid warming devices - A review. Acta Ophthalmologica. 2022;**100**(5):499-510. DOI: 10.1111/aos.15052

[6] The Definition and Classification Subcommittee of the International Dry Eye WorkShop. The definition and classification of dry eye disease: Report of the Definition and Classification Subcommittee of the International Dry Eye WorkShop (2007). The Ocular Surface. 2007;**5**(2):75-92. DOI: 10.1016/S1542-0124(12)70081-2

[7] Gipson IK. The ocular surface: The challenge to enable and protect vision. Investigative Ophthalmology and Visual Science. 2007;**48**(10):4390-4398. DOI: 10.1167/iovs.07-0770

[8] Chen Y et al. Prevalence and risk factors of exposure keratopathy among critically ill patients: A systematic review and meta-analysis. Nursing Open. 2023;**11**(1):e2061. DOI: 10.1002/nop2.2061

[9] Saritas TB et al. Ocular surface disorders in intensive care unit patients. The Scientific World Journal. 2013;**2013**:182038. DOI: 10.1155/2013/182038

[10] Andrew D. Bacterial conjunctivitis. EyeRounds.org. University of Iowa Department of Ophthalmology and Visual Sciences; 2008. Available from: https://eyerounds.org/atlas/pages/bacterial-conjunctivitis.html [Accessed: May 16, 2025]

[11] Pflugfelder SC, Stern ME. Biological functions of tear film. Experimental Eye Research. 2020;**197**:108115. DOI: 10.1016/j.exer.2020.108115

[12] Sanghi P et al. Ocular complications in the prone position in the critical care setting: The COVID-19 pandemic. Journal of Intensive Care Medicine. 2021;**36**(3):361-372. DOI: 10.1177/0885066620959031

[13] Mercieca F et al. Ocular surface disease in intensive care unit patients. Eye (London, England). 1999;**13**(Pt 2):231-236. DOI: 10.1038/eye.1999.57

[14] Reinstein DZ et al. Epithelial thickness in the Normal cornea: Three-dimensional display with Artemis very high-frequency digital ultrasound. Journal of Refractive Surgery (Thorofare,

N.J.: 1995). 2008;**24**(6):571-581. DOI: 10.3928/1081597X-20080601-05

[15] Sridhar MS. Anatomy of cornea and ocular surface. Indian Journal of Ophthalmology. 2018;**66**(2):190-194. DOI: 10.4103/ijo.IJO_646_17

[16] Heilman J. Allergic conjunctivitis showing conjunctival edema [photograph]. Wikimedia Commons; 14 Nov 2013. Available from: https://commons.wikimedia.org/wiki/File:Allergicconjunctivitis.jpg. [Accessed: May 16, 2025]

[17] Ezra DG, Lewis G, Healy M, Coombes A. Preventing exposure keratopathy in the critically ill: A prospective study comparing eye care regimes. British Journal of Ophthalmology. 2005;**89**(8):1068-1069. DOI: 10.1136/bjo.2004.062406

[18] Płaszewska-Żywko L et al. Risk factors of eye complications in patients treated in the intensive care unit. International Journal of Environmental Research and Public Health. 2021;**18**(21):11178. DOI: 10.3390/ijerph182111178

[19] The Royal College of Ophthalmologists, Intensive Care Society. Eye Care in the Intensive Care Unit (ICU): Ophthalmic Services Guidance. London: The Royal College of Ophthalmologists; 2020. Available from: https://www.rcophth.ac.uk/wp-content/uploads/2021/01/Eye-Care-in-the-Intensive-Care-Unit-2020.pdf [Accessed: April 24, 2025]

[20] Merle DA et al. Automated measurement and three-dimensional fitting of corneal ulcerations and erosions via AI-based image analysis. Current Eye Research. 2024;**49**(8):835-842. DOI: 10.1080/02713683.2024.2344197

[21] Zucco L, Webb C. Improving the documentation of the daily review of patients in general intensive care. BMJ Quality Improvement Reports. 2014;**3**(1):u539.w496. DOI: 10.1136/bmjquality.u539.w496

[22] Larkin G, McHugh J, Montgomery H, Hingorani M; The Royal College of Ophthalmologists' Quality and Safety Group; The Intensive Care Society; The Faculty of Intensive Care. Eye Care in the Intensive Care Unit. Royal College of Ophthalmologists; Apr 2020. Available from: https://www.rcophth.ac.uk/wp-content/uploads/2021/01/Eye-Care-in-the-Intensive-Care-Unit-2020.pdf [Accessed: May 7, 2025]

[23] Mahani M, A et al. The effect of polyethylene cover intervention on ocular surface disorder of intensive care unit patients: A systematic review and meta-analysis. BMC Ophthalmology. 2024;**24**(1):109. DOI: 10.1186/s12886-024-03360-6

[24] Vislisel J. Punctate epithelial erosions (PEE) secondary to exposure keratopathy. Eye Forum Atlas. University of Iowa Department of Ophthalmology and Visual Sciences. Available from: https://webeye.ophth.uiowa.edu/eyeforum/atlas/pages/Punctate-epithelial-erosions/index.htm [Accessed: May 9, 2025]

[25] Imanaka H et al. Ocular surface disorders in the critically ill. Anesthesia and Analgesia. 1997;**85**(2):343-346. DOI: 10.1097/00000539-199708000-00018

[26] Hernandez EV, Mannis MJ. Superficial keratopathy in intensive care unit patients. American Journal of Ophthalmology. 1997;**124**(2):212-216. DOI: 10.1016/s0002-9394(14)70786-x

[27] Hartford JB et al. Prevalence and risk factors of exposure keratopathy across different intensive care units.

Cornea. 2019;**38**(9):1124. DOI: 10.1097/ICO.0000000000001961

[28] Liesegang TJ. Contact lens-related microbial keratitis: Part I: Epidemiology. Cornea. 1997;**16**(2):125-131

[29] Al-Mujaini A et al. Bacterial keratitis: Perspective on epidemiology, Clinico-pathogenesis, diagnosis and treatment. Sultan Qaboos University Medical Journal. 2009;**9**(2):184-195

[30] Vislisel J. Fungal keratitis. Eye Forum Atlas. University of Iowa Department of Ophthalmology and Visual Sciences; 2017. Available from: https://webeye.ophth.uiowa.edu/eyeforum/atlas/pages/fungal-keratitis/index.htm [Accessed: May 7, 2025]

[31] Risma JM, Syed NA. Exposure keratopathy in the critically ill: A case report, discussion, and systems-based intervention. EyeRounds.org. University of Iowa Department of Ophthalmology and Visual Sciences; 1 Jul 2014. Available from: https://eyerounds.org/cases/189-exposure-keratopathy.htm [Accessed: May 16, 2025]

[32] Mela EK et al. Ocular surface bacterial colonisation in sedated intensive care unit patients. Anaesthesia and Intensive Care. 2010;**38**(1):190-193. DOI: 10.1177/0310057X1003800129

[33] Parkin B et al. Bacterial keratitis in the critically ill. The British Journal of Ophthalmology. 1997;**81**(12):1060-1063. DOI: 10.1136/bjo.81.12.1060

[34] Mercieca F, Suresh P, Morton A, Tullo A. Ocular surface disease in intensive care unit patients. Eye (Lond). 1999;**13**(Pt 2):231-236. DOI: 10.1038/eye.1999.57

[35] Grixti A, Sadri M, Datta AV. Uncommon ophthalmologic disorders in intensive care unit patients. Journal of Critical Care. 2012;**27**(6):746.e9-746.22. DOI: 10.1016/j.jcrc.2012.07.013

[36] Grixti A et al. Common ocular surface disorders in patients in intensive care units. The Ocular Surface. 2012;**10**(1):26-42. DOI: 10.1016/j.jtos.2011.10.001

[37] Breazzano MP et al. Utility of ophthalmologic screening for patients with Candida bloodstream infections: A systematic review. JAMA Ophthalmology. 2019;**137**(6):698-710. DOI: 10.1001/jamaophthalmol.2019.0733

[38] Danielescu C et al. The diagnosis and treatment of fungal endophthalmitis: An update. Diagnostics. 2022;**12**(3):679. DOI: 10.3390/diagnostics12030679

[39] Panchabhai TS et al. Acute ischemic optic neuropathy with extended prone position ventilation in a lung transplant recipient. International Journal of Critical Illness and Injury Science. 2016;**6**(1):45-47. DOI: 10.4103/2229-5151.177367

[40] Petsas A, Chapman G, Stewart R. Acute angle closure glaucoma – A potential blind spot in critical care. Journal of the Intensive Care Society. 2017;**18**(3):244-246. DOI: 10.1177/1751143717701946

[41] Fox A et al. A multidisciplinary educational curriculum for the management of orbital compartment syndrome. The American Journal of Emergency Medicine. 2020;**38**(6):1278-1280. DOI: 10.1016/j.ajem.2019.12.002

[42] Kam R et al. National survey of protective eye care practices in the critically ill. Critical Care. 2011;**15**(Suppl. 1):P538. DOI: 10.1186/cc9958

[43] Sevgi M et al. Improving eye care in an intensive care unit. Journal of the Intensive Care Society. 2024;**25**(3):346-349. DOI: 10.1177/17511437241228587

[44] Gungor S, Andı S, Akçoban S, Tosun B. Knowledge, attitudes and practices of intensive care nurses regarding eye care. Journal of Clinical Nursing. 9 Mar 2025. DOI: 10.1111/jocn.17733

[45] Mehrjardi ZM et al. Effect of training eye care clinical guideline for ICU patients on clinical competence of eye care in nurses. Critical Care Research and Practice. 2021;**2021**:6669538. DOI: 10.1155/2021/6669538

Chapter 7

Pharmacological Safety in Neonatal Care: A Focus on Clinical Pharmacy Intervention

Norhan Attia Ahmed

Abstract

Neonates in neonatal intensive care units (NICUs) are at high risk for drug-related problems (DRPs) due to their rapid physiological changes, complex pharmacotherapy, and lack of neonatal-specific formulations. Reported DRP incidences range widely from 33.6% to 89.6%, with treatment effectiveness being the most common issue, followed by drug safety concerns and incomplete prescriptions. Among the leading causes, dose selection errors account for over 50%, increasing the risk of toxicity or therapeutic failure. Factors such as high clinical workloads, knowledge gaps, and manual prescription processes further contribute to medication errors in this vulnerable population. Clinical pharmacists play a critical role in optimizing medication safety and resolving DRPs in NICUs. In this study, pharmacists primarily intervened at the drug level (69.2%), with additional interventions at the prescriber level (13.8%). The acceptance rate of pharmacist interventions was exceptionally high (98.8%), demonstrating strong interdisciplinary collaboration and trust in their expertise. Furthermore, 99.7% of pharmacist interventions had a positive impact on patient safety, efficacy, and overall quality of life. These findings highlight the essential role of clinical pharmacists in NICUs, reinforcing the need for structured pharmacist-led interventions, individualized dosing strategies, and enhanced prescribing protocols to minimize medication errors and optimize neonatal outcomes.

Keywords: neonatal intensive care unit (NICU), drug-related problems (DRPs), clinical pharmacy, pharmaceutical interventions, patient outcomes

1. Introduction

Drug-related problems (DRPs) are a significant concern in the healthcare sector, with over half of the harm to patients being preventable [1, 2]. According to the Pharmaceutical Care Network of Europe (PCNE) classification, a drug-related problem (DRP) has been defined as "an event or circumstance involving drug therapy that actually or potentially interferes with desired health outcomes" [3].

An increased risk of medication errors is prevalent in critically ill ICU patients, with neonatal infants being a particularly vulnerable subset of this population.

A neonate is a "child under 28 days of age" [4]; the Neonatal Intensive Care Unit (NICU) is a complex clinical setting that often leads to undesirable outcomes and medical errors [5]. In this high-risk environment, where complicated regimens are present, the incidence and impact of DRPs can be serious. There are numerous differences between neonates in comparison to adults and pediatrics regarding the treatment [6]. A medication dosage for an adolescent can be up to a 100 times higher than that for a preterm neonate. While a pediatric dose might be one-tenth of an adult's dose, it could still be ten times the appropriate dose for a preterm neonate. These variations significantly contribute to the risk of medication errors in this population [7]. The neonates are considered "unique drug recipient" due to rapid changes that affect their body composition and organ function [8, 9]. The processes of absorption, distribution, metabolism, and elimination vary with age and significantly impact the pharmacological effects of drugs.

Neonates, especially the preterm ones, often cannot receive medications or nutrients orally for varying durations after birth. This poses a challenge in providing essential medical support and nutrition. Consequently, the intravenous route offers a solution by allowing parenteral administration of necessary formulations to meet their needs.

Three factors contribute to an increased risk of DRPs in NICU patients compared to other populations:

1. NICU patients experience higher exposure to medications from the time of admission.

2. There is a lack of clinical trials on pharmacotherapies in neonates due to ethical considerations.

3. There is a lack of specific formulations for neonates, as the majority of drugs used to treat newborns are either not licensed for this age group or used off-label (for unapproved indications, doses, or administration routes). This often requires dilution before administration, increasing the potential for dosage errors [10, 11].

The doses are calculated based on weight. Errors in decimal placement during prescribing can result in 10-fold or larger dosing errors, underscoring the crucial importance of accuracy [11]. The drug formulary used in the NICU is relatively limited compared to that used in other patient populations. Consequently, there is a constant need to modify drug formulations to suit the needs of neonatal patients [11]. A study performed on hospitalized children found that the highest incidence of ADEs occurred in the NICU compared to other wards (pediatric medical ward, pediatric surgical ward, and postnatal ward) [12].

2. Incidence and types of drug-related problems in NICUs

2.1 Prevalence of DRPs

Limited research has explored the prevalence of DRPs in NICUs, revealing significant variability in reported rates, ranging from 33.6% to 89.6% [13–20].

These variations likely stem from differences in patients' clinical conditions and illness severity. Key factors influencing DRP detection include NICU infrastructure, staffing levels, availability of clinical pharmacists, adoption of electronic health records, and adherence to medication safety protocols. NICUs equipped with comprehensive resources and dedicated medication safety programs tend to report lower incidence rates due to proactive management practices.

For instance, an observational prospective study conducted from October 2015 to October 2016 at an NICU in a women's health hospital in Brazil, focusing on neonates undergoing antimicrobial therapy for suspected early sepsis, reported a DRP incidence of 33.6% [13]. Similarly, another observational prospective study on septic neonates in Ethiopia, conducted from May to August 2018, reported a higher DRP incidence of 48.8% (95% CI 41.7–55.9%) [16]. This variation in incidence rates could be attributed to differences in NICU resources, local healthcare practices, antimicrobial stewardship protocols, and population demographics, which may affect the detection and management of drug-related issues in clinical settings.

An exploratory study conducted in Brazil between October 2013 and June 2014 on extremely low birth weight (ELBW) neonates in an NICU recruited 33 neonates and showed a higher incidence of DRPs at 39.4% [14]. This higher incidence can be explained by the increased care standards required for low birth weight neonates, who often need more complex and individualized treatment regimens, leading to a greater potential for drug-related issues.

A cross-sectional study conducted in Brazil aimed to identify the incidence and types of DRPs in neonates with heart diseases. The study, conducted from January 2014 to December 2016, included 122 neonates and found a DRP incidence of 74.6% (95% CI 65.9–82%) [15]. This high incidence is explainable, as the presence of heart disease increases the complexity of treatment.

Two observational studies conducted in the NICUs of teaching hospitals in Brazil recruited 600 neonates. The studies, carried out between January 2014 and November 2016 and April 2014 and January 2017, showed higher incidences of DRPs, with rates of 59.8% (95% CI 55.8–63.8%) and 60.5%, respectively [18, 19]. These high incidence rates can be attributed to the complexity of cases typically managed in teaching hospitals, where critically ill neonates often require more intensive and varied pharmacological interventions, increasing the likelihood of encountering DRPs.

A prospective descriptive study was conducted in the NICU of a tertiary children's teaching hospital in Egypt over a 4-month period (August–November 2023). The study recruited 316 neonates and reported a high incidence of drug-related problems (DRPs), reaching 89.6% [20].

Another cross-sectional study conducted in a tertiary hospital in India over an 18-month period also reported a DRP incidence of 55.6% [17].

These variations underscore the challenges in standardizing DRP detection and management across NICUs, potentially impacting treatment outcomes and patient safety. Ensuring consistent adherence to medication safety protocols and enhancing resource allocation in NICUs may help mitigate these disparities and improve overall patient care.

2.2 Common types and causes of DRPs in NICUs

Drug-related problems (DRPs) are a significant concern in neonatal intensive care units (NICUs), with treatment effectiveness emerging as the most prevalent issue across multiple studies. In a study conducted by Ahmed et al., treatment effectiveness accounted for 46.4% of DRPs [20], a finding that aligns with other research, including a study on cardiac neonates, which reported a similar incidence of 49% [15]. Furthermore, a study in Brazil identified treatment effectiveness as the primary issue in 54.2% of the cases [19]. However, even higher rates have been observed in some settings. For instance, a study from India reported an incidence of 87.8% [17], while another investigation focusing on neonates receiving antimicrobial therapy found treatment effectiveness problems in 84.8% of the cases [13].

The predominance of treatment effectiveness issues can be attributed to the dynamic physiological changes that occur in neonates. Rapid fluctuations in body weight [21], along with significant pharmacokinetic and pharmacodynamic variations, play a crucial role in determining drug efficacy. Neonatal growth is accompanied by substantial shifts in body composition, including changes in total body water and fat distribution, which directly affect drug absorption and distribution. Additionally, the maturation of metabolic pathways, particularly hepatic and renal enzyme systems, significantly influences drug clearance, necessitating careful dose adjustments. These pharmacodynamic and pharmacokinetic changes contribute to the complexity of achieving optimal therapeutic outcomes in neonates, underscoring the need for individualized dosing strategies and rigorous monitoring to ensure safe and effective medication use. Standardized dosing guidelines often fail to account for these rapid developmental changes, emphasizing the importance of tailored pharmacotherapy in this vulnerable population [22].

In addition to treatment effectiveness concerns, drug safety represents another critical category of DRPs in NICUs. In the study by Ahmed et al., safety-related DRPs accounted for 26.4% of the cases [20]. However, studies from Brazil have documented much higher incidences, with safety-related issues reported in 54.4% [19] and 41.4% of the cases [15]. Conversely, other investigations have found significantly lower rates; for example, studies in India and among neonates receiving antimicrobial therapy identified safety-related DRPs in only 2.7% [17] and 15.2% of the cases [13], respectively.

A third category of DRPs, classified under the "other domain," was identified in 27.2% of the cases in Ahmed et al.'s study, with "unclear problems" accounting for 20.2% [20]. This rate is notably higher than those reported in previous research. For example, an Indian study found that issues within this category accounted for only 9.5% of DRPs [17], while two separate studies from Brazil reported even lower rates of 9.8% [15] and 3.6% [19], respectively. One of the primary contributors to the "unclear problems" category in this study was incomplete prescriptions, a recurring challenge in NICU settings. Physicians are responsible for prescribing and calculating medication doses for neonates, a process that requires precision and careful consideration of each infant's rapidly changing clinical parameters. However, the high workload and time constraints faced by healthcare providers may increase the likelihood of incomplete or ambiguous prescriptions.

Incomplete prescriptions have been identified as a major concern in multiple healthcare settings. A Malaysian study conducted on pediatric patients reported that "treatment safety" was the most frequently observed DRP (34.3%), followed by "unclear problems" (28.3%), which were primarily related to incomplete prescriptions. In the same study, treatment effectiveness issues were documented in 23.2% of the cases, with "unoptimized drug treatment" accounting for 17.7% [23]. These findings underscore the widespread nature of prescription-related challenges, which persist across different patient populations and healthcare environments. The root causes of incomplete prescriptions often include high clinical workloads, insufficient time for thorough documentation, and the absence of standardized protocols for prescription verification. Addressing these issues requires the implementation of targeted interventions, such as electronic prescribing systems, enhanced pharmacist involvement, and structured medication review processes to minimize errors and improve the completeness of prescriptions [20].

2.3 Clinical pharmacists' interventions and acceptance rates in NICUs

Beyond the classification of DRPs, an analysis of their underlying causes revealed that dose selection errors were the leading contributor, accounting for over 50% of all identified issues. This aligns with findings from studies conducted in Brazil [19], and by Nunes et al. [13], which similarly identified dose selection as a primary source of DRPs. Errors in neonatal dosing can result in significant clinical consequences, including toxicity due to overdose or therapeutic failure due to suboptimal drug levels. Since neonatal dosing is largely weight-based, the risk of calculation errors is inherently higher than in adult populations. These challenges are compounded by factors such as knowledge gaps, limited clinical experience, inadequate staffing, and high workloads among junior physicians and nurses [24].

Clinical pharmacists play a crucial role in optimizing medication therapy and addressing drug-related problems (DRPs) in neonatal intensive care units (NICUs). A study conducted by Ahmed et al. [20] examined pharmacist-led interventions and their impact on patient care. The study found that pharmacists performed a total of 2149 interventions, with the majority 69.2% occurring at the drug level, followed by 17% classified as other interventions and 13.8% at the prescriber level. This distribution was influenced by the study's methodological approach, which categorized all medication-related interventions comprehensively under the drug level. Notably, a significant proportion of these interventions involved dosage modifications, aligning with the predominant DRP type—dose selection errors. These findings differ from research in India [17], where a greater proportion of interventions were directed at the prescriber level.

The acceptance rate of pharmacist interventions is a critical indicator of interdisciplinary collaboration and the perceived value of clinical pharmacy services in NICUs. The study by Norhan et al. reported an exceptionally high acceptance rate of 98.8%, with 93% of interventions fully implemented. Similarly, research from Brazil on neonates in critical care settings has shown acceptance rates exceeding 90% [15, 19].

However, variations exist across different healthcare settings. A study among extremely low birth weight (ELBW) neonates has reported acceptance rates above 80% [14], while research from Brazil focusing on neonates undergoing antimicrobial therapy for suspected sepsis indicated an acceptance rate of 81% [13].

The remarkably high acceptance rate in the NICU setting examined by Ahmed et al. and other studies highlights the integral role of pharmacists in neonatal care and the strong collaboration between pharmacists and physicians. This partnership enhances communication, ensures prompt resolution of medication-related issues, and ultimately contributes to improved patient safety and therapeutic outcomes. Given the vulnerability of neonates and the complexity of their pharmacotherapy, the involvement of clinical pharmacists is essential in minimizing medication errors and optimizing treatment efficacy.

2.4 Impact of clinical pharmacists' interventions on patient outcomes

Of the 2149 interventions provided in this study by Ahmed et al., 99.7% were found to enhance safety, efficacy, and overall quality of life for neonates, with only

0.3% having no impact on patient outcomes [20]. These findings align with those from other studies, such as one involving extremely low birth weight (ELBW) neonates, where 97.3% of pharmacist interventions were reported to have a positive effect on patient outcomes [14]. Similarly, research by Strong and Tsang [25] found that 93% of interventions for pediatric patients had a beneficial impact.

These results surpass those of a study utilizing a modified version of Overhage et al.'s scale, which reported that 78.6% of pharmacist interventions significantly improved patient outcomes [26]. Additionally, a study focusing on adolescent patients documented an 86% positive impact rate [27]. These comparisons highlight that pharmacist-led interventions in our NICU setting contribute to an even greater enhancement of patient care, further emphasizing the critical role of clinical pharmacy services in neonatology.

3. Conclusion

Clinical pharmacists play a crucial role in neonatal intensive care units (NICUs) by optimizing medication therapy and preventing drug-related problems (DRPs). This chapter highlights that selection errors are the most common DRPs, emphasizing the importance of pharmacist interventions in improving medication safety. With an exceptionally high acceptance rate, these interventions demonstrate strong collaboration between pharmacists and healthcare providers, leading to enhanced patient outcomes. Given the complexity of neonatal pharmacotherapy, integrating clinical pharmacy services is essential for minimizing medication errors and ensuring optimal treatment. Expanding pharmacists' roles in NICUs can further improve patient safety and healthcare efficiency.

Author details

Norhan Attia Ahmed
Faculty of Pharmacy, Assiut University, Assiut, Egypt

*Address all correspondence to: norhan_attia@pharm.aun.edu.eg

References

[1] Panagioti M, Khan K, Keers RN, Abuzour A, Phipps D, Kontopantelis E, et al. Prevalence, severity, and nature of preventable patient harm across medical care settings: Systematic review and meta-analysis. The BMJ. 2019;**366**

[2] Hodkinson A, Tyler N, Ashcroft DM, Keers RN, Khan K, Phipps D, et al. Preventable medication harm across health care settings: A systematic review and meta-analysis. BMC Medicine. 2020;**18**(1):313

[3] Pharmaceutical Care Network Europe Drug Related Problem Classification. Available from: https://www.pcne.org/upload/files/417_PCNE_classification_V9-1_final.pdf

[4] Muhe LM. Newborn health. In: Raviglione MCB, Tediosi F, Villa S, Casamitjana N, Plasència A, editors. Global Health Essentials. Cham: Springer; 2023. pp. 43-45

[5] Stavroudis TA, Miller MR, Lehmann CU. Medication errors in neonates. Clinics in Perinatology. 2008;**35**(1):141-161

[6] Krzyzaniak N, Bajorek B. Medication safety in neonatal care: A review of medication errors among neonates. Therapeutic Advances in Drug Safety. 2016;**7**(3):102-119

[7] Grissinger M. Medication errors affecting pediatric patients: Unique challenges for this special population. Pennsylvania Patient Safety Advisory. 2015;**12**(3):96-102

[8] Morselli PL. Clinical pharmacokinetics in neonates. Clinical Pharmacokinetics. 1976;**1**(2):81-98

[9] Milsap RL, Jusko WJ. Pharmacokinetics in the infant. Environmental Health Perspectives. 1994;**102**(suppl 11):107-110. DOI: 10.1289/ehp.94102s11107

[10] Sorrentino E, Alegiani C. Medication errors in the neonate. The Journal of Maternal-Fetal & Neonatal Medicine: The Official Journal of the European Association of Perinatal Medicine, the Federation of Asia and Oceania Perinatal Societies, the International Society of Perinatal Obstetricians. 2012;**25**(Suppl 4):91-93

[11] Holmes APTATT. NICU Primer for Pharmacists. NV-1 o. Bethesda, Maryland: ASHP publications; 2016

[12] Kunac DL, Kennedy J, Austin N, Reith D. Incidence, preventability, and impact of adverse drug events (ADEs) and potential ADEs in hospitalized children in New Zealand: A prospective observational cohort study. Pediatric Drugs. 2009;**11**(2):153-160

[13] Nunes BM, Xavier TC, Martins RR. Antimicrobial drug-related problems in a neonatal intensive care unit. Revista Brasileira de Terapia Intensiva. 2017;**29**:331-336

[14] Loureiro CV, Fonteles MM, Mascarenhas MB, Chaves EF, Firmino PY. Medication follow-up in newborns with extremely low birth-weight. Pharmacy Practice (Granada). 2019;**17**(4)

[15] do Nascimento ARF, RWD L, dos Santos MET, da Costa TX, Martins RR. Drug-related problems in cardiac neonates under intensive care. Revista Paulista de Pediatria. 2020;**38**:e2018134

[16] Awoke M, Melaku T, Beshir M. Drug-related problems and its determinant among hospitalized neonates with sepsis at Jimma University Medical Center, Ethiopia: A prospective observational study. Journal of Pharmaceutical Health Care and Sciences. 2021;**7**:1-8

[17] Dwivedi P, Sah SK, Murthy S, Ramesh M. Identification and resolution of drug-related problems among neonates in neonatal intensive care unit (NICU): A prospective longitudinal observational study. Clinical Epidemiology and Global Health. 2024;**29**:101728

[18] Leopoldino RD, Santos MT, Costa TX, Martins RR, Oliveira AG. Risk assessment of patient factors and medications for drug-related problems from a prospective longitudinal study of newborns admitted to a neonatal intensive care unit in Brazil. BMJ Open. 2019;**9**(7):e024377

[19] Leopoldino RD, Santos MT, Costa TX, Martins RR, Oliveira AG. Drug related problems in the neonatal intensive care unit: Incidence, characterization and clinical relevance. BMC Pediatrics. 2019;**19**:1-7

[20] Ahmed NA, Fouad EA, El-Asheer OM, Ghanem ASM. Pharmaceutical interventions for drug-related problems in the neonatal intensive care unit: Incidence, types, and acceptability. Frontiers in Pharmacology. 2024;**15**:1-14

[21] Wilbaux M, Fuchs A, Samardzic J, Rodieux F, Csajka C, Allegaert K, et al. Pharmacometric approaches to personalize use of primarily renally eliminated antibiotics in preterm and term neonates. The Journal of Clinical Pharmacology. 2016;**56**(8):909-935

[22] De Rose DU, Cairoli S, Dionisi M, Santisi A, Massenzi L, Goffredo BM, et al. Therapeutic drug monitoring is a feasible tool to personalize drug administration in neonates using new techniques: An overview on the pharmacokinetics and pharmacodynamics in neonatal age. International Journal of Molecular Sciences. 2020;**21**(16):5898

[23] Hon MY, Chua XY, Premakumar CM, Mohamed SN. Drug-related problems in a general paediatric ward of a tertiary care hospital in Malaysia. International Journal of Clinical Pharmacy. 2020;**42**(3):948-955

[24] Lesar TS, Briceland L, Stein DS. Factors related to errors in medication prescribing. Journal of the American Medical Association. 1997;**277**(4):312-317

[25] Strong DK, Tsang GWY. Focus and impact of pharmacists' interventions. Canadian Journal of Hospital Pharmacy. 1993;**46**(3):101-108

[26] Fernández-Llamazares CM, Calleja-Hernandez MA, Manrique-Rodriguez S, Pérez-Sanz C, Duran-García E, Sanjurjo-Saez M. Impact of clinical pharmacist interventions in reducing paediatric prescribing errors. Archives of Disease in Childhood. 2012;**97**(6):564-568

[27] Virani A, Crown N. The impact of a clinical pharmacist on patient and economic outcomes in a child and adolescent mental health unit. Canadian Journal of Hospital Pharmacy. 2003;**56**(3):158-162

Chapter 8

Withdrawal/Withholding of Life-Sustaining Therapies in the Intensive Care Unit

Ángel Becerra-Bolaños, Raúl Vega-Rodríguez, Héctor Trujillo-Morales, Nazario Ojeda-Betancor and Aurelio Rodríguez-Pérez

Abstract

Limitations of life-sustaining therapies in the Intensive Care Unit (ICU) are usually applied when therapeutic measurements are considered futile. Withholding and withdrawal therapies are then applied because therapies cannot achieve the desired outcomes. When implemented, several aspects should be taken into consideration, such as cultural, sociological, or personal preferences regarding end-of-life care. Withholding is the decision not to start or increase a treatment if the benefit is not clear, and is the most common measure applied, including orders such as do-not-resuscitate, do-not-intubate, or non-renal-replacement therapies. Withdrawal is a less frequent approach, and it is defined as the decision to stop a treatment. Decision-making should be multidisciplinary and consensual. It must respect the wishes of the patient and/or their relatives. These decisions usually carry a substantial emotional burden, especially for healthcare professionals, who might consider limitation of life-sustaining therapies as a failure, even though this perception should evolve. In addition, the implementation of these measures may lead to stressful situations for professionals, which need to be addressed to avoid a negative impact. Mortality is the most common outcome that emerges from the use of these measures. However, a significant number of patients survive to hospitalization. Survival can have consequences that may affect the patient's subsequent quality of life. Due to the potential concerns, the difficulty of implementation, and the challenges in the decision-making process, communication between healthcare professionals, patients, and families/relatives is an important issue when it comes to limiting life-sustaining therapies.

Keywords: intensive care unit, life-sustaining therapies, futility, limitation of therapeutic effort, withholding, withdrawal, advance directives, end-of-life, frailty, ethics

1. Introduction

Every country is facing an increase in the size and the proportion of elderly in their population [1]. Improved society and healthcare have resulted in more elderly patients in intensive care units (ICUs) [2], leading to higher multimorbidity and frailty. These conditions contribute to poorer clinical outcomes and higher healthcare costs [3, 4]. Cognitive and technological advances have made it possible to replace vital functions during critical situations, and have shifted therapeutic efforts toward managing the worsening of chronic conditions [5, 6]. However, patients' baseline status is often suboptimal, and ICU admission may lead to devastating consequences [7].

The primary objective of ICU treatment is to preserve life while avoiding unnecessary suffering or the prolongation of the dying process [8]. Therefore, evaluating the appropriateness of ongoing treatment is crucial to avoid therapeutic obstinacy and to focus on preserving the patient's dignity, in alignment with the bioethical principles of autonomy, beneficence, justice, and non-maleficence [9].

1.1 Futility

A treatment is deemed futile when physicians determine that achieving the desired outcome is highly improbable, based on clinical practice, shared experiences, or empirical data. It is also important to differentiate between the effect on a specific part and the overall benefit to the patient [10]. A futile treatment is one that fails to achieve its intended objectives, either because it does not provide a reasonable chance of survival, proves to be clinically ineffective, does not improve the patient's quality of life, or does not align with the patient's goals [11].

The definition of *medical* futility is based on two criteria involving independent variables: quantitative and qualitative criteria. *Quantitative* or *physiological* futility refers to the numerical probability that a medical intervention will achieve the desired effect. Since it relates to alterations in organ function, its assessment presents relatively few challenges or debates among physicians. On the other hand, *qualitative* futility refers to the probability that the physiological effect will provide meaningful benefit to the patient [12], making its assessment more holistic and significantly more complex [13]. The overall futility of a treatment can be calculated as the product of quantitative and qualitative futility. Both components are essential in determining the futility of a therapy. If the chance of a treatment influencing one of the two components (qualitative or quantitative) approaches zero, the medical intervention is considered futile [14].

The perception of the futility of a therapy can be influenced by physicians' goals, sociocultural and religious values, and characteristics of both doctors and patients [15]. However, continuing ineffective treatment affects patients, their families, other patients, healthcare professionals, and systems negatively, increasing the economic costs [16]. Thus, futility justifies limiting life-sustaining therapies that offer no patient benefit while potentially increasing suffering.

1.2 Definition of limitation of life-support therapies

The limitation of life-sustaining therapies can be applied in two modalities: withholding and withdrawal. Withholding refers to the decision not to initiate additional life-sustaining measures, whereas withdrawal involves discontinuing previously implemented supportive interventions. Although both approaches are ethically equivalent, they may be perceived differently by healthcare professionals, especially those less experienced with end-of-life care in the ICU setting. Withdrawal is often seen as a more direct action leading to the patient's death. Nevertheless, both strategies are recognized as ethically sound alternatives to therapeutic obstinacy, striving to achieve a balance between the quantity and quality of life [17].

The primary challenge in implementing limitations on life-sustaining therapies lies in the fact that determining the futility of a therapy is not always clear-cut. While clinicians may estimate the likely course of an illness, accurately predicting a precise prognosis is often elusive. This uncertainty can lead to conflicts among professionals or between healthcare providers and the patient's family members [9]. Besides, surveys conducted among ICU professionals highlight the challenges in determining which treatment goals are realistically achievable and what constitutes an unfavorable risk-benefit balance [18].

If it is justified to not start a treatment, then it is also justified to stop that same treatment, assuming the patient's condition and values remain consistent. Certain clinical conditions define an irreversible dying process, such as progressive multi-organ failure with no prospect of successful treatment of the underlying cause, or the possibility of adequately and durably replacing organ function. Other scenarios include potentially fatal diseases or complications leading to complete loss of vital functions, as well as the terminal stage of chronic or malignant diseases that can no

Withholding	Decision made not to start or increase a life-sustaining intervention
Withdrawal	Decision made to actively stop an intervention already given
Active shortening of the dying process	Circumstance in which someone performs an act with the intention of shortening the dying process
Palliative care	Specialized medical care for people with a serious illness, focused on providing relief from the symptoms and stress associated with the illness. It is aimed at improving quality of life for both the patients and their families
End-of-life care	Includes the decision-making as to the limitation of life-sustaining therapies and the physical, emotional, social, and spiritual support for patients and their families
Advanced directives	Legal document that states a person's wishes about receiving medical care if that person is no longer able to make medical decisions; it may also give a person the authority to make medical decisions for another person when the patient can no longer make decisions (power of attorney)
Conflict	Dispute, disagreement, incompatibility, opposition, or difference of opinion related to the patient's management
Appropriate care	A patient care proportional to his/her expected survival and quality of life and in line with the patient's and relatives' values
Burnout	A psychological syndrome arising in response to chronic emotional and interpersonal stressors on the job, characterized by three different features: emotional exhaustion, depersonalization, and lack of personal and professional completion
Decision-making	A stepwise practice of gathering and interpreting information, weighing different options, and ultimately making a shared, evidence-based, and personalized decision

Adapted from the European Society of Intensive Care Medicine Guidelines on end-of-life and palliative care in the intensive care unit [24].

Table 1.
Definitions.

longer be managed [8]. However, this is not solely a technical judgment. It is also essential to assess the current circumstances and consequences, considering the patient's values and the available resources [19].

The interaction between personal and professional spheres in decision-making regarding the limitation of life-sustaining therapies imposes a significant psychological burden on both healthcare professionals and the patient's family and loved ones. This process may evoke feelings of guilt or regret [20]. Therefore, the implementation of these measures should be approached in an individualized and holistic manner. To prevent conflicts in their application, recommendations have been made for hospitals and medical centers to establish mechanisms that support this decision-making process [21].

Although the limitation of life-sustaining therapies is widely accepted by professionals, it is sometimes perceived as a form of euthanasia [22]. Euthanasia involves an explicit and repeated request from the patient for an act intended to cause death to prevent further suffering [23]. However, during the limitation of life-sustaining therapies, it is the underlying disease that causes the patient's death, not the actions of healthcare professionals. Some key definitions relevant to this topic are presented in **Table 1**.

The objective of this chapter is to provide a guide to limiting life-sustaining therapies, acknowledging that a universal approach is not feasible, and that individualized decision-making must be the basis of these measures.

2. Limitation of life-sustaining therapies

2.1 Epidemiology

There is wide variability in the limitation of life-sustaining therapies, ranging from 5 to 15% of patients admitted to ICUs [6, 17, 25–27]. The frequency of these practices varies depending on geographic region and the healthcare setting in which the facility is located [28]. A study conducted across 199 ICUs in 36 countries demonstrated that the practice of limiting life-sustaining therapies differs significantly among regions [29]. Contextual factors contribute to the regional variation in decisions regarding withholding or withdrawing treatment in critically ill patients. A multicenter study conducted in Poland on ICU patients over the age of 80 reported an incidence of limitation of life-sustaining therapies of 17.9% [30]. This percentage was lower than the 24.6% observed in a German cohort [31] and significantly lower than the 41.9% reported in a Norwegian cohort [32].

Issues related to the patient's pathology or the type of unit in which the study is carried out also influence the frequency and epidemiology of these measures. In 4671 critically ill patients with COVID-19 admitted to the ICU between February and May 2020, the prevalence of limitation of long-term therapies was 14.5% [33]. In patients who received cardiopulmonary resuscitation maneuvers after out-of-hospital cardiac arrest, its prevalence was 30.7% [34], while a study carried out in septic patients detected an incidence higher than 35% [35]. On the other hand, ICUs with a greater number of post-surgical patients generally have lower rates of limitation of life-support therapies than ICUs with a higher number of patients with decompensated medical pathologies [25].

The percentage of limitation of life-support measures increases between 43 and 81% of patients who die in the ICU [17, 36].

2.2 Factors associated with the limitation of life-support therapies

The variables associated with the implementation of life-sustaining therapy limitation measures are multifaceted, including medical, ethical, and individual factors [6]. The most frequently reported factors are:

- Age: Older patients are more likely to be prescribed limitation of life-sustaining therapies [36, 37]. Age over 80 years is significantly associated with the decision to limit life-sustaining therapies [6, 26, 30]. Paradoxically, in a sub-analysis conducted across 12 ICUs participating in a multicenter study, the clinical characteristics of patients for whom these decisions were made revealed a profile of individuals younger than 70 years [38]. However, early decision-making is often associated with the patient's age and chronic poor health [39].

- Functional status: Functional dependence, assessed by the Barthel index, is also an important variable. Patients with total dependence (Barthel index less than or equal to 20) are more likely to be subject to limitation of life-sustaining therapies [40].

- Comorbidities: The Charlson Comorbidity Index has also been associated with the probability of limiting life-sustaining therapies [37]. This index is quite useful, given its correlation with the expected 10-year survival rate of the patient. Cardiovascular comorbidities were present in more than half of the patients who underwent limitation of life-sustaining therapies in a multicenter study carried out in Spanish ICUs [38].

- Frailty: A syndrome defined by increased vulnerability due to decreased physiological reserve. It affects the ability to adapt to stressors, such as acute illness [41]. Patients who undergo life-sustaining therapy are often frailer [37]. Assessment of frailty using tools such as the Clinical Frailty Scale has been associated with increased 30-day mortality [32], reinforcing the importance of considering this variable in the decision-making process.

- Quality of life: A poorer quality of life prior to ICU admission also increases the likelihood of a decision to limit life-sustaining therapies [6, 26]. Considering quality of life prior to admission is controversial, since patients' perception does not usually coincide with professionals' perceptions, who tend to underestimate it [42]. A survey showed that 85% of physicians and 93% of nurses agreed that it was important to consider quality of life after ICU admission to establish limitation of therapeutic effort [43]. Currently, quality of life after ICU admission is one of the main determinants [44]. Since it is related to mortality after discharge [45], the application of an objective tool for its evaluation could shed light on a patient's prognosis.

- Severity of illness leading to ICU admission: Scales such as Glasgow Coma Scale, Acute Physiology and Chronic Health Evaluation II (APACHE II), Sequential Organ Failure Assessment (SOFA), Simplified Acute Physiology Score II (SAPS II), and Mortality Probability Model II (MPM II) help evaluate survival probability and reduce prognostic uncertainty in decisions regarding life-sustaining therapy limitations [26, 30, 36, 37, 46, 47]. Both the SOFA score and disease progression within the first 5 days after ICU admission have been associated with 100% mortality rate [48]. APACHE-II score is also an independent predictor of mortality [49]. Other scales, such as Nine Equivalents of Nursing Manpower Use Score (NEMS), have shown association with life-support therapies limitation [6]. In patients over 60 years old who suffer from traumatic brain injury, the Extended Glasgow Outcome Scale (EOS) score lower than 5 has been associated with an unfavorable neurological outcome [50]. So, this scale could be used in these patients to decide on limiting life-support therapies. Poor prognosis [34] along with the perception of patient suffering are determining factors in many of the proposals for limiting therapies [44].

- Admission characteristics: Patients admitted due to decompensations of medical conditions have a higher likelihood of limiting life-sustaining therapies [25]. This may be because patients with medical decompensations tend to have greater severity at the time of ICU admission and a poorer quality of life. Consequently, these patients are often considered to have a lower likelihood of improvement. Additionally, there is a perception that surgical treatment may be curative, fully resolving the condition that led to ICU admission. Decision-making for surgical patients also requires the surgeon's agreement, and surgeons may be more reluctant to withdraw therapy [6], as this could be perceived as a failure of the surgical intervention. Furthermore, patients who are subjected to therapeutic effort limitation are frequently admitted for non-elective reasons [51].

- Other patient- or disease-related variables identified include ICU length of stay and duration of mechanical ventilation. These factors may be interrelated or associated with age, the presence of comorbidities or frailty, poorer baseline status, or greater disease severity [20, 30, 52, 53].

- External and organizational factors: Socioeconomic factors may influence decision-making regarding life-sustaining therapy limitations. In the United States, decisions to limit life-sustaining therapies are made earlier for uninsured trauma patients compared to those with private health insurance [54]. Inequities in healthcare provision not only accelerate withdrawal of life-sustaining treatment but also impact overall mortality in patients with traumatic brain injury [55]. Additionally, financial constraints within families may lead caregivers to discharge critically ill children from the hospital against treating physicians' recommendations. This affects 1.4 to 5.7% of pediatric patients in low-income countries and leads to almost certain death of the patient [56], during which the comfort and care of the patient's symptoms or family are not assured. For this reason, it is essential to establish international standards to minimize geographic and economic variability in providing optimal end-of-life care.

- Given the influence of ethical and individual factors, it is important to highlight that some of the most decisive elements in decision-making process include both the patient's family and healthcare professionals. Studies have shown that patient desires influenced the decision in 2–63% of cases, while families were involved in 2–90%. Regarding healthcare professionals, in emergency departments, decisions were made jointly with at least one other physician in 80% of cases, while nursing staff participated in up to 30% of cases [20]. Regarding religious factors, a study conducted in Lebanon showed that both Christian and Muslim

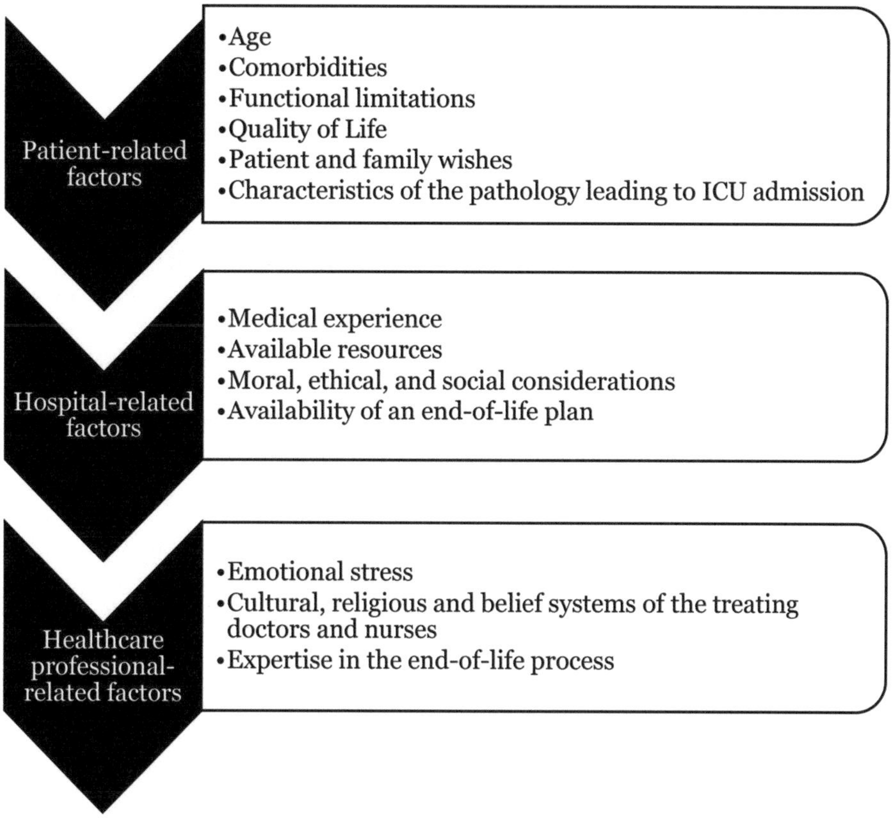

Figure 1.
Key factors influencing decisions.

physicians accepted both withholding and withdrawing life-sustaining therapies when appropriate [57].

Therefore, decisions are mainly influenced by factors related to the patient and disease, factors related to the hospital, and factors related to the healthcare professionals (**Figure 1**) [20, 58].

2.3 Decision-making

2.3.1 Advance directives

Advance directives are legal documents that state the will of the patient, safeguarding the bioethical principle of autonomy. Autonomy is the right of individuals to make decisions about their health and illness without coercion and with all the necessary information. It therefore implies knowledge of the different treatment options available and the consequences of using or not using them [9]. It is estimated that only 1.6% of patients have advance directives in Spanish ICUs. However, up to 62% of patients would accept limitations on life-sustaining therapies in cases of a poor prognosis or a significant decline in quality of life [59]. This is confirmed in other countries, where the patient's wishes are unknown in more than 40% of cases [60].

These documents allow patients to express their personal preferences regarding future medical treatments in the event that they are unable to communicate their wishes actively [61]. The content of an advance directive depends on the patient's condition, varying based on whether the individual is healthy, has chronic illnesses, or faces an advanced disease with an imminent risk of death [62]. When completed under favorable prognostic conditions, advance directives are frequently modified over time [63]. Conversely, advance directives completed within the last 3 months of life are associated with a greater likelihood of opting for aggressive care [64]. However, the presence of an acute, potentially reversible condition can impair the patient's capacity to make decisions. Despite the limitations of advance directives, understanding a patient's previously expressed wishes—regardless of how distant they may be from the circumstances leading to ICU admission—is invaluable, if not essential, in the current decision-making process. Therefore, these directives should not only be considered, but should also serve as the guiding framework to uphold patient autonomy when the patient is unable to exercise it. In such cases, this responsibility often falls to family members and close contacts.

The clinical condition during ICU admission, due to the underlying pathology or the effects of administered medications, often prevents patients from rationally expressing their preferences regarding ICU management. This situation becomes particularly challenging when it is unclear whether the patient has fully understood physicians' explanations about their prognosis. Whenever possible, decisions regarding the limitation of life-sustaining therapies should involve all individuals responsible for the patient's treatment and care [8], while considering the patient's potential wishes as perceived by those who know them best and their prior lifestyle before the critical illness.

The physician overseeing the patient's clinical management likely has the most comprehensive perspective on patient's condition, recent progression, and short- to medium-term prognosis based on the course of the disease. Although the "physician in charge" of the patient management must have the necessary tools to coordinate the conversation regarding their own proposal or that of the patient or their family members, the decision must always be discussed with the healthcare team and aligned with the explicit wishes of the patient's family [65]. Empowering those close to the patient in decision-making can be considered surrogate decision-making. This can extend the autonomy of the incapacitated person, allowing professionals to understand their previously expressed values and preferences. However, it is not easy to distinguish between the choices family members would make for themselves and those they are asked to make on behalf of someone else [66].

2.3.2 When to make the proposal

The timing of the proposal to limit life-sustaining therapies is influenced by several factors, including the state of mind of the professionals, their previous experience with death, or their knowledge of how to cope with extreme experiences. It is essential that both patients and their representatives are well informed about the prognosis of the current situation and the available therapeutic options [22]. This will allow them to consider what type of consequences they are willing to accept and at what risk. An interprofessional approach that involves both physicians and nurses in decision-making helps to maintain consistent messages and reduces moral distress among healthcare providers [67].

Proposing the limitation of life-sustaining therapies too early may be perceived by family members or close contacts as an abandonment of responsibility or as a consequence of deficiencies in the healthcare system. However, considering the possibility of limiting life-support measures early after ICU admission can reduce anxiety for both the patient and their family [37]. It is therefore crucial to identify the appropriate moment to initiate discussions leading to a shared decision-making process. Deciding within the first 48 hours of ICU admission that a patient is not a candidate for cardiopulmonary resuscitation has been associated with fewer interventions, reduced suffering, and a lower likelihood of loss of dignity as perceived by nurses. Additionally, nurses were less likely to perceive that the patient was in distress or not peaceful in cases where the patient ultimately died in the ICU. Importantly, such early decisions did not accelerate death compared to cases where the decision was made later [68]. Thus, delaying such discussions longer than necessary should be avoided. However, decision-making should be started only after gathering sufficient information regarding the patient's pre-existing conditions and the factors leading to ICU admission. This period also allows for the initiation of therapeutic measures and provides both the patient and their family an opportunity to recognize a worsening evolution. Time-limited trials recognize clinical uncertainties and prevent the extension of invasive interventions in the ICU.

End-of-life discussions have been shown to offer benefits for both patients and caregivers without significantly increasing emotional distress or psychiatric disorders [69]. Training healthcare teams in communication strategies is essential to prevent stress disorders and improve decision-making. Standardized interventions aim to reduce stress among family members and improve communication skills among healthcare professionals [70]. In addition, the entire process and the characteristics of the decision-making should be adequately recorded in the patient's medical record.

2.3.3 Conflicts that may arise

Conflicts may arise among the members of the medical team, who may consider a treatment futile, and the patient's representatives, who insist on maintaining all possible measures. A lack of understanding of the patient's current clinical situation by the patient's relatives is often the consequence of poor communication between them and the medical team. This opposition can lead healthcare professionals to fear potential legal action [71]. In such cases, it is crucial to interrupt the discussion and assess the root causes of the conflict. Conducting an appropriate differential diagnosis can help resolve potential issues and allow the focus to remain on providing appropriate care for the patient. These conflicts may stem from factors related to the family, the physician, or the healthcare organization [72].

Families may experience conflict due to a lack of understanding of the situation. This may result from insufficient psychological preparation to hear patient's diagnosis or prognosis, considering that bad news is often poorly processed. Additionally, the traditional communication style of physicians may contribute to misunderstandings or lead families to seek information from other sources. Even when families understand and acknowledge the situation, their decisions may also be influenced by feelings of guilt or secondary gains [73].

Physicians may also feel uncomfortable with prognostic uncertainty, leading them to approach these conversations either hesitantly or with excessive confidence. Additionally, they may be overburdened with work, fatigue, frustration, or stress. Discussing end-of-life matters may also be perceived as a professional failure. It is essential for healthcare professionals to foster honest dialog, actively listening to patients or representatives, and incorporating this input as a crucial factor in proposing appropriate actions [74].

Social and organizational factors contributing to decision-making conflicts extend beyond the lack of financial compensation for discussions that are time-consuming. Restrictions on visiting hours limit contact between families and patients, hindering communication about end-of-life issues and preventing families from fully understanding the patient's condition [75]. Once a differential diagnosis of the conflict's reason has been established, it is necessary to develop interventions aimed at addressing and preventing these conflicts. Such measures promote better understanding between families and healthcare professionals, ultimately facilitating a consensual decision on the most appropriate course of action based on the patient's current condition.

Once it becomes clear that the patient's improvement is unlikely and that death may be approaching, conversation should continue. So, efforts can be redirected toward clarifying the patient's priorities and optimizing pain and symptom management [76].

2.4 Implementation: Withdrawal or withholding?

From an ethical standpoint, the decision to withdraw life-sustaining therapies is no different from the decision not to initiate or escalate them [77]. Although withdrawing interventions may seem more aggressive, as it involves the removal of all support and inevitably influences a potentially fatal outcome, a study revealed that life-sustaining interventions were withdrawn in nearly half of the cases [27]. From a practical perspective, withholding and withdrawing therapies can be considered equivalent. In fact, there may be uncertainty about whether a decision falls into one category or the other, and this distinction may not lead to any significant changes in the overall management of the patient. According to the Canadian Critical Care Society, legal and psychological differences between withholding and withdrawing life-sustaining treatment should not be overstated, as there may be no clinically significant differences between discontinuing an intervention and choosing not to escalate it [78].

2.4.1 Withholding

Withholding refers to the decision not to administer a life-sustaining treatment to a patient for whom it is unlikely to provide a clear benefit. This form of limitation is the most frequently used in surgical ICUs [25]. The rate of withholding-based limitations tends to be higher in studies conducted in Southern Europe compared to those involving hospital in Northern Europe, reinforcing the impact of cultural differences on these decisions. In Spain and Portugal, withholding was practiced in 63–83% of patients receiving end-of-life care, whereas these percentages were lower in other European multicenter studies [6, 25, 26, 29].

The most commonly used withholding measures are included in **Figure 2** [79]. Most publications exploring the application of withholding focus on the decision to forgo cardiopulmonary resuscitation [49]. This measure is common in end-of-life care, as cardiopulmonary resuscitation may cause more harm than benefit. Do-not-resuscitate orders are primarily indicated in three scenarios: patients who will not benefit from cardiopulmonary resuscitation, patients for whom resuscitation may

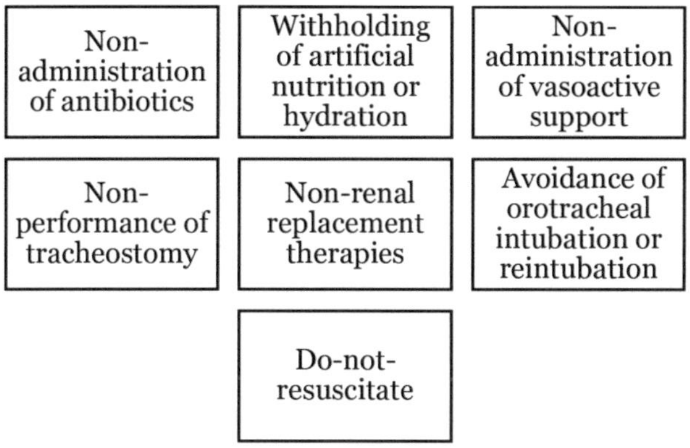

Figure 2.
Commonly employed withholding measures.

result in permanent harm or loss of consciousness, and patients with poor quality of life for whom recovery after resuscitation is unlikely [80]. This measure was significantly applied during the COVID-19 pandemic due to poor prognosis of these patients at a moment when healthcare-system demand exceeded available resources [81].

Respiratory failure accounts for nearly one-third of ICU admissions, making invasive mechanical ventilation a cornerstone of treatment for these patients. In these cases, decision-making is influenced not only by the patient's or physician's judgment but also by external factors. For example, ICU overcrowding forced many hospitals to forgo intubation in some patients due to a lack of resources during the COVID-19 pandemic [82]. The decision not to perform orotracheal intubation is generally associated with increased mortality and, in many cases, is closely aligned with a do-not-resuscitate order. The main criteria under this decision include advanced age, severe cognitive impairment, prolonged immobility, short life expectancy, limited functional capacity, or the presence of advance directives. The frequency of this decision varies across countries and published studies [82, 83]. However, up to 25% of patients for whom intubation was not performed were successfully treated with noninvasive mechanical ventilation [84].

The recommendation regarding do-not-resuscitate and do-not-intubate orders is that these directives should always be implemented in alignment with clearly defined treatment goals, ensuring consistency with the overall care plan. According to consensus guidelines, these decisions should always involve the patient, their family, and the healthcare team [24, 82]. These principles are also applicable to surgical airway management, as evidence suggests that proper palliative and end-of-life care can reduce the need for tracheostomies [85].

The complex hemodynamic and inflammatory conditions seen in ICU patients frequently lead to impaired renal function. The indication for renal replacement therapies in the ICU must distinguish between two different scenarios: patients experiencing acute kidney injury requiring renal replacement therapy due to their current condition, and those already enrolled in chronic dialysis programs who are admitted to the ICU for an intercurrent illness. These two groups have different implications when considering withholding renal replacement therapies. Only 21% of nephrologists in the United States are aware of the existence of a clinical guideline for limiting dialysis in patients with acute kidney injury and chronic kidney disease [86, 87]. The expected benefit must be considered. Despite currently increasing patient tolerance to continuous therapies, it is important to recognize that renal replacement therapies should not be offered to all patients [86]. Among patients receiving continuous renal replacement therapy in the ICU, in-hospital mortality reached 61% for those with acute kidney injury and 54% for those with chronic kidney disease. However, renal function recovery occurred in 41–82% of survivors, with long-term outcomes being difficult to determine [88–90]. In this context, another relevant factor is the temporal window for therapeutic intervention in acute kidney injury, which is significantly shorter in patients with chronic kidney disease. The absence of advance directives further shortens this timeframe, necessitating discussions with families that, although often perceived by nephrologists as a bilateral agreement, do not always result in consensus [91]. Therefore, decisions regarding the limitation of renal replacement therapies should be made early, and the use of advance directives is particularly recommended for patients enrolled in chronic dialysis programs. One approach suggested by clinical guidelines is a trial of renal replacement therapy with predefined outcomes and duration, after which, if no improvement is observed, withdrawal may be considered [86, 87]. Additionally, dialysis withdrawal in elderly patients is generally well accepted by many physicians, even in cases where patients oppose the decision [92], despite it being a common cause of death in patients with chronic kidney disease [93]. The general acceptance of dialysis withdrawal may be attributed to the association between renal replacement therapies and a poorer quality of life.

Intravenous treatments are also frequently limited in critically ill patients with a poor prognosis, especially antibiotics and vasoactive support. To properly determine when to prescribe or withdraw an antibiotic in critically ill patients, it may sometimes be necessary to involve palliative care specialists in the patient assessment. In a cohort of 1177 cancer patients who died in the ICU, palliative care consultation led to fewer antibiotic prescriptions, a higher deprescription rate, and a lower rate of antibiotic treatment escalation [94]. Antibiotic deprescription most commonly occurs less than a day before death. In this context, the goal of end-of-life care is to improve comfort and alleviate suffering. Guidelines recommend antibiotic administration for symptomatic infections, with the aim of relieving symptoms, although there is little consensus on its usefulness in lower respiratory tract infections. Furthermore, broad-spectrum antibiotic therapy can cause patients to become reservoirs of multidrug-resistant microorganisms, with subsequent epidemiological and clinical implications. Therefore, if prolonging survival is not the primary objective, withholding antibiotics should be considered. Due to evidence of reduced symptoms and suffering, even in pneumonia, antibiotic treatment should be administered orally when possible [95–97].

Vasopressor treatment should be evaluated separately from the indication of no cardiopulmonary resuscitation and no orotracheal intubation, despite their close relationship. The administration of vasoactive drugs in patients with a poor prognosis can unnecessarily prolong life, so it should be considered as an initial measure to be limited [98]. Actually, vasopressor therapies are usually limited before more invasive therapies, such as mechanical ventilation. On the other hand, measures that must be ultimately suspended should be parenteral nutrition and hydration, since they are considered non-therapeutic measures, but rather support measures, without curative intent, that seek relief [99]. In addition, the suspension of artificial hydration and feeding has been associated with intestinal discomfort, diarrhea, and aspiration. Hence, the decision to suspend them must be made preserving the comfort and dignity of the patient, in consensus with the patient and her/his families [80].

2.4.2 Withdrawal

Withdrawal of life-sustaining treatments is a complex process that requires careful consideration of several factors, which are taken into account when organic support is considered futile [58, 100]. In this case, a treatment that is unlikely to provide any benefit to the patient is stopped. This decision should be based on an ethical assessment that considers the patient's rights, needs, and wishes. However, involving family members in the process helps mitigate emotional stress and facilitates a smoother transition [70]. Although, as previously noted, withholding and withdrawal decisions are equivalent, on a practical level, carrying out withdrawal entails a greater emotional burden for health professionals, since culturally the moral equivalence between not starting treatment and stopping treatment has not been reached [101].

The futility of cardiopulmonary resuscitation in critically ill patients is a complex issue. Only 17–22% of patients with in-hospital cardiac arrest survive to hospital discharge, and a significant percentage of these patients are prone to suffer any associated neurological dysfunction [102]. Therefore, the precise moment to stop resuscitation remains a matter of debate. According to clinical guidelines, discontinuation of cardiopulmonary resuscitation maneuvers should be considered in the absence of return of spontaneous circulation after an adequate period of resuscitation and advanced life support. Retrospective studies have shown that the probability of survival is less than 1% when resuscitation is prolonged beyond 39 minutes, and that significant neurological recovery is unlikely if cardiopulmonary resuscitation is prolonged beyond 32 minutes [103, 104]. However, recent medical advances, such as the use of cardiopulmonary bypass systems, have allowed documented cases in which return of spontaneous circulation has been achieved after more than 150 minutes of cardiopulmonary resuscitation. Therefore, it is essential to evaluate each case individually before deciding to discontinue the maneuvers [105].

Patients frequently reach the end of life while connected to invasive mechanical ventilation. When the situation is irreversible, withdrawal of mechanical ventilation should be considered. Ventilatory support can be removed in two ways: terminal weaning (consists of gradually reducing the dose of oxygen and ventilatory support) or terminal extubation (cessation of ventilatory support and removing the endotracheal tube in a single time). These two methods are often used, either together or separately, and there is no evidence as to which one is better [106]. However, dyspnea is predictable in ventilator-dependent patients in the process of weaning, especially at the end of life. Dyspnea is a common and distressing symptom that should be managed appropriately to ensure patient comfort [107]. The pharmacological and non-pharmacological measures for maintaining comfort after weaning are difficult to achieve. Many patients who are weaned off ventilation can be treated with noninvasive ventilation or high-flow oxygen therapy [108]. Patients with signs of respiratory distress in whom it is decided to withdraw mechanical ventilation are usually treated with morphine or fentanyl [107]. The most frequent causes reported for disconnection of ventilatory support were the physician's decision as the survival expectancy is less than 10%, the prediction of a severe cognitive function deficit, and the perception that the patient does not want advanced life support. Given the characteristics of invasive mechanical ventilation, this decision is usually made by consensus with the family, without the patient's participation [109, 110]. The published literature suggests that terminal extubation was associated with higher rates of airway obstruction, gasping, and a higher behavioral pain scale score, whereas terminal weaning involved more opioids, hypnotics, and neuromuscular blocking agents, suggesting more active comfort management. Although both methods were similar in time to patient death [111], contrasting results have been reported regarding the psychological impact of these interventions on both families and healthcare professionals. Families tended to show high levels of satisfaction with the management of the situation in both cases, but ICU staff showed higher levels of stress with immediate extubation. The fact that this modality was associated with higher rates of gasping may indicate the need for better palliative management in this type of patient [111]. Pain is the most frequently reported distressing symptom in patients at high risk of death [112], so it is usually the main objective and continuous attention is usually given to it.

In developed countries, dialysis withdrawal is a cause of mortality in 15–22% of patients who die while on renal replacement therapy. In the ICU, stopping renal replacement therapy is one of the most frequent decisions to limit therapeutic effort at the end of life [113, 114]. The cessation of dialysis therapy and transition to palliative care is recommended for those patients with poor quality of life and poor prognosis [115].

Vasopressors and comfort medications should be withdrawn gradually, ensuring that the patient receives adequate treatment of pain and other symptoms so that he/she is comfortable [100]. General well-being is multidimensional and encompasses symptoms other than pain.

The timing of withdrawal of life support is influenced by several factors, which are crucial for setting expectations, managing resources, and considering organ donation possibilities. This process must be carefully planned and executed. This includes mechanical ventilation, administration of vasoactive support, and the use of extracorporeal assist devices. Measures that may seem simpler should be considered equivalent to organ support measures, but any therapeutic measure that is no longer justified on medical grounds should be discontinued. Thus, from an ethical and legal point of view, each of the measures shown in **Figure 3** should be considered equivalent in relation to the fact that the process of irreversible death should not be prolonged [8].

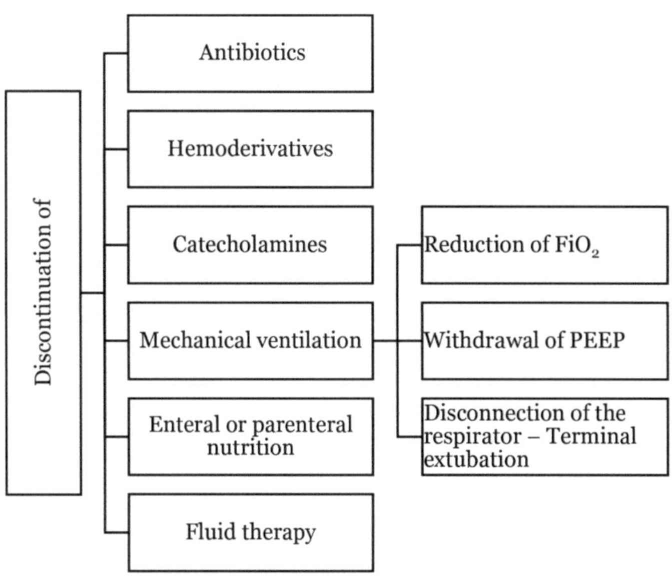

Figure 3.
Withdrawal.

Predicting the time to asystole from the withdrawal of life support is important for setting expectations and planning resource use. Some factors, such as deteriorating oxygenation or the absence of reflexes, are indicators that asystole is imminent [100]. Although the process should last long enough for the family to be able to accept the outcome, it should not be prolonged unnecessarily. The unpredictability of the dying process is a challenge for families and healthcare providers [116]. The following factors influence the withdrawal process's duration:

- Physiologic indicators: In adults, impending asystole (considered within the first 60 minutes) is associated with impaired oxygenation, absence of corneal and cough reflexes, decreased blood pressure, and the use of vasopressors and analgesics [100]. It is difficult to make accurate predictions in children because the physiological process is less well understood [116].

- Predictive models: Several predictive models exist for estimating time to asystole in adults. However, their generalizability and accuracy vary, and further validation is needed [100]. Few tools are available for pediatric patients.

- Emotional and logistical considerations: The unpredictability of the patient's time to death can cause emotional distress for families and healthcare professionals, affecting the potential organ donation after death [116]. Healthcare providers should assist families with logistics, medications, and setting expectations during the process [117].

- Cultural and ethical tensions: There might be tensions between maintaining a dignified dying process and therapeutic interventions, and between the role of healthcare professionals and the wishes of families [118].

2.5 Implications of implementation

The implementation of limiting life-sustaining therapies in the ICU is complex, infrequent, emotionally charged, and usually occurs at a point when various therapeutic interventions have been exhausted and futility has been demonstrated. Despite being the group in closest contact with the critically ill patient, nurses recognize that the decision to initiate life-sustaining interventions is usually made by the physician and feel that their opinion is almost never considered [71]. Although the physician may be the appropriate person to lead discussions about initiating the withholding or withdrawal of life-sustaining therapies, it is advisable to involve the entire team of professionals responsible for the patient's care (nurses, physiotherapists). In addition, families should feel involved in any changes in the patient's treatment, as both healthcare professionals and family members play a fundamental role in these situations [119]. The importance of involving all personnel responsible for the patient's care is that the decision to withdraw life-sustaining treatment can raise a moral dilemma for the nursing staff, who are often the ones responsible for withdrawing these therapies [120]. However, despite an obvious imbalance between medical and nursing staff decision-making, ICU nurses report relief when implementing life-sustaining therapy limitation measures [121].

The implementation of decisions can be interpreted by many professionals as a professional failure, as it is usually followed by the death of the patient [22]. This can affect emotional and professional well-being [58, 121]. The main effects of these decisions on ICU staff are included in **Table 2**.

Emotional stress and ethical dilemmas	Nurses may experience ethical conflicts due to disagreements among medical teams and the perception that physicians prolong unnecessary treatments rather than allowing for a dignified death. They acknowledge that physicians occasionally avoid applying irreversibility criteria, opting instead to extend interventions in an effort to defeat death, rather than facilitate a peaceful end-of-life process [71]. As a result, staff members often struggle to balance their duty to preserve life against the recognition of the patient's suffering [22, 58].
Feelings of frustration and powerlessness	Professionals may feel frustrated when their opinions are not considered in the decision-making process. This can lead to a sense of professional devaluation and make it more difficult for them to engage in a care plan they do not feel a part of [71, 122]. Poor communication can increase anxiety and depression among both professionals and the patient's relatives [70, 123].
Difficulty in withdrawing treatments	The discontinuation of previously prescribed treatments often adds stress to the decision-making process [71].
Risk of burnout and moral distress	Providing futile treatments can cause moral distress, emotional exhaustion, and even lead to a desire to leave the profession [58]. The emotional burden associated with limiting life-sustaining therapies combined with the high demands of the ICU environment increase the risk of burnout [122].
Need to provide comfort and relief	Nurses focus on ensuring patient comfort and relief during the end-of-life process, with the aim of securing a "good death." This includes creating a dignified and respectful environment, ensuring the presence of family, and alleviating pain and distress [71].

Table 2.
Effects of implementation on ICU staff.

Before implementing any decisions, it is advisable to avoid confusion between limiting life-sustaining therapies and euthanasia. Clearly distinguishing between these two concepts enables healthcare providers to make sound decisions that can benefit the patient during moments of great uncertainty [22]. Training in bioethics and the creation of spaces for reflection and dialog can help healthcare professionals face these challenges. Furthermore, emotional support and inclusion in the decision-making process are essential to mitigating the negative impact of limiting life-sustaining therapies on staff and family's well-being [19].

2.6 Outcomes

Despite the vast amount of medical information that intensive care physicians handle, significant uncertainty remains in clinical practice. This inevitably leads to differing outcomes among patients despite limited therapeutic measures, and consequently, a range of different results that can be obtained after implementing these decisions [124]. Clinical consequences after implementing life-sustaining therapies limitation may include survival, disability, or death—in the ICU, during the hospital stay, or after hospital discharge.

Mortality is probably the most common and sometimes most expected outcome. However, a causal relationship between the limitation of measures and patient death has not been clearly defined. During the COVID-19 pandemic, it was found that withholding was associated with a 75% mortality rate in ICU patients, while withdrawal was associated with a 95% mortality rate. In British ICUs, a study that included almost 800,000 patients found a 26% higher mortality difference in those patients who were withheld or withdrawn compared to those who were not [29, 33, 124, 125].

Healthcare professionals often associate this decision-making with mortality [29]. However, patient death is not always the outcome. One in five ICU admissions where therapeutic effort limitation measures are applied survives the hospitalization. Paradoxically, in a study of a cohort of over one million patients, those hospitals with higher rates of end-of-life treatment had slightly better survival rates [126].

Thus, after limiting life-sustaining treatment, ICU survival remains high (22%), with hospital survival at 16% [60]. Limitation of life-sustaining therapies does not always result in the patient's death. In up to 20% of cases, the implementation of these measures is associated with clinical improvement. This may be due to reversible diseases, misdiagnoses, a positive outcome from treatments administered prior to the decision, or because the decision involved limiting interventions that the patient ultimately did not need. For example, establishing a therapeutic ceiling by not initiating renal replacement therapies in patients who do not experience acute kidney failure during their hospital stay [29].

Patients who survive ICU admission suffer numerous complications and marked deterioration, which makes it difficult to regain pre-admission functional capacity. This may be exacerbated in patients who have undergone limited life-sustaining therapies, who tend to be more fragile, with multiple comorbidities and a worse prognosis [29]. For example, patients undergoing mechanical ventilation in the ICU experience a loss of up to 40% in their ability to perform some activities of daily living after admission. Cognitive impairment, brain fog, muscle weakness, fatigue, anxiety, and depression are some of the other symptoms that patients often present with upon discharge from the ICU [127]. Therefore, it is expected that patients who have received withholding or withdrawal of life-support measures will also experience a deterioration in their quality of life after discharge from the unit.

Limiting life-sustaining therapies often allows for earlier transitions to palliative care, which reduces ICU congestion [128] and costs without compromising the ethics of care [129]. Furthermore, when care goals are aligned and decision-making is consensual, ICU teams function more cohesively and with less internal conflict.

The implementation of structured approaches, such as time-limited trials, reduces the duration and intensity of non-beneficial treatments and the length of ICU stays without affecting overall mortality, improving the quality of experience for the families of critically ill patients [130]. Families generally appreciate honest and empathetic communication and sharing decision-making. Furthermore, clear communication reduces anxiety and improves the grieving experience [131], as they are more likely to feel that the patient died with dignity and that their values were respected [69]. Fear of legal liability and accusations of unethical behavior are common concerns among healthcare professionals, as observed in a Polish cross-sectional study [132]. However, when decision-making is well documented and agreed upon, legal risks are minimal [133].

It is mandatory to emphasize that the limitation on life-sustaining therapies does not imply the abandonment of the patient. Awareness of this principle can bring relief and comfort both to the professionals carrying out these practices and to the families of the patients involved. The fundamental components of a dignified death include ensuring the patient is free from pain, suffering, and distress, and is accompanied by family members throughout the process [71]. In the final stages of life, opioids are the most commonly used analgesics, with morphine the most frequent, followed by fentanyl. Among benzodiazepines, midazolam is the most used sedative. The average doses of analgesics and sedatives tend to increase both before and after the withdrawal of life support [134]. Patients admitted to the ICU typically have intravenous access and continuous monitoring in place. The intravenous administration of both opioids and sedatives is often the most efficient route for effective symptom management. The use of continuous intravenous drug infusion allows for a stable blood concentration that can be adjusted according to the infusion rate. This rate can be increased as needed to alleviate discomfort during the end-of-life process [66].

3. Conclusions

When a therapy is found to be futile, limiting life-sustaining therapies that do not benefit the patient should be considered. Both withholding and withdrawing therapies already given are equally valid ways of avoiding unnecessary prolongation of ICU stay and, eventually, life. However, the use of one of these methods depends on certain patient-related, cultural, or clinician-related factors. The decision should be multidisciplinary, taking into account the wishes of the patient and family in accordance with the principle of autonomy. Decision-making should begin as soon as sufficient information has been gathered to know the patient's prognosis, to avoid unnecessary delays, and to facilitate the active involvement of families to prevent stress and reduce uncertainty. Adequate and compassionate communication will prevent conflicts between families and doctors or among health professionals.

Withholding refers to the decision not to provide life-sustaining treatment to a patient for whom it is unlikely to provide clear benefit. Withdrawing refers to the discontinuation of a treatment that is unlikely to benefit the patient. The implementation of both methods can be complex, emotionally charged, and have consequences for healthcare professionals. In addition, the clinical consequences often lead to the patient's death, requiring active support with pharmacological and non-pharmacological therapies to facilitate end-of-life care. Sometimes the patient survives despite the limitation of life-sustaining therapies because of reversible diseases, misdiagnosis, a positive outcome of treatments administered prior to the decision, or because the decision involved limiting interventions that the patient may not need. In these cases, the possibility of complications or disability after discharge is a possibility that will affect the quality of life of the patient and their caregivers.

Conflict of interest

The authors declare no conflict of interest.

Thanks

We would like to thank Peter Mangiaracina and Bruno Rodríguez-Reveggino for their assistance in preparing this chapter.

Author details

Ángel Becerra-Bolaños[1,2]*, Raúl Vega-Rodríguez[1], Héctor Trujillo-Morales[1], Nazario Ojeda-Betancor[1] and Aurelio Rodríguez-Pérez[1,2]

1 Hospital Universitario de Gran Canaria Doctor Negrín, Las Palmas de Gran Canaria, Spain

2 Universidad de Las Palmas de Gran Canaria, Las Palmas de Gran Canaria, Spain

*Address all correspondence to: angbecbol@gmail.com

References

[1] WHO. Ageing and Health. 2024. Available from: https://www.who.int/news-room/fact-sheets/detail/ageing-and-health [Accessed: February 28, 2025]

[2] Ruiz C, Díaz MÁ, Zapata JM, Bravo S, Panay S, Escobar C, et al. Características y evolución de los pacientes que ingresan a una Unidad de Cuidados Intensivos de un hospital público [Characteristics and evolution of patients admitted to a public hospital intensive care unit]. Revista Médica de Chile. 2016;**144**(10):1297-1304. DOI: 10.4067/S0034-98872016001000009

[3] Hoogendijk EO, Afilalo J, Ensrud KE, Kowal P, Onder G, Fried LP. Frailty: Implications for clinical practice and public health. Lancet. 2019;**394**(10206):1365-1375. DOI: 10.1016/S0140-6736(19)31786-6

[4] Becerra-Bolaños Á, Hernández-Aguiar Y, Rodríguez-Pérez A. Preoperative frailty and postoperative complications after non-cardiac surgery: A systematic review. The Journal of International Medical Research. 2024;**52**(9):3000605241274553. DOI: 10.1177/03000605241274553

[5] Patrícia KR, Lenise PM, do, Almeida Cabral Patrícia Fernanda de, Jatobá de Souza Ana Izabel, Anders Jane Cristina. El cuidado y la tecnología en las unidades de cuidados intensivos. Index de Enfermería. 2013;**22**(3):156-160. Available from: http://scielo.isciii.es/scielo.php?script=sci_arttext&pid=S1132-12962013000200009&lng=es. DOI: 10.4321/S1132-12962013000200009

[6] Iribarren-Diarasarri S, Latorre-García K, Muñoz-Martínez T, Poveda-Hernández Y, Dudagoitia-Otaolea JL, Martínez-Alutiz S, et al. Limitación del esfuerzo terapéutico tras el ingreso en una Unidad de Medicina Intensiva. Análisis de factores asociados [limitation of therapeutic effort after ICU admission. Analysis of related factors]. Medicina Intensiva. 2007;**31**(2):68-72. DOI: 10.1016/s0210-5691(07)74778-2

[7] Boelens YFN, Melchers M, van Zanten ARH. Poor physical recovery after critical illness: Incidence, features, risk factors, pathophysiology, and evidence-based therapies. Current Opinion in Critical Care. 2022;**28**(4):409-416. DOI: 10.1097/MCC.0000000000000955

[8] Valentin A, Druml W, Steltzer H, Wiedermann CJ. Recommendations on therapy limitation and therapy discontinuation in intensive care units: Consensus paper of the Austrian associations of intensive care medicine. Intensive Care Medicine. 2008;**34**(4):771-776. DOI: 10.1007/s00134-007-0975-6

[9] García MÁG, Arenas MÁR, Cornejo AM. Bioethics in critical care patients. In: Reflections on Bioethics. London, UK: InTech; 2018. DOI: 10.5772/intechopen.75565

[10] Schneiderman LJ. Defining medical futility and improving medical care. The Journal of Bioethical Inquiry. 2011;**8**(2):123-131. DOI: 10.1007/s11673-011-9293-3

[11] Jecker NS, Pearlman RA. Medical futility. Who decides? Archives of Internal Medicine. 1992;**152**(6):1140-1144

[12] Schneiderman LJ, Jecker NS, Jonsen AR. Medical futility: Its meaning and ethical implications. Annals of

Internal Medicine. 1990;**112**(12):949-954. DOI: 10.7326/0003-4819-112-12-949

[13] Aghabarary M, Dehghan NN. Medical futility and its challenges: A review study. The Journal of Medical Ethics and History of Medicine. 2016;**9**:11

[14] Bernat JL. Medical futility: Definition, determination, and disputes in critical care. Neurocritical Care. 2005;**2**(2):198-205. DOI: 10.1385/NCC:2:2:198

[15] Cardona-Morrell M, Kim J, Turner RM, Anstey M, Mitchell IA, Hillman K. Non-beneficial treatments in hospital at the end of life: A systematic review on extent of the problem. International Journal for Quality in Health Care. 2016;**28**(4):456-469. DOI: 10.1093/intqhc/mzw060

[16] Aksoy E, Ilkilic I. Medical futility at the end of life: The first qualitative study of ethical decision-making methods among Turkish doctors. BMC Medical Ethics. 2024;**25**(1):122. DOI: 10.1186/s12910-024-01120-1

[17] McPherson K, Carlos WG 3rd, Emmett TW, Slaven JE, Torke AM. Limitation of life-sustaining care in the critically ill: A systematic review of the literature. Journal of Hospital Medicine. 2019;**14**(5):303-310. DOI: 10.12788/jhm.3137

[18] Jox RJ, Schaider A, Marckmann G, Borasio GD. Medical futility at the end of life: The perspectives of intensive care and palliative care clinicians. Journal of Medical Ethics. 2012;**38**(9):540-555. DOI: 10.1136/medethics-2011-100479

[19] Hernando P, Diestre G, Baigorri F. Limitación del esfuerzo terapéutico: "cuestión de profesionales o también de enfermos?" [limitation of therapeutic effort: A "question for professionals or for patients as well?"]. Anales del Sistema Sanitario de Navarra. 2007;**30**(Suppl. 3):129-135. DOI: 10.23938/ASSN.0207

[20] Walzl N, Sammy IA, Taylor PM, Smith JE, Lowe DJ. Systematic review of factors influencing decisions to limit treatment in the emergency department. Emergency Medicine Journal. 2022;**39**(2):147-156. DOI: 10.1136/emermed-2019-209398

[21] Bosslet GT, Pope TM, Rubenfeld GD, Lo B, Truog RD, Rushton CH, et al. An official ATS/AACN/ACCP/ESICM/SCCM policy statement: Responding to requests for potentially inappropriate treatments in intensive care units. American Journal of Respiratory and Critical Care Medicine. 2015;**191**(11):1318-1330. DOI: 10.1164/rccm.201505-0924ST

[22] González-Castro A, Azcune O, Peñasco Y, Rodríguez JC, Domínguez MJ, Rojas R. Opinión de los profesionales de una unidad de cuidados intensivos sobre la limitación del esfuerzo terapéutico [Opinion of professionals in an intensive care unit on the limitations of therapeutic effort]. Revista de Calidad Asistencial. 2016;**31**(5):262-266. DOI: 10.1016/j.cali.2015.12.007

[23] Pantoja ZL. Problemas éticos al final de la vida:¿ todo es eutanasia? Seminarios de la Fundación Española de Reumatología. 2009;**10**:128-131

[24] Kesecioglu J, Rusinova K, Alampi D, Arabi YM, Benbenishty J, Benoit D, et al. European Society of Intensive Care Medicine guidelines on end of life and palliative care in the intensive care unit. Intensive Care Medicine. 2024;**50**(11):1740-1766. DOI: 10.1007/s00134-024-07579-1

[25] Becerra-Bolaños Á, Ramos-Ahumada DF, Herrera-Rodríguez L,

Valencia-Sola L, Ojeda-Betancor N, Rodríguez-Pérez A. Withdrawal/withholding of life-sustaining therapies: Limitation of therapeutic effort in the intensive care unit. Medicina (Kaunas, Lithuania). 2024;**60**(9):1461. DOI: 10.3390/medicina60091461

[26] Monteiro NF, Simões I, Gaspar I, Carmo E. Do-not-resuscitate and treatment limitation decisions - six years of experience from a Portuguese general intensive care unit. Revista da Associacao Medica Brasileira (1992). 2019;**65**(9):1168-1173. DOI: 10.1590/1806-9282.65.9.1168

[27] Feldman C, Sprung CL, Mentzelopoulos SD, Pohrt A, Hartog CS, Danbury C, et al. Richards GA; Ethicus-2 study group. Global comparison of communication of end-of-life decisions in the ICU. Chest. 2022;**162**(5):1074-1085. DOI: 10.1016/j.chest.2022.05.007

[28] Löfmark R, Nilstun T, Cartwright C, Fischer S, van der Heide A, Mortier F, et al. Physicians' experiences with end-of-life decision-making: Survey in 6 European countries and Australia. BMC Medicine. 2008;**6**:4. DOI: 10.1186/1741-7015-6-4

[29] Avidan A, Sprung CL, Schefold JC, Ricou B, Hartog CS, Nates JL, et al. Variations in end-of-life practices in intensive care units worldwide (Ethicus-2): A prospective observational study. The Lancet Respiratory Medicine. 2021;**9**(10):1101-1110. DOI: 10.1016/S2213-2600(21)00261-7

[30] Pasieka P, Surówka A, Fronczek J, Skwara E, Czuczwar M, Borys M, et al. Prevalence of life-sustaining treatment limitations in polish very old intensive care patients (VIPs). A post-hoc analysis of two prospective observational studies. Journal of Critical Care. 2024;**79**:154439. DOI: 10.1016/j.jcrc.2023.154439

[31] Bruno RR, Wernly B, Beil M, Muessig JM, Rahmel T, Graf T, et al. Therapy limitation in octogenarians in German intensive care units is associated with a longer length of stay and increased 30 days mortality: A prospective multicenter study. Journal of Critical Care. 2020;**60**:58-63. DOI: 10.1016/j.jcrc.2020.07.024

[32] Andersen FH, Ariansen Haaland Ø, Klepstad P, Flaatten H. Frailty and survival in elderly intensive care patients in Norway. Acta Anaesthesiologica Scandinavica. 2021;**65**(8):1065-1072. DOI: 10.1111/aas.13836

[33] Giabicani M, Le Terrier C, Poncet A, Guidet B, Rigaud JP, Quenot JP, et al. COVID-ICU study investigators. Limitation of life-sustaining therapies in critically ill patients with COVID-19: A descriptive epidemiological investigation from the COVID-ICU study. Critical Care. 2023;**27**(1):103. DOI: 10.1186/s13054-023-04349-1

[34] Naito H, Sakuraya M, Hongo T, Takada H, Yumoto T, Yorifuji T, et al. Prevalence, reasons, and timing of decisions to withhold/withdraw life-sustaining therapy for out-of-hospital cardiac arrest patients with extracorporeal cardiopulmonary resuscitation. Critical Care. 2023;**27**(1):252. DOI: 10.1186/s13054-023-04534-2

[35] Chang YC, Fang YT, Chen HC, Lin CY, Chang YP, Chen YM, et al. Effect of do-not-resuscitate orders on patients with sepsis in the medical intensive care unit: A retrospective, observational and propensity score-matched study in a tertiary referral hospital in Taiwan. BMJ Open. 2019;**9**(6):e029041. DOI: 10.1136/bmjopen-2019-029041

[36] López González UA, Bautista Rentero D, Crespo Gómez M, Cárcamo

Ibarra P, Míguez Santiyán AM. Factors associated with limitation of life support: Post-ICU mortality case study of a tertiary hospital. Revista española de anestesiología y reanimación (English edition). 2024;**71**(5):387-393. DOI: 10.1016/j.redare.2024.02.007

[37] Lacoste-Palasset T, Sutterlin L, M'Rad A, Modestin L, Mourman V, Pepin-Lehalleur A, et al. Impact of early limitation of therapeutic effort in elderly COVID-19 patients admitted to the intensive care unit-a cohort study. Journal of Personalized Medicine. 2022;**12**(9):1501. DOI: 10.3390/jpm12091501

[38] Estella Á, Lagares C, Furones MJ, Martínez López P, Lázaro Martín NI, Estebánez B, et al. Limitation of life support treatments in Spanish intensive care units: Analysis of the ETHICUS II study. Medicina Intensiva (English Edition). 2024;**48**(5):247-253. DOI: 10.1016/j.medine.2024.02.013

[39] Adamski J, Weigl W, Musialowicz T, Lahtinen P, Reinikainen M. Predictors of treatment limitations in Finnish intensive care units. Acta Anaesthesiologica Scandinavica. 2022;**66**(4):526-538. DOI: 10.1111/aas.14035

[40] Toyas Miazza C, Martínez-Álvarez RM, Díez-Manglano J, Ezpeleta Galindo AI, Laín Miranda ME, Aspiroz SC. Limitación del esfuerzo terapéutico en pacientes con bacteriemia [limitation of therapeutic effort in patients with bacteremia]. Revista Española de Geriatría y Gerontología. 2018;**53**(5):262-267. DOI: 10.1016/j.regg.2018.02.005

[41] Hernández-Aguiar Y, Becerra-Bolaños Á, Rodríguez-Pérez A. Preoperative diagnosis of frailty. The Journal of International Medical Research. 2024;**52**(5):3000605241251705. DOI: 10.1177/03000605241251705

[42] Spanish Group for the Epidemiological Analysis of Critical Patients (PAEEC), Mata GV. Quality of life: A tool for decision-making in the ICU. Intensive Care Medicine. 1994;**20**(4):251-252. DOI: 10.1007/BF01708958

[43] Abizanda R, Almendros Corral L, Balerdi PB. Aspectos éticos de la medicina intensiva. Resultados de una encuesta de opinión [Ethical aspects of intensive medicine. Results of an opinion survey]. Medicina Clínica (Barcelona). 1994;**102**(14):521-526

[44] Bueno Muñoz MJ. Limitación del esfuerzo terapéutico: aproximación a una visión de conjunto [Limitation of therapeutic effort: Approach to a combined view]. Enfermería Intensiva. 2013;**24**(4):167-174. DOI: 10.1016/j.enfi.2013.04.003

[45] Rivera-Fernández R, Sánchez-Cruz JJ, Abizanda-Campos R, Vázquez-Mata G. Quality of life before intensive care unit admission and its influence on resource utilization and mortality rate. Critical Care Medicine. 2001;**29**(9):1701-1709. DOI: 10.1097/00003246-200109000-00008

[46] Teres D, Lemeshow S, Avrunin JS, Pastides H. Validation of the mortality prediction model for ICU patients. Critical Care Medicine. 1987;**15**(3):208-213. DOI: 10.1097/00003246-198703000-00005

[47] White DB, Pope TM. Medical futility and potentially inappropriate treatment. In: Youngner AJ, Arnold RM, editors. The Oxford Handbook of Ethics at the End of Life. New York, USA: Oxford University Press; 2016

[48] Cabré L, Mancebo J, Solsona JF, Saura P, Gich I, Blanch L, et al. Multicenter study of the multiple organ

dysfunction syndrome in intensive care units: The usefulness of sequential organ failure assessment scores in decision making. Intensive Care Medicine. 2005;**31**(7):927-933. DOI: 10.1007/s00134-005-2640-2

[49] Wang AY, Ma HP, Kao WF, Tsai SH, Chang CK. Characteristics and outcomes of "do not resuscitate" patients admitted to the emergency department-intensive care unit. Journal of the Formosan Medical Association. 2019;**118**(1 Pt 2):223-229. DOI: 10.1016/j.jfma.2018.03.016

[50] Launey Y, Coquet A, Lasocki S, Dahyot-Fizelier C, Huet O, Le Pabic E, et al. Factors associated with an unfavourable outcome in elderly intensive care traumatic brain injury patients. A retrospective multicentre study. BMC Geriatrics. 2022;**22**(1):1004. DOI: 10.1186/s12877-022-03651-x

[51] Ramos JGR, Tourinho FC, Borrione P, Azi P, Andrade T, Costa V, et al. Effect of a palliative care program on trends in intensive care unit utilization and do-not-resuscitate orders during terminal hospitalizations. An Interrupted Time Series Analysis. Rev Bras Ter Intensiva. 2018;**30**(3):308-316. DOI: 10.5935/0103-507X.20180042

[52] Brunker LB, Boncyk CS, Rengel KF, Hughes CG. Elderly patients and management in intensive care units (ICU): Clinical challenges. Clinical Interventions in Aging. 2023;**18**:93-112. DOI: 10.2147/CIA.S365968

[53] Muscedere J, Waters B, Varambally A, Bagshaw SM, Boyd JG, Maslove D, et al. The impact of frailty on intensive care unit outcomes: A systematic review and meta-analysis. Intensive Care Medicine. 2017;**43**(8):1105-1122. DOI: 10.1007/s00134-017-4867-0

[54] Hoit G, Wijeysundera DN, Hamad DM, Nauth A, Atrey A, Halai M, et al. Insurance type and withdrawal of life-sustaining therapy in critically injured trauma patients. JAMA Network Open. 2024;**7**(7):e2421711. DOI: 10.1001/jamanetworkopen.2024.21711

[55] Malhotra AK, Shakil H, Essa A, Mathieu F, Taran S, Badhiwala J, et al. Influence of health insurance on withdrawal of life sustaining treatment for patients with isolated traumatic brain injury: A retrospective multi-center observational cohort study. Critical Care. 2024;**28**(1):251. DOI: 10.1186/s13054-024-05027-6

[56] Feleke H, Moges T. Critical insights into pediatric care: Unveiling trends and outcomes of discharge against medical advice at Ethiopia's premier hospital: A retrospective cross-sectional survey. The Ethiopian Journal of Pediatrics and Child Health. 2023;**18**(2):149-161

[57] El Jawiche R, Hallit S, Tarabey L, Abou-Mrad F. Withholding and withdrawal of life-sustaining treatments in intensive care units in Lebanon: A cross-sectional survey of intensivists and interviews of professional societies, legal and religious leaders. BMC Medical Ethics. 2020;**21**(1):80. DOI: 10.1186/s12910-020-00525-y

[58] Choi HR, Ho MH, Lin CC. Futile life-sustaining treatment in the intensive care unit - nurse and physician experiences: Meta-synthesis. BMJ Supportive & Palliative Care. 2024;**14**(1):36-46. DOI: 10.1136/spcare-2023-004640

[59] Muñoz Camargo JC, Hernández-Martínez A, Rodríguez-Almagro J, Parra-Fernández ML, Prado-Laguna MDC, Martín M. Perceptions of patients and their families regarding limitation of therapeutic effort in the intensive care unit. Journal of Clinical Medicine.

2021;**10**(21):4900. DOI: 10.3390/jcm10214900

[60] Denke C, Jaschinski U, Riessen R, Bercker S, Spies C, Ragaller M, et al. End-of-life practices in 11 German intensive care units: Results from the ETHICUS-2 study. Medizinische Klinik – Intensivmedizin und Notfallmedizin. 2023;**118**(8):663-673. DOI: 10.1007/s00063-022-00961-1

[61] Orentlicher D. From the Office of the General Counsel. Advance Medical Directives. JAMA. 1990;**263**(17):2365-2367. DOI: 10.1001/jama.263.17.2365

[62] Sedini C, Biotto M, Crespi Bel'skij LM, Moroni Grandini RE, Cesari M. Advance care planning and advance directives: An overview of the main critical issues. Aging Clinical and Experimental Research. 2022;**34**(2):325-330. DOI: 10.1007/s40520-021-02001-y

[63] Wong HJ, Seow H, Gayowsky A, Sutradhar R, Wu RC, Lim H. Advance directives change frequently in nursing home residents. Journal of the American Medical Directors Association. 2024;**25**(8):105090. DOI: 10.1016/j.jamda.2024.105090

[64] Enguidanos S, Ailshire J. Timing of advance directive completion and relationship to care preferences. Journal of Pain and Symptom Management. 2017;**53**(1):49-56. DOI: 10.1016/j.jpainsymman.2016.08.008

[65] Melltorp G, Nilstun T. Decisions to forego life-sustaining treatment and the duty of documentation. Intensive Care Medicine. 1996;**22**(10):1015-1019. DOI: 10.1007/BF01699221

[66] Tanaka Gutiez M, Efstathiou N, Innes R, Metaxa V. End-of-life care in the intensive care unit. Anaesthesia. 2023;**78**(5):636-643. DOI: 10.1111/anae.15908

[67] Blythe JA, Kentish-Barnes N, Debue AS, Dohan D, Azoulay E, Covinsky K, et al. An interprofessional process for the limitation of life-sustaining treatments at the end of life in France. Journal of Pain and Symptom Management. 2022;**63**(1):160-170. DOI: 10.1016/j.jpainsymman.2021.06.016

[68] Ouyang DJ, Lief L, Russell D, Xu J, Berlin DA, Gentzler E, et al. Timing is everything: Early do-not-resuscitate orders in the intensive care unit and patient outcomes. PLoS One. 2020;**15**(2):e0227971. DOI: 10.1371/journal.pone.0227971

[69] Wright AA, Zhang B, Ray A, Mack JW, Trice E, Balboni T, et al. Associations between end-of-life discussions, patient mental health, medical care near death, and caregiver bereavement adjustment. Journal of the American Medical Association. 2008;**300**(14):1665-1673. DOI: 10.1001/jama.300.14.1665

[70] Termoz A, Subtil F, Drouin P, Marchal M, Verroul M, Langlois C, et al. Evaluating the impact of a standardised intervention for announcing decisions of withholding and withdrawing life-sustaining treatments on the stress of relatives in emergency departments (DISCUSS): Protocol for a stepped-wedge randomised controlled trial. BMJ Open. 2024;**14**(9):e087444. DOI: 10.1136/bmjopen-2024-087444

[71] Paredes Escobar MC. Limitación del esfuerzo terapéutico en la práctica clínica: Percepciones de profesionales médicos y de enfermería de unidades de pacientes críticos de un hospital público de adultos en la Región Metropolitana. Acta bioeth. 2012;**18**(2):163-171. DOI: 10.4067/S1726-569X2012000200004. Available from: http://www.scielo.cl/scielo.

php?script=sci_arttext&pid=S1726-569X2012000200004&lng=es

[72] Goold SD, Williams B, Arnold RM. Conflicts regarding decisions to limit treatment: A differential diagnosis. Journal of the American Medical Association. 2000;**283**(7):909-914. DOI: 10.1001/jama.283.7.909

[73] Ness DE, Ende J. Denial in the medical interview, Recognition and Management. JAMA. 1994;**272**(22):1777-1781

[74] Heyland DK, Dodek P, Rocker G, Groll D, Gafni A, Pichora D, et al. What matters most in end-of-life care: Perceptions of seriously ill patients and their family members. CMAJ. 2006;**174**(5):627-633. DOI: 10.1503/cmaj.050626

[75] Rosenczweig C. Should relatives witness resuscitation? Ethical issues and practical considerations. CMAJ. 1998;**158**(5):617-620

[76] Quill TE. Perspectives on care at the close of life. Initiating end-of-life discussions with seriously ill patients: Addressing the "elephant in the room". Journal of the American Medical Association. 2000;**284**(19):2502-2507. DOI: 10.1001/jama.284.19.2502

[77] Cabré Pericas L, Solsona Durán JF. Limitación del esfuerzo terapéutico en medicina intensiva. Medicina Intensiva. 2002;**26**(6):304-311

[78] Canadian Critical Care Society Ethics Committee, Bandrauk N, Downar J, Paunovic B. Withholding and withdrawing life-sustaining treatment: The Canadian critical care society position paper. Canadian Journal of Anaesthesia. 2018;**65**(1):105-122. DOI: 10.1007/s12630-017-1002-1

[79] Penders YWH, Bopp M, Zellweger U, Bosshard G, Swiss Medical End-of-Life Decisions Study Group. Continuing, withdrawing, and withholding medical treatment at the end of life and associated characteristics: A mortality follow-back study. Journal of General Internal Medicine. 2020;**35**(1):126-132. DOI: 10.1007/s11606-019-05344-5

[80] Pan H, Shi W, Zhou Q, Chen G, Pan P. Palliative care in the intensive care unit: Not just end-of-life care. Intensive Care Research. 2022;**3**:77-82. DOI: 10.1007/s44231-022-00009-0

[81] Oliveira HC, Sauthier M, Silva MMD, Crespo MDCA, Seixas APR, Campos JF. Do-not-resuscitate order in COVID-19 times: Bioethics and professional ethics. Revista Gaúcha de Enfermagem. 2021;**42**(spe):e20200172. DOI: 10.1590/1983-1447.2021.20200172

[82] Wilson ME, Mittal A, Karki B, Dobler CC, Wahab A, Curtis JR, et al. Do-not-intubate orders in patients with acute respiratory failure: A systematic review and meta-analysis. Intensive Care Medicine. 2020;**46**(1):36-45. DOI: 10.1007/s00134-019-05828-2

[83] Vilaça M, Aragão I, Cardoso T, Dias C, Cabral-Campello G. The role of noninvasive ventilation in patients with "do not intubate" order in the emergency setting. PLoS One. 2016;**11**(2):e0149649. DOI: 10.1371/journal.pone.0149649

[84] Levy M, Tanios MA, Nelson D, Short K, Senechia A, Vespia J, et al. Outcomes of patients with do-not-intubate orders treated with noninvasive ventilation. Critical Care Medicine. 2004;**32**(10):2002-2007. DOI: 10.1097/01.ccm.0000142729.07050.c9

[85] Hsu NC, Huang CC, Hsu CH, Wang TD, Sheng WH. Does hospitalist care enhance palliative care and reduce

aggressive treatments for terminally ill patients? A propensity score-matched study. Cancers (Basel). 2023;**15**(15):3976. DOI: 10.3390/cancers15153976

[86] Claure-Del Granado R, Mehta RL. Withholding and withdrawing renal support in acute kidney injury. Seminars in Dialysis. 2011;**24**(2):208-214. DOI: 10.1111/j.1525-139X.2011.00832.x

[87] Patel SS, Holley JL. Withholding and withdrawing dialysis in the intensive care unit: Benefits derived from consulting the renal physicians association/American society of nephrology clinical practice guideline, shared decision-making in the appropriate initiation of and withdrawal from dialysis. Clinical Journal of the American Society of Nephrology. 2008;**3**(2):587-593. DOI: 10.2215/CJN.04040907

[88] Allegretti AS, Steele DJ, David-Kasdan JA, Bajwa E, Niles JL, Bhan I. Continuous renal replacement therapy outcomes in acute kidney injury and end-stage renal disease: A cohort study. Critical Care. 2013;**17**(3):R109. DOI: 10.1186/cc12780

[89] Chen JCY, Hu B, Frank RD, Kashani KB. Inpatient kidney function recovery among septic shock patients who initiated kidney replacement therapy in the hospital. Nephron. 2020;**144**(8):363-371. DOI: 10.1159/000507999

[90] Stevens JS, King KL, Robbins-Juarez SY, Khairallah P, Toma K, Alvarado Verduzco H, et al. High rate of renal recovery in survivors of COVID-19 associated acute renal failure requiring renal replacement therapy. PLoS One. 2020;**15**(12):e0244131. DOI: 10.1371/journal.pone.0244131

[91] van Biesen W, van de Luijtgaarden MW, Brown EA, Michel JP, van Munster BC, Jager KJ, et al. Nephrologists' perceptions regarding dialysis withdrawal and palliative care in Europe: Lessons from a European renal best practice survey. Nephrology, Dialysis, Transplantation. 2015;**30**(12):1951-1958. DOI: 10.1093/ndt/gfv284

[92] Clement R, Chevalet P, Rodat O, Ould-Aoudia V, Berger M. Withholding or withdrawing dialysis in the elderly: The perspective of a western region of France. Nephrology, Dialysis, Transplantation. 2005;**20**(11):2446-2452. DOI: 10.1093/ndt/gfi012

[93] Chan S, Marshall MR, Ellis RJ, Ranganathan D, Hawley CM, Johnson DW, et al. Haemodialysis withdrawal in Australia and New Zealand: A binational registry study. Nephrology, Dialysis, Transplantation. 2020;**35**(4):669-676. DOI: 10.1093/ndt/gfz160

[94] Kim JH, Yoo SH, Keam B, Heo DS. Antibiotic prescription patterns during last days of hospitalized patients with advanced cancer: The role of palliative care consultation. The Journal of Antimicrobial Chemotherapy. 2023;**78**(7):1694-1700. DOI: 10.1093/jac/dkad156

[95] Barlam TF, Cosgrove SE, Abbo LM, MacDougall C, Schuetz AN, Septimus EJ, et al. Implementing an antibiotic stewardship program: Guidelines by the infectious diseases society of America and the society for healthcare epidemiology of America. Clinical Infectious Diseases. 2016;**62**(10):e51-e77. DOI: 10.1093/cid/ciw118

[96] van der Steen JT, Ooms ME, van der Wal G, Ribbe MW. Pneumonia: The demented patient's best friend? Discomfort after starting or withholding antibiotic treatment.

Journal of the American Geriatrics Society. 2002;**50**(10):1681-1688. DOI: 10.1046/j.1532-5415.2002.50460.x

[97] van der Steen JT, Pasman HR, Ribbe MW, van der Wal G, Onwuteaka-Philipsen BD. Discomfort in dementia patients dying from pneumonia and its relief by antibiotics. Scandinavian Journal of Infectious Diseases. 2009;**41**(2):143-151. DOI: 10.1080/00365540802616726

[98] Ramazzotti D, Clardy P, Celi LA, Stone DJ, Rudin RS. Withholding or withdrawing invasive interventions may not accelerate time to death among dying ICU patients. PLoS One. 2019;**14**(2):e0212439. DOI: 10.1371/journal.pone.0212439

[99] Morgan CK, Varas GM, Pedroza C, Almoosa KF. Defining the practice of "no escalation of care" in the ICU. Critical Care Medicine. 2014;**42**(2):357-361. DOI: 10.1097/CCM.0b013e3182a276c9

[100] Nicolson C, Burke A, Gardiner D, Harvey D, Munshi L, Shaw M, et al. Predicting time to asystole following withdrawal of life-sustaining treatment: A systematic review. Anaesthesia. 2024;**79**(6):638-649. DOI: 10.1111/anae.16222

[101] Aita K, Kai I. Physicians' psychosocial barriers to different modes of withdrawal of life support in critical care: A qualitative study in Japan. Social Science and Medicine. 2010;**70**(4):616-622. DOI: 10.1016/j.socscimed.2009.10.036

[102] Beck K, Vincent A, Cam H, Becker C, Gross S, Loretz N, et al. Medical futility regarding cardiopulmonary resuscitation in in-hospital cardiac arrests of adult patients: A systematic review and meta-analysis. Resuscitation. 2022;**172**:181-193. DOI: 10.1016/j.resuscitation.2021.11.041

[103] Okubo M, Komukai S, Andersen LW, Berg RA, Kurz MC, Morrison LJ, et al. Duration of cardiopulmonary resuscitation and outcomes for adults with in-hospital cardiac arrest: Retrospective cohort study. BMJ. 2024;**384**:e076019. DOI: 10.1136/bmj-2023-076019

[104] Panchal AR, Bartos JA, Cabañas JG, Donnino MW, Drennan IR, Hirsch KG, et al. Part 3: Adult basic and advanced life support: 2020 American Heart Association guidelines for cardiopulmonary resuscitation and emergency cardiovascular care. Circulation. 2020;**142**(16 suppl. 2):S366-S468. DOI: 10.1161/CIR.0000000000000916

[105] Kim YS, Choi W, Hwang J. Resuscitation of prolonged cardiac arrest from massive pulmonary embolism by extracorporeal membrane oxygenation. European Journal of Cardio-Thoracic Surgery. 2017;**51**(6):1206-1207. DOI: 10.1093/ejcts/ezw413

[106] Orr S, Efstathiou N, Baernholdt M, Vanderspank-Wright B. ICU clinicians' experiences of terminal weaning and extubation. Journal of Pain and Symptom Management. 2022;**63**(5):e521-e528. DOI: 10.1016/j.jpainsymman.2022.01.016

[107] Obarzanek L, Campbell ML. Withholding and withdrawal of life support in critically ill patients at the end of life: Pain is not the only symptom to manage. Intensive Care Medicine. 2021;**47**(4):489-490. DOI: 10.1007/s00134-020-06345-3

[108] Nava S, Ferrer M, Esquinas A, Scala R, Groff P, Cosentini R, et al. Palliative use of non-invasive ventilation in end-of-life patients with solid tumours: A randomised feasibility trial. The Lancet Oncology. 2013;**14**(3):219-227. DOI: 10.1016/S1470-2045(13)70009-3

[109] Cook D, Rocker G, Marshall J, Sjokvist P, Dodek P, Griffith L, et al. Withdrawal of mechanical ventilation in anticipation of death in the intensive care unit. The New England Journal of Medicine. 2003;**349**(12):1123-1132. DOI: 10.1056/NEJMoa030083

[110] Chen YC, Fan HY, Curtis JR, Lee OK, Liu CK, Huang SJ. Determinants of receiving palliative care and ventilator withdrawal among patients with prolonged mechanical ventilation. Critical Care Medicine. 2017;**45**(10):1625-1634. DOI: 10.1097/CCM.0000000000002569

[111] Robert R, Le Gouge A, Kentish-Barnes N, Cottereau A, Giraudeau B, Adda M, et al. Terminal weaning or immediate extubation for withdrawing mechanical ventilation in critically ill patients (the ARREVE observational study). Intensive Care Medicine. 2017;**43**(12):1793-1807. DOI: 10.1007/s00134-017-4891-0

[112] Puntillo KA, Arai S, Cohen NH, Gropper MA, Neuhaus J, Paul SM, et al. Symptoms experienced by intensive care unit patients at high risk of dying. Critical Care Medicine. 2010;**38**(11):2155-2160. DOI: 10.1097/CCM.0b013e3181f267ee

[113] Neto MJA, Moura AFS, Suassuna JHR. Renouncement of renal replacement therapy: Withdrawal and refusal. Jornal Brasileiro de Nefrologia. 2017;**39**(3):312-322. DOI: 10.5935/0101-2800.20170054

[114] Metaxa V, Lavrentieva A. End-of-life decisions in burn intensive care units - an international survey. Burns. 2015;**41**(1):53-57. DOI: 10.1016/j.burns.2014.05.018

[115] Ramakrishnan C, Widjaja N, Malhotra C, Finkelstein E, Khan BA, Ozdemir S, et al. Unravelling complex choices: Multi-stakeholder perceptions on dialysis withdrawal and end-of-life care in kidney disease. BMC Nephrology. 2024;**25**(1):6. DOI: 10.1186/s12882-023-03434-5

[116] Francoeur C, Hornby L, Silva A, Scales NB, Weiss M, Dhanani S. Paediatric death after withdrawal of life-sustaining therapies: A scoping review protocol. BMJ Open. 2022;**12**(9):e064918. DOI: 10.1136/bmjopen-2022-064918

[117] Francoeur C, Silva A, Hornby L, Wollny K, Lee LA, Pomeroy A, et al. Pediatric death after withdrawal of life-sustaining therapies: A scoping review. Pediatric Critical Care Medicine. 2024;**25**(1):e12-e19. DOI: 10.1097/PCC.0000000000003358

[118] Choi HR, Ho MH, Lin CC. Navigating tensions when life-sustaining treatment is withdrawn: A thematic synthesis of nurses' and physicians' experiences. Journal of Clinical Nursing. 2024;**33**(6):2337-2356. DOI: 10.1111/jocn.17059

[119] Pérez Pérez FM. Adecuación del esfuerzo terapéutico, una estrategia al final de la Vida [the suitability of therapeutic effort: An end-of-life strategy]. SEMERGEN. 2016;**42**(8):566-574. DOI: 10.1016/j.semerg.2015.11.006

[120] Birchley G. Angels of mercy? The legal and professional implications of withdrawal of life-sustaining treatment by nurses in England and Wales. Medical Law Review. 2012;**20**(3):337-361. DOI: 10.1093/medlaw/fws007

[121] Velarde-García JF, Luengo-González R, González-Hervías R, Cardenete-Reyes C, Álvarez-Embarba B, Palacios-Ceña D. Limitation of therapeutic effort experienced by intensive care nurses.

Nursing Ethics. 2018;**25**(7):867-879. DOI: 10.1177/0969733016679471

[122] Restrepo BD, Cossio C, Ochoa JFL, Jaramillo JC, Bedoya J, Duque D, et al. Conocimientos, actitudes y prácticas frente a la limitación de esfuerzos terapéuticos en personal de salud de un hospital universitario. Persona y Bioética. 2013;**17**(2):216-226

[123] Douplat M, Jacquin L, Frugier S, Tazarourte K, Le Coz P. Difficulty of the ethical decision-making process in withholding and withdrawing life-sustaining treatments in French EDs during COVID pandemic. Scandinavian Journal of Trauma, Resuscitation and Emergency Medicine. 2020;**28**(1):78. DOI: 10.1186/s13049-020-00772-3

[124] Maharaj R, Harrison DA, Rowan K. The association between the decision to withdraw life-sustaining therapy and patient mortality in U.K. ICUs. Critical Care Medicine. 2022;**50**(4):576-585. DOI: 10.1097/CCM.0000000000005306

[125] Azoulay E, Pochard F, Garrouste-Orgeas M, Moreau D, Montesino L, Adrie C, et al. Decisions to forgo life-sustaining therapy in ICU patients independently predict hospital death. Intensive Care Medicine. 2003;**29**(11):1895-1901. DOI: 10.1007/s00134-003-1989-3

[126] Lin CY, Farrell MH, Lave JR, Angus DC, Barnato AE. Organizational determinants of hospital end-of-life treatment intensity. Medical Care. 2009;**47**(5):524-530. DOI: 10.1097/MLR.0b013e31819261bd

[127] Rosa RG, Teixeira C, Piva S, Morandi A. Anticipating ICU discharge and long-term follow-up. Current Opinion in Critical Care. 2024;**30**(2):157-164. DOI: 10.1097/MCC.0000000000001136

[128] Halpern NA, Pastores SM. Critical care medicine in the United States 2000-2005: An analysis of bed numbers, occupancy rates, payer mix, and costs. Critical Care Medicine. 2010;**38**(1):65-71. DOI: 10.1097/CCM.0b013e3181b090d0

[129] Khandelwal N, Curtis JR. Economic implications of end-of-life care in the ICU. Current Opinion in Critical Care. 2014;**20**(6):656-661. DOI: 10.1097/MCC.0000000000000147

[130] Chang DW, Neville TH, Parrish J, Ewing L, Rico C, Jara L, et al. Evaluation of time-limited trials among critically ill patients with advanced medical illnesses and reduction of nonbeneficial ICU treatments. JAMA Internal Medicine. 2021;**181**(6):786-794. DOI: 10.1001/jamainternmed.2021.1000

[131] Heyland DK, Rocker GM, Dodek PM, Kutsogiannis DJ, Konopad E, Cook DJ, et al. Family satisfaction with care in the intensive care unit: Results of a multiple center study. Critical Care Medicine. 2002;**30**(7):1413-1418. DOI: 10.1097/00003246-200207000-00002

[132] Damps M, Gajda M, Kowalska M, Kucewicz-Czech E. Limitation of futile therapy in the opinion of nursing staff employed in polish hospitals-results of a cross-sectional study. International Journal of Environmental Research and Public Health. 2022;**19**(24):16975. DOI: 10.3390/ijerph192416975

[133] White DB, Curtis JR, Lo B, Luce JM. Decisions to limit life-sustaining treatment for critically ill patients who lack both decision-making capacity and surrogate decision-makers. Critical Care Medicine. 2006;**34**(8):2053-2059. DOI: 10.1097/01.CCM.0000227654.38708.C1

[134] Laserna A, Durán-Crane A, López-Olivo MA, Cuenca JA, Fowler C, Díaz DP, et al. Pain management during the withholding and withdrawal of life support in critically ill patients at the end-of-life: A systematic review and meta-analysis. Intensive Care Medicine. 2020;**46**(9):1671-1682. DOI: 10.1007/s00134-020-06139-7

Chapter 9

Brain Stem Death

Hana Elamin, Ahmad M. Obeidat, Ashish Kumar, Mojahid Mohammed Khalid Alhussein, Mohammad Ataur Rahman, Zia Mahmood, Fernando Ruiz Gonzalez, Sanghamitra Padhy, Prabu Bhuvanendran and Sohel M.G. Ahmed

Abstract

This chapter gives an overall picture of brain death, showing how ideas about it have changed over time, from initial assumptions to modern diagnostic criteria. It shows how definitions of death have evolved from cardiopulmonary to neurological criteria because of improvements in organ transplantation and critical care, with important contributions from the Harvard Committee in 1968 and later global recommendations. The chapter goes into detail about the physical and physiological reasons for brain death, focusing on how brain and brainstem processes stop permanently. To be brain dead, all brain and brainstem functions must be permanently lost, as shown by clinical exams, apnea tests, and other tests like EEG and angiography. The chapter covers important diagnostic protocols such as clinical exams, apnea tests, as well as their limitations and how they differ from country to country. There are also special considerations for certain categories of people, like pregnant women, children, and patients on extracorporeal membrane oxygenation (ECMO). There are discrepancies in international procedures, such durations of observations last, how tests are done, and which further tests are preferred. Religious and cultural views affect how people feel about brain death; therefore, it is important to communicate carefully. The chapter concludes with thoughts on the future, such as how biomarkers and artificial intelligence can help make brain death diagnoses more accurate. This chapter makes it clear that we need to reach a global agreement on how to deal with differences in determining brain death while considering the medical, ethical, and legal issues that come up.

Keywords: brain stem, death, guidelines, ancillary tests, future perspectives

1. Introduction

Traditionally, death is defined as the cessation of cardiac and pulmonary function. This became challenging with advances in critical care support mechanisms, as bodily functions could now be performed artificially with ventilators and extracorporeal machines, long after intrinsic function had ceased [1]. This has led to the inclusion of other criteria to diagnose death based on the irreversible cessation of brain stem functions [2, 3].

In 1954, neurologist Robert Schwab of Massachusetts General Hospital encountered this dilemma firsthand when treating a comatose patient with a massive intracranial hemorrhage on a respirator [4]. Five years later, Wertheimer and Jouvet reached a similar conclusion, referring to the phenomenon as "death of the nervous system" [5, 6]. In 1959, French physicians Maurice Mollaret and Stanley Goulon coined the term coma dépassé (beyond coma). They viewed coma dépassé as a prognosis of imminent death rather than death itself [7]. In 1963, aiming to address uncertainty surrounding the "death of the nervous system," neurologist Robert Schwab proposed a set of criterion to declare death "in spite of cardiac action" [8]. Schwab later applied these criteria to 90 patients, who subsequently died, and were found at autopsy to have extensive brain necrosis (**Table 1**) [9].

In 1968, the Harvard Medical School Ad Hoc Committee, chaired by Henry Beecher, advanced Schwab's earlier neurological criteria for determining death [10–12]. The committee's definition of brain death established the irreversible loss of brain function, as a criterion for diagnosing death. The committee's findings provided a crucial legal aspect for assessing death (**Table 2**). Concurrently, the transition from a cardiopulmonary to a brain-based definition of death paralleled the emergence of modern organ transplantation [13, 14].

Harvard Criteria have been critiqued for their conceptual uncertainty and ethical concerns. Critics claimed that the criteria were created to focus on facilitating organ transplantation more than focusing on providing a clear definition of brain death [15–17]. In 1976, the United Kingdom formally adopted the concept of brainstem death, as endorsed by the Conference of the Medical Royal Colleges and their faculties [18], declaring that loss of brainstem function equaled death [19]. However, this meant that patients with preserved cortical electrical activity by EEG could be considered dead in the United Kingdom but alive in the United States.

	Robert Schwab criteria for death 1963
1	Fixed, dilated pupils, absence of brainstem reflexes; and no spontaneous movements
2	Apnea (no respiratory effort)
3	isoelectric (flat line) EEG

Table 1.
Death Criteria by Robert Schwab in 1963.

1	Presence of specific clinical signs (ex. Unresponsive coma)
2	Absence of brain reflexes
3	Lack of spontaneous movement following 1 hour of observation
4	Apnea for at least 3 minutes after disconnection from mechanical ventilator
5	Isoelectric (Flat line) EEG
6	Exclusion of reversible conditions (ex. Hypothermia, CNS depressants)
7	Repetition of clinical assessments within 24 h

Table 2.
Brain death criteria determined by Harvard Ad Hoc committee.

To address the need for uniformity, the Uniform Determination of Death Act (UDDA) was proposed in 1980 [20]. This act granted legal equivalence to both cardiovascular and neurological criteria for death, but did not standardize the neurological criteria.

Further efforts to clarify brain death determination were made by the American Academy of Neurology (AAN) in 1995, which issued clinical guidelines that became the foundation for diagnostic protocols worldwide [21]. These guidelines were further revised in 2010 [22].

On a global level, the World Health Organization (WHO) in 2014 defined human death as *"the permanent loss of capacity for consciousness and all brainstem functions, as a consequence of permanent cessation of circulation or catastrophic brain injury"* [23]. In 1987, the American Academy of Pediatrics issued its first guidelines for brain death determination in children [24], which were updated in 2011 [25, 26].

One of the central ongoing debates in the field of brain death involves the terminology used to define it, with terms such as "whole brain death" and "brainstem death" frequently used interchangeably, most experts advocate for the use of the term brain death (BD) or death by neurological criteria (DNC) [27].

This chapter aims to address critical aspects of brain death. Explore key differences between brain death and vegetative state. Furthermore, reviewing international legal differences in brain death definitions and the diagnostic approach in specific cohorts.

2. Anatomy and the blood supply of the brain

Brain anatomy and brain functions are crucial parts in understanding the mechanism and the clinical presentation of brain insult (**Figure 1**) [28]. The major division of the brain consists of cerebrum, cerebellum, and the brain stem.

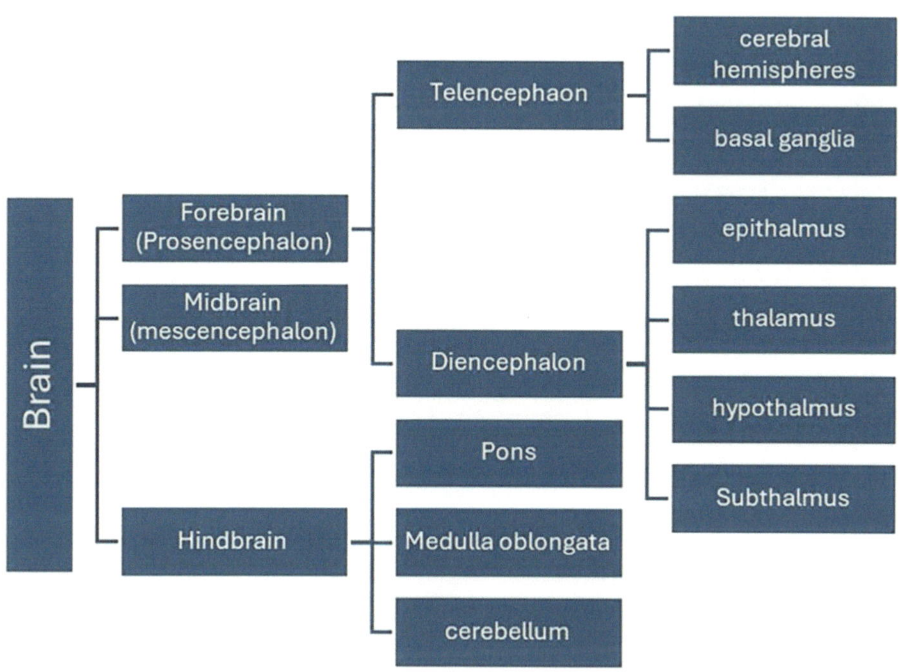

Figure 1.
Major parts of the brain.

Lobe	Anatomical location and description	Function	Frontal lobe
Located in front of the *central sulcus* and above the *lateral sulcus*.	It is responsible for voluntary motor control, decision-making, personality, and speech production (Broca's area).	Parietal lobe	Positioned behind the *central sulcus* and above the *lateral sulcus*.
It processes somatosensory information such as touch, temperature, and proprioception.	Occipital lobe	Situated posterior to the *parieto-occipital sulcus*.	This lobe is the primary center for visual processing.
Temporal lobe	Located below the *lateral sulcus*.	It is involved in auditory processing, memory, and language comprehension (Wernicke's area).	

Table 3.
Major cerebral lobes and their anatomical locations.

The cerebrum is the largest part of the brain and consists of two cerebral hemispheres. Each hemisphere extends from the frontal to the occipital bone, and the two hemispheres are separated by a deep cleft: the longitudinal fissure and falx cerebri, they are interconnected by a mass of white matter called the corpus callosum. Within each cerebral hemisphere, there is a cavity known as the lateral ventricle, which communicates with the third ventricle through the interventricular foramina [29, 30]. The brain's outer surface of each hemisphere is the cortex, which consists of gray matter. The cerebral cortex is structured into folds (gyri), which are separated by fissures (sulci). Several large sulci sub-split the surface of each hemisphere into lobes (**Table 3**) [2, 30–33].

The cerebral cortex is divided into four main lobes, each with different anatomical landmarks and functional specialization (**Figure 2**). The cerebellum lies within the posterior crania fossa beneath the tentorium cerebellum. It is situated posterior to the pons and the medulla oblongata. It consists of two hemispheres connected by a median portion, the vermis [29]. It is connected to the midbrain by the superior cerebellar peduncle, to the pons by the middle cerebellar peduncles, and to the medulla

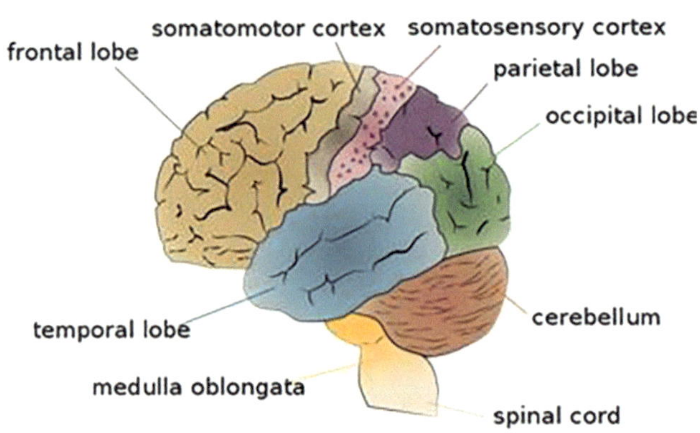

Figure 2.
Cerebral lobes.

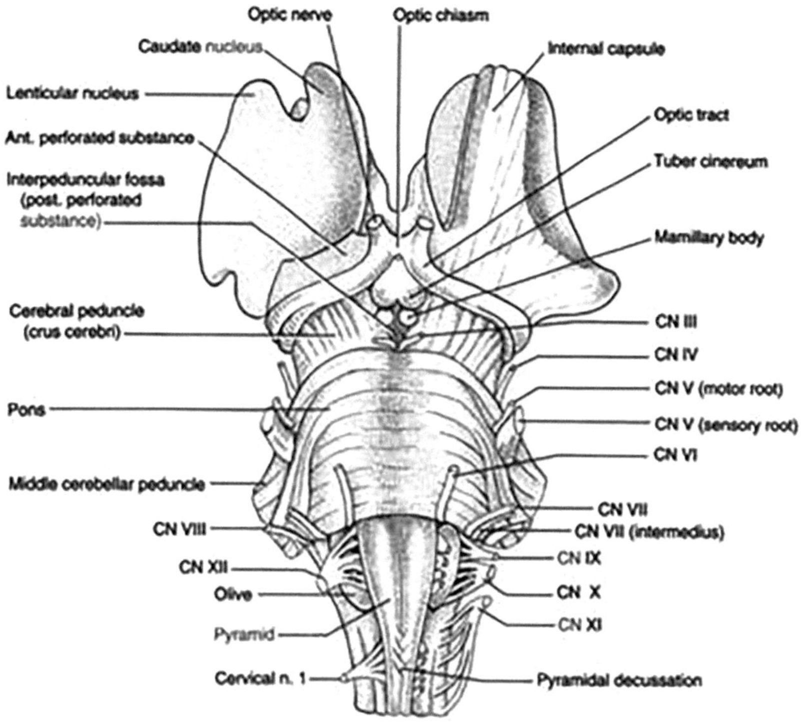

Figure 3.
Anatomy of brain stem.

by the inferior cerebellar peduncles. The brain stem consists of the midbrain, pons, and medulla oblongata (**Figure 3**). The brainstem gives rise to 10 of the 12 cranial nerves (**Table 4**).

The gray matter within the brainstem consists of nerve cell bodies and forms many important brainstem nuclei. The white matter tracts of the brainstem include axons of nerves traversing their course to different structures; the axons originate from cell bodies located elsewhere within the central nervous system (CNS) (**Table 5**) [34].

The midbrain connects the pons to the diencephalon. It communicates with the cerebellum *via* the superior cerebellar peduncle. It consists of two lateral halves called cerebral peduncles. Each peduncle is divided into an anterior part, the crus cerebri. The narrow cavity of the midbrain is cerebral aqueduct [29].

The pons is situated on the anterior surface of the cerebellum below the midbrain and above the medulla oblongata. It is composed of nerve fibers which connect the two halves of the cerebellum. The pons contains the ascending and descending fibers connecting the forebrain, midbrain, and the spinal cord [29].

Conical in shape, the medulla oblongata connects the pons above to the spinal cord below. It consists of a median fissure on the anterior surface and on each side, called the pyramids. They are bundles of nerve fibers originating from large nerve cells of precentral gyrus. The pyramids taper below, and here most of the descending nerve fibers cross to the opposite side of the body, forming decussation of the pyramids [29]. **Figure 4** illustrates the flow of the cerebrospinal fluid (CSF), **Figure 5** the blood supply to the brain, and **Table 6** the brain stem reflexes.

Cranial nerve (CN)	Name	Origin from brainstem	Function
CN III	Oculomotor	Midbrain	Eye movement, pupil constriction
CN IV	Trochlear	Midbrain (dorsally)	Eye movement (superior oblique muscle)
CN V	Trigeminal	Pons	Facial sensation, chewing
CN VI	Abducens	Pontomedullary junction	Eye movement (lateral rectus muscle)
CN VII	Facial	Pontomedullary junction	Facial expression, taste (anterior 2/3 tongue)
CN VIII	Vestibulocochlear	Pontomedullary junction	Hearing and balance
CN IX	Glossopharyngeal	Medulla	Taste (posterior 1/3 tongue), swallowing
CN X	Vagus	Medulla	Parasympathetic to thorax and abdomen
CN XI	Accessory (Spinal)	Medulla/spinal cord	Shoulder and neck muscles (sternocleidomastoid, trapezius)
CN XII	Hypoglossal	Medulla	Tongue movement

Table 4.
Cranial nerves and its functions.

Brainstem part	Anatomical location and description	Function
Midbrain	Uppermost part, below thalamus	Visual and auditory reflexes, motor coordination (*via* substantia nigra)
Pons	Middle part	Bridges cerebrum and cerebellum, regulates breathing
Medulla Oblongata	Lowest part, continues into spinal cord	This lobe is the primary center for visual processing

Table 5.
Anatomical description and function of brain stem part.

3. Differentiating brain death vs. coma vs. persistent vegetative state

3.1 Brain death (BD)

Brain death (BD) is the irreversible cessation of all functions of the entire brain, including the brainstem. It is legally and medically recognized as death [35–37]. Key Features of diagnosing BD include:

- No brain activity: All parts of the brain, including the brainstem, have stopped functioning [38].
- No consciousness or awareness.
- No brainstem reflexes [39].

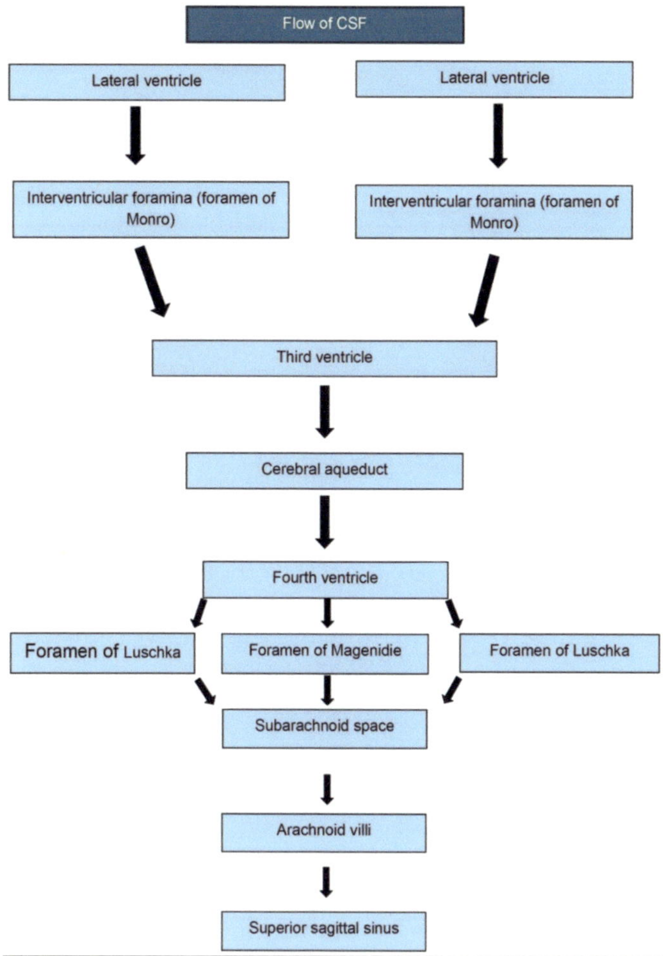

Figure 4.
Flow of CSF.

- No spontaneous breathing: patient is dependent on a ventilator [39].

Irreversible-recovery is impossible [39].

It is paramount that a clear catastrophic cause leading to brain damage must be established. The cause must have led to irreversible loss of all brain and brainstem function (**Table** 7) [38, 39].

3.2 Coma

Coma is a disorder of consciousness that is characterized by a state of profound irresponsiveness and a lack of awareness that persists for more than 1 hour. There is no wakefulness or awareness [37].Key features of a coma include:

- Unarousable unconsciousness: The patient cannot be awakened and shows no purposeful response to stimuli.

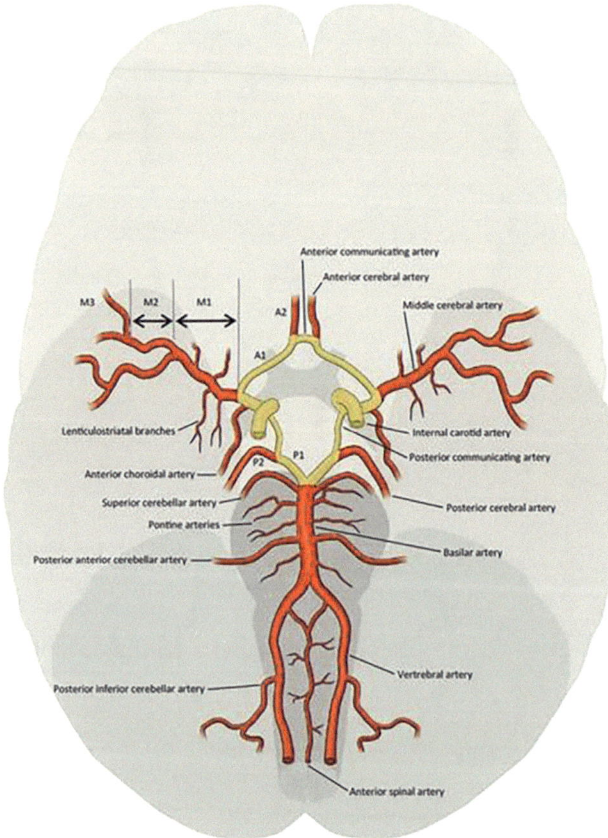

Figure 5.
Blood supply to the brain.

- Some brainstem reflexes may be preserved (e.g., pupils may react to light) [39].
- Breathing is often present without mechanical support.
- Brain activity is present but depressed; EEG shows some function [38, 39].

Potential for recovery or progression to other states (e.g., vegetative state or brain death) [40].Coma results from diffuse or focal brain injury [36, 39]. It is diagnosed based on clinical examination, including assessment of responsiveness, reflexes, and imaging to rule out reversible causes. The prognosis of coma is variable; recovery depends on cause, severity, and duration [40].

A vegetative state is a condition of wakefulness without awareness, typically following coma. The patient may open their eyes and display sleep-wake cycles but lacks evidence of conscious awareness [39–42]. Vegetative state is broadly classified into:

- Persistent Vegetative State: Lasts more than 1 month
- Permanent Vegetative state: Irreversible: typically, after 3 months (non-traumatic) or 12 months (traumatic)

Brainstem reflex tests				
Test	**Cranial nerve**		**Test details (brainstem level)**	**Response in brainstem death**
	Sensory (Afferent)	**Motor (Efferent)**		
Pupillary response	II	III	A bright light shone into each eye in turn. Direct and consensual reflexes should be sought (mid brain)	Absence of pupillary constriction
Corneal reflexes	V	VII	The cornea is brushed lightly with a swab (pons)	No blinking
Oculo-vestibular reflexes	VIII	III, IV, VI	50 ml of ice cold saline is instilled into the external auditory meatus over 1 min. The tympanic membrane should be visualized by otoscopy before testing. Both sides should be tested though inability to perform the test on one side does not invalidate the test (pons)	No eye movement
Response to painful stimulus	V	VII	Painful stimulus is applied to the supra orbital ridge (pons), and also to the limbs and trunk	No motor response in the cranial distribution
Gag reflex	IX	X	The pharynx is stimulated with a spatula or similar device (medulla)	No gag or pharyngeal contractions
Cough reflex	X	X	A bronchial catheter is passed to the carina (medulla)	No cough

Table 6.
Brain stem reflex tests.

Feature	Brain death	Coma	Vegetative state
Consciousness	Absent	Absent	Absent
Wakefulness	Absent	Absent	Present (sleep-wake cycles)
Brainstem Reflexes	Absent	May be present	Present
Spontaneous Breathing	Absent	Usually, present	Present
EEG Activity	None	Depressed but present	Variable, may be present
Recovery Possible	Never	Sometimes	Rarely
Legal Status	Dead	Alive	Alive
Prognosis	Fatal	Variable	Poor, rarely improves

Table 7.
Comparison table.

The key features of vegetative state include:

- No awareness of self or environment.
- Sleep-wake cycles are present; eyes may open spontaneously.

- Basic brainstem functions are preserved.
- Reflexive or spontaneous movements may occur, but not purposeful.
- Some patients may recover partially, but most remain severely disabled.

Vegetative state often follows coma when there is severe damage to the cerebral cortex but sparing of the brainstem, allowing for autonomic and sleep-wake functions to persist.

4. Clinical criteria for brain death determination: Prerequisites and neurological examination

There is a worldwide variance in methods used in the determination of BD/DNC [23, 43–46]. In 2023, the American Academy of Neurology, American Academy of Pediatrics, Child Neurology Society, and Society of Critical Care Medicine published the most up-to-date Guideline for Pediatric and Adult BD/DNC Determination (**Table 8**). However, it is always advised to follow national protocols.

Components	
Age	• >37 weeks corrected gestational age
Etiology	• Establish the presence of a catastrophic, permanent brain injury caused by an identified mechanism known to lead to BD/ DNC in the absence of confounders. • Do not perform a BD/DNC evaluation if there is any evidence of consciousness, preservation of any brainstem reflex, motor movements mediated by the brain/brainstem, or spontaneous breathing. • Conduct further diagnostic evaluation and do not evaluate for BD/DNC if a patient is comatose, is apneic, and has no brainstem reflexes, but there is no identified mechanism of brain injury known to lead to BD/DNC.
Observation period after brain injury and before initiating the BD/ DNC evaluation	• Observe for at least 48 h after acute brain injury before initiating BD/DNC evaluation in patients younger than 24 months. • Observe for at least 24 h after hypoxic-ischemic brain injury before initiating BD/DNC evaluation in patients 24 months or older. • Observe for enough time (based on the pathophysiology of the brain injury) after brain injury before initiating BD/DNC evaluation to ensure that there is no potential for recovery. • Observe for enough time (based on the pathophysiology of the brain injury and the findings on neuroimaging) after medical or surgical interventions to treat elevated intracranial pressure before initiating BD/DNC evaluation to ensure that there is no potential for recovery.
Severity of brain injury	• Establish that brain injury is permanent (function is lost and will not resume spontaneously and medical interventions will not be used to attempt to restore function).
Neuroimaging results	• Ensure that neuroimaging is consistent with the mechanism and severity of brain injury. • Ensure that neuroimaging shows evidence of catastrophic supratentorial injury before BD/ DNC evaluation in patients with primary posterior fossa injury.

Components	
Temperature	• Core temperature $>36^{\circ}C$ • Wait at least 24 h after rewarming to $36^{\circ}C$ before BD/DNC evaluation if core body.
Blood pressure	• Ensure that systolic blood pressure is $\geq 100\, mm\ Hg$ and mean arterial pressure is $\geq 75\, mm\ Hg$ (only the mean arterial pressure goal is applicable on veno-arterial extracorporeal membrane oxygenation) in adults. • Ensure that systolic and mean arterial pressure are $\geq 5th$ percentile for age (only the mean arterial pressure goal is applicable on veno-arterial extracorporeal membrane oxygenation) in children. • Target a systolic and mean arterial pressure that approximates the known chronic baseline for patients who have a baseline blood pressure that varies significantly from their age-based normal.
Exclude intoxication	• Exclude intoxication by any substance that can depress the central nervous system by i. Ensuring blood and urine drug screen are negative (if clinically indicated). ii. Ensuring the serum level is therapeutic or subtherapeutic and not considered to contribute to the neurologic state. iii. Waiting at least 5 half-lives, taking hepatic or renal dysfunction, body mass index, body temperature (hypothermia), and age into consideration (pharmacokinetic table provided for common drugs that depress the central nervous system). • Ensure the pentobarbital level is <5ug/mL or below the lower limit of detection for the laboratory (if administered) • Ensure blood alcohol level is <80 mg/dL
Exclude pharmacologic paralysis	Exclude pharmacologic paralysis, if administered or suspected, using a train-of-four stimulator or demonstration of deep tendon reflexes.
Laboratory parameters	• Exclude severe metabolic, acid-base or endocrine disturbance. • Evidence of neuroendocrine function does not preclude BD/DNC evaluation.
Other considerations	• Pregnancy is not a contraindication for BD/DNC evaluation.

Table 8.
2023 American Academy of Neurology, American Academy of Pediatrics, Child Neurology Society, and Society of Critical Care Medicine Guideline for Pediatric and Adult BD/DNC Determination.

4.1 Minimal clinical criteria for determination of BD/DNC

Diagnosing brain death (BD) or death by neurologic criteria (DNC) is a clinical decision requiring meticulous evaluation. A comprehensive assessment of the patient's clinical history, underlying etiology, and neuroimaging must confirm a permanent catastrophic brain, consistent with BD/DNC criteria. All potential confounding factors-including metabolic imbalances, drug intoxication, or hypothermia-must be systematically excluded. Repeated evaluations or ancillary testing (e.g., TCD or scintigraphy and angiography) are critical when ambiguities arise, as numerous documented instances of reversible BD have been reported [47–65]. Multiple case reports of situations falsely suggesting BD/DNC have been published in the literature [66–70].

Before initiating the determination of BD/DNC, it must be confirmed that the patient has a well-established neurologic diagnosis of a type and severity that can cause a permanent loss of consciousness, permanent absence of all brainstem reflexes, and an irreversible inability to breathe spontaneously in response to elevated carbon dioxide and acidosis. Before testing for BD/DNC, one of the following must be present:

- Neuroimaging evidence of intracranial hypertension, such as severe cerebral edema and herniation,or
- Intracranial pressure measurements that are equal to or greater than the mean arterial pressure.

If neuroimaging does not show evidence of herniation, it is recommended to proceed with caution when considering an evaluation for BD/DNC.

4.1.1 Prerequisites before proceeding with an evaluation for BD/DNC

- The patient's core temperature should be at least 36°C.
- Adults must have a systolic blood pressure of at least 100 mm Hg and a mean arterial pressure of at least 75 mm Hg; pediatric patients should meet age-appropriate blood pressure targets.

4.1.2 Confounding factors that must be excluded before performing brain stem testing

- Pharmacologic paralysis.
- The effects of central nervous system (CNS) depressant drugs and toxins.
- Blood alcohol level must be 80 mg/dL or lower.
- Severe metabolic, acid-base or endocrine disturbances that could affect the neurologic exam must be corrected. If these cannot be fully corrected ancillary testing should be used to confirm the diagnosis.

4.1.3 Interventions and observation periods

Interventions to reduce intracranial pressure should be performed only when clinically necessary. A sufficient observation period should be considered before proceeding with clinical testing for BD/DNC:

For anoxic brain injury following resuscitated cardiac arrest, at least 24 hours of observation after rewarming is recommended.

For other types of brain injury, the optimal observation period is not clearly defined and should be determined by clinical judgment.

4.1.4 Clinical testing

It is universally agreed that the clinical evaluation for determination of BD/DNC includes an assessment for coma and an evaluation for brainstem areflexia to demonstrate that:

1. There should be no motor responses originating from the brain.

2. There should be no pupillary reaction to bright light, with the pupils typically found in a mid-position (approximately 4–6 mm). Although pupils may initially be dilated in cases of brain death due to a surge of adrenal catecholamines, they generally return to a mid-position after several hours.

3. Corneal reflexes must be absent. This is assessed by gently touching the cornea with a cotton swab or by applying drops of water or saline solution, which is preferred for repeated testing to reduce the risk of corneal abrasion.

4. Absent oculocephalic reflex

5. There should be no cough response when the trachea is suctioned

6. Absent sucking or rooting reflexes in <6 months old.

7. Apnea as demonstrated by apnea test [44, 71–74].

4.2 Indications for ancillary testing

In most instances, brain death (BD) or death by neurological criteria (DNC) is diagnosed through a clinical evaluation, and extra tests are rarely needed. However, extra tests are needed when clinical exams or apnea testing cannot be done or are inconclusive. This can happen when the patient has suffered a head or neck injury that makes it hard to properly assess brainstem reflexes, apnea testing cannot be conducted safely because of the risk of hypoxia, when neurological signs are inconclusive, or when their metabolic imbalances are not easily corrected.

4.3 Spinal cord reflexes in brain stem death testing

Spinal cord reflexes may occur in response to certain stimuli. These reflexes may get weaker with repeated stimulation (habituation) and occur as a reflex and are not purposeful. Polysynaptic spinal reflexes and automatisms usually do not show up until after brain death, but when they do, they are seen as proof of brain death as they occur after spinal shock sets in. Most of these reflexes happen within 24 hours of brain death and do not last longer than 72 hours.

Spinal cord reflexes represent primitive motor patterns that become unmasked when the brainstem and neocortex no longer exert control over the spinal cord. They are thought to result from hypoxia and hypercapnia-induced activation of cervical spinal cord neurons that are isolated from higher brain regions. Mechanical factors, such as stretching of the spinal roots or compression of the spinal cord – triggered by noxious stimuli or neck flexion – may also contribute to these movements.

About 33–75% of brain-dead patients show spinal reflexes and automatisms, which can occur spontaneously or triggered by touch [75–77]. Some common examples are facial twitching (myokymia), eye tremors, changes in the pupils that happen in cycles, and autonomic responses like sweating or a fast heart rate. Neck flexion might produce more complicated reflexes like the Lazarus sign, in which the patient's trunk and limbs move in sync. Other movements include bending the fingers, the

1. Locked-in syndrome	
2. High C-spine injury	
3. Hypothermia	
4. Drug intoxication	• Tricyclic antidepressants • Lidocaine • Baclofen • Sedatives, especially barbiturates • Paralytics • Anticholinergics • Bupropion • Valproic acid • Organophosphate intoxication
5. Neuromuscular paralysis, as found in severe, acute polyneuropathies such as	Guillain-Barré syndrome (some may also have autonomic dysfunction, including pupillary areflexia) or with neuromuscular blocking agents, such as botulism

Table 9.
Brain death mimics.

triple flexion response, moving the toes in a wave-like pattern, posturing, myoclonus, opening the eyelids, turning the head, and even breathing-like movements. This can happen in the first 24 hours and rarely last more than 72 hours [78–80]. **Table 9** examines some condition which mimic brain death.

5. Apnea test in the diagnosis of brain death

Confirmation of the irreversible loss of all brain functions, including the respiratory centers of the brainstem, is necessary for the clinical diagnosis of brain death. By confirming that there is no respiratory drive despite hypercapnia and acidosis—conditions that typically stimulate breathing *via* medullary centers—the apnea test plays a crucial role [81, 82]. The respiratory centers are strongly activated when arterial $PaCO_2$ rises to ≥60 mm Hg (or by ≥20 mm Hg above baseline) because CO_2 diffuses into the inefficiently buffered cerebrospinal fluid very quickly. The apnea test is only conducted after all other criteria for brain death have been met to prevent complications such as hypoxemia or cardiovascular collapse [83].

The number of tests needed varies; for adults, one apnea test is enough, but pediatric patients require two tests, each following a different neurological examination [81].

Patients at high risk of cardiopulmonary decompensation, such as those with severe hypoxia, hypotension, or arrhythmias, are contraindications for the apnea test. In these situations, an ancillary study should be utilized in place of the test [81].

Since motor output may be compromised despite intact brainstem function, other conditions such as neuromuscular disorders (e.g., GuillainBarré and myasthenia gravis) or high cervical spinal cord injuries may invalidate the apnea test [83]. However, ancillary testing is necessary to confirm brain death in these situations, and the neurological examination and apnea test should be carried out as thoroughly as possible [84].

5.1 Prerequisites for performing the apnea test

Deviation from the prerequisites, such as hypotension or inadequate preoxygenation, or electrolytes or acid-base abnormalities or arrhythmias, can lead to complications during apnea test. A study by Goudreau et al. [85] showed that complications occurred in approximately one in four apnea tests, occurring significantly more often in patients who had unfavorable conditions before the apnea test (39%) than in those without these unfavorable factors (only 15%) [85]. Therefore, it is of the utmost importance to meet the following criteria before beginning:

- Core temperature ≥ 36°C.
- Systolic blood pressure ≥ 100 mmHg and mean arterial pressure ≥ 75 mmHg.
- PaO_2 > 200 mmHg after preoxygenation.
- pH in normal limits, 7.35–7.45.
- Normovolemia (usually aiming for positive balance in the previous 6 hours).
- Acceptable electrolyte levels.

5.2 Preparation for apnea testing

1. Preoxygenation for ≥10 minutes with FiO_2 100% on the ventilator (and through the membrane lung, for patients on extracorporeal membrane oxygenation) to achieve PaO_2 ≥ 200 mmHg. Supplying 100% O_2, effectively washes out nitrogen from the lungs, increasing the oxygen reservoir and thereby prolonging the safe apnea time [86, 87].

2. Adjustment of ventilatory rate and tidal volume to achieve normocapnia ($PaCO_2$ 35–45 mmHg). In CO_2 retainers, target the chronic baseline $PaCO_2$ if the baseline $PaCO_2$ is known, or the estimated chronic baseline if the baseline $PaCO_2$ is unknown.

3. Arterial line is recommended for continuous BP monitoring, pressor titration, and quick extraction of blood gases.

5.3 Standard procedure for apnea test

The first step in the apnea test is to expose the chest and abdomen and watch for spontaneous breathing while the ventilator is disconnected. Apneic oxygenation is maintained by using an insufflation catheter that is less than 70% the diameter of the endotracheal tube, delivering 100% oxygen at a rate of 4–6 L per minute. Increased flows could lengthen the test and partially clear CO_2 [83] or a Continuous Positive Airway Pressure (CPAP) on a ventilator set to the previous PEEP level (**Table 10**).

Abdominal or chest movements that produce sufficient tidal volume are indicative of true breathing. Respiratory-like movements, such as shoulder elevation, back arching, or intercostal expansion without significant tidal volume, can emerge later in the test and may be confused with actual breathing, even though spontaneous respirations

Concern	Risk	Solution
Auto-triggering	Cardiac oscillations mimicking effort	Disable triggering/adjust sensitivity
Machine breath delivery	Apnea backup mode	Backup rate = 0, PS = 0
Test ambiguity	False interpretation of spontaneous effort	Alarms off, careful observation

Table 10.
The use of ventilator CPAP is safe and acceptable if configured properly.

usually occur early. A spirometer can verify the lack of tidal volume in situations where there is uncertainty [84]. Attention should be paid to auto-triggering brought on by condensation or cardiac oscillations might mistakenly imply breathing [81].

5.4 Apnea test interpretation

The test is positive (i.e., confirms brain death) if no respiratory movements are observed while the following occur simultaneously [81]:

1. $PaCO_2 \geq 60$ mmHg

2. Increase of $PaCO_2 \geq 20$ mmHg from baseline

3. pH < 7.30

The test is negative if any respiratory movement is perceived during the observation period, that is, the patient does not meet criteria for BD/DNC.

Apnea test is considered inconclusive if:

1. The test duration is insufficient to reach the required thresholds. This may happen in patients with:

   i. Low baseline $PaCO_2$ (e.g., chronic hyperventilation or respiratory alkalosis).

   ii. Severely impaired gas exchange, where CO_2 rise is slow or O_2 desaturation occurs early.

3. The test is technically feasible but physiologically unreliable due to impaired respiratory motor output, regardless of brainstem function (e.g., high cervical spine cord injury and neuromuscular diseases).

4. The test is aborted because of any complications, such as

   i. ≥1 breath (the test is negative, i.e., the patient does not meet criteria for BD/DNC)

   ii. Systolic blood pressure < 100 mm Hg or mean arterial pressure < 75 mmHg in adults or < 5th percentile for age in children despite titration of vasopressors, inotropes, and/or intravenous fluids

iii. Progressive decrease in O_2 saturation < 85%

iv. Cardiac arrhythmia with hemodynamic instability

6. Ancillary methods to diagnose brainstem death

Since ancillary methods provide objective proof of irreversible brainstem failure, they are crucial for diagnosing brainstem death (BSD) in situations where clinical exams are unclear or confusing. Important standardized assessments include:

i. Electroencephalography (EEG) as a supplement rather than a stand-alone test because it measures cortical activity and electrocerebral silence indicates BSD.

ii. Somatosensory Evoked Potentials (SSEPs) and Brainstem Auditory Evoked Potentials (BAEPs), which are technically difficult but advised by the UK Academy of Medical Royal Colleges (AoMRC), aid in the detection of severe brain dysfunction and brainstem failure, respectively [88].

iii. Transcranial Doppler (TCD) as an ancillary test shows cerebral circulatory arrest with waveforms and has been shown to be 98% specific for BSD [89, 90].

iv. Four-vessel angiography is the invasive gold standard for detecting the absence of intracranial blood flow, while CTA and MRA are alternatives that are less invasive is angiography [91].

v. Radionuclide scintigraphy, which uses technetium-99 m scans to confirm BSD by demonstrating no intracranial uptake [90].

With four-vessel angiography as the gold standard and multimodal techniques like TCD and scintigraphy being extremely specific, ancillary tests complement clinical diagnosis but do not replace it; the decision is based on local legal and clinical expertise.

7. Legal frameworks variability in national and institutional guidelines

The diagnosis of brainstem death (BSD) is a critical and irreversible determination with profound medical, legal, and ethical implications. Recent guidelines from major international societies—including the European Society of Intensive Care Medicine (ESICM), the American Academy of Neurology (AAN), the UK Academy of Medical Royal Colleges (AoMRC), and the Australian and New Zealand Intensive Care Society (ANZICS) provide standardized protocols for BSD diagnosis. While these guidelines share core principles, key differences exist in ancillary testing, prerequisites, and procedural details (**Table 11**).

7.1 Differences in prerequisites for BSD testing

Before beginning brainstem death (BSD) testing, all major guidelines require that confounding factors such as sedation, hypothermia, and metabolic disturbances

Criteria	ANZICS (2023)	ESICM (2022)	AAN (2010)	UK AoMRC (2025)
Prerequisites				
Observation period	$\geq 4h$ (adults); 24 h (children)	12–24 h (injury-dependent)	$\geq 6h$ (adults)	$\geq 6h$ (adults); 24 h (children)
Anoxic injury delay	24 h	72 h	24 h	24 h
Clinical examination				
Examiners	2 ICU/neuro consultants	2 physicians (1 intensivist)	1 neurologist +1 physician	2 senior consultants
Apnea test	Mandatory ($PaCO_2 \geq 60$ mmHg)	Mandatory	Mandatory	Optional if ancillary test used
Exam intervals	$\geq 4h$ (with ancillary test)	Single exam + ancillary test	$\geq 6h$	$\geq 6h$
Ancillary test				
First-line	Angiography/scintigraphy	TCD/CTA	Scintigraphy/angiography	Scintigraphy
Second-line	EEG	EEG	EEG	TCD/CTA
Excluded	TCD	—	—	—
Special populations				
Children	3 exams +24 h observation	2 exams +24 h observation	Deferred to pediatric protocols	2 exams +24 h observation
Pregnancy	Explicit fetal monitoring	Not addressed	Not addressed	Not addressed
Legal	Independent 2nd team confirmation	No explicit witness requirement	No explicit witness requirement	Second consultant con

Table 11.
Comparison of international BSD guidelines.

be ruled out. A 12- to 24-hour observation period following injury is advised by the ESICM prior to testing; this period is further prolonged for anoxic brain injury treated with therapeutic hypothermia [90]. The AAN mandates two clinical examinations spaced at least 6 hours apart but does not specify an observation period. According to the AoMRC, senior clinicians must conduct two examinations 6 hours apart for adults and 24 hours apart for children [88]. Adults may undergo expedited testing as soon as 4 hours following an injury, according to ANZICS guidelines.

7.2 Differences in clinical examination criteria

To diagnose brain death, the ESICM, AAN, AoMRC, and ANZICS all concur that an apnea test with $PaCO_2$ ≥60 mmHg or a 20 mmHg increase from baseline is necessary, as is confirmation of absent brainstem reflexes. But when clinical examinations are not conclusive, they diverge in ancillary testing: Transcranial Doppler (TCD) or CT angiography (CTA) is preferred by ESICM, with EEG as a backup; EEG, cerebral angiography, or scintigraphy are equally recommended by AAN; radionuclide scintigraphy or TCD is preferred by AoMRC, with CTA as a backup; and four-vessel angiography or scintigraphy is recommended first by ANZICS, excluding TCD because of operator dependence and using EEG as a backup [92]. AAN employs a particular pediatric protocol, ESICM and AoMRC demand 24–48 hours of observation for pediatric brain death, and ANZICS adheres to ESICM/AoMRC timing but requires three tests. In hypoxic-ischemic injury cases, ESICM advises longer waiting (72 hours) versus AAN's 24 hours.

8. Evaluation of brain death in special groups

8.1 Brain death in pregnancy

The assessment of brain death in pregnant individuals is particularly very challenging as it intertwines medical and ethical factors, compounded by legal issues within the critical care domain. Though the core neurological criteria for diagnosing brain death stay uniform across different groups, pregnancy carries distinct physiological and ethical challenges that necessitate a tailored approach for protocols leading to collaborative management strategies [46, 93, 94]. Medical literature is documenting a rising trend of prolonged maternal physiological support following brain death (MPS-BD) in pregnant individuals declared brain-dead at gestational stages far below the threshold of fetal viability. Current research indicates that the standard criteria for diagnosing brain death can be effectively applied to pregnant patients, although certain adjustments to testing procedures may be required to ensure the safety of the fetus; the apnea test should not be performed; other means, such as radiologic absence of cranial blood flow, should be utilized for the formulation of the diagnosis of BD [95].

8.1.1 Clinical management and somatic support challenges

Pregnant women rarely experience brain death; according to one study, only 5 out of 252 brain-dead patients (2.8%) were pregnant women between the ages of 15 and 45 [96]. A minimum gestational age for supporting a brain-dead mother and her fetus is not universally agreed upon, but after 24 weeks, the chances of survival improve dramatically, rising from roughly 20–30% at 24 weeks to nearly 98% at 32 weeks, with a decline in the likelihood of severe disability [97]. Other factors that affect survival include the age of the mother and any underlying brain pathology [92]. In such cases, prolonged somatic support frequently results in severe complications, such as infections, hormone imbalances, and cardiac problems, that necessitate critical care [98, 99]. According to the American Academy of Neurology, families should be well-informed about legal issues and fetal outcomes are considered when deciding whether to continue or stop support, while considering the patient's and family's desires, legal considerations, possible fetal brain damage, and fetal viability [100].

Because decisions must weigh the interests of the brain-dead mother and the viable fetus, guided by bioethical principles like autonomy, beneficence, nonmaleficence, and justice, brain death during pregnancy presents difficult ethical and legal issues [99]. While removing support ends the fetus's life, promoting fetal development may clash with upholding the deceased's dignity. Legally speaking, most hospital policies are vague about who has the power to make decisions for the fetus, which leaves room for involvement from a variety of sources, including family members, medical professionals, ethics committees, and government representatives [99]. Region-specific laws vary, with some relying on court decisions and others having particular statutes.

8.2 Pediatric/neonatal brain death

Due to limited data and developmental differences in the neonatal and pediatric population, brain stem assessments must be carefully modified for neonates (≥36 weeks of gestation to 30 days old), infants, and children up to 18 years old [25, 26, 73, 79, 101]. While ancillary tests such as EEG or radionuclide cerebral blood flow studies are not usually necessary, they may aid in the diagnosis in cases where clinical examinations or apnea tests cannot be conducted with reliability.

Two sets of clinical examinations and apnea tests are advised for pediatric BD/DNC, 12 to 24 hours apart, to verify irreversibility. Patients should be kept in an unresponsive coma for at least 24 hours before testing, particularly following asphyxia or hypothermia-induced rewarming. For younger patients, tracheal insufflation should be avoided, and age-appropriate targets must be used. Transcranial Doppler is not yet approved for use in children, but ancillary tests like EEG or radionuclide imaging are acceptable if necessary. Standardized checklists are recommended to increase consistency and accuracy in diagnosing BD/DNC in children, and testing must be performed by certified pediatric specialists. **Table 12** outlines brain death criteria in infants.

8.3 Apnea test in ECMO patients

Up to 25% of patients receiving extracorporeal membrane oxygenation may develop BD/DNC, and the apnea test (AT) is essential for neurological evaluation to confirm brain death or death by neurological criteria. AT should still be carried out, though, unless it is dangerous [102]. In patients receiving ECMO, hypercapnia is essential for a reliable AT. Circuit configurations and patient-specific variables affect CO_2 levels. As blood flows along one side of the membrane oxygenator, gas exchange takes place, with sweeping gas moving in the opposite direction to remove CO_2 and add oxygen. The ability of modern oxygenators to efficiently remove CO_2 makes it difficult to induce hypercapnia and prolongs tests [3, 27, 102, 103].

Criterion	Requirement
Age	Term newborn (>37 weeks) to <1 year
Prerequisites	Correct hypothermia, hypotension, metabolic/drug effects
Clinical exams	2 exams by different physicians
Observation period	24 h (newborns to 30 d) 12 h (>30 d to 18y)
Brainstem reflexes	Absent Absent
Apnea test	Required, with adequate CO_2 stimulus
Neuroimaging	Evidence of irreversible CNS injury
Temperature	$>35^{\circ}C\left(95^{\circ}F\right)$

These criteria are based on consensus guidelines from the American Academy of Pediatrics, American Academy of Neurology, and other international bodies.

Table 12.
Brain death criteria in infants.

Maintaining patient oxygenation is essential during an AT. A PaO_2 above 200 mmHg is the goal, and this is accomplished by giving 100% oxygen *via* the ventilator and ECMO circuit for at least 10 minutes. The extracorporeal circuit is necessary for oxygenation in veno-venous (VV) ECMO, but differential hypoxia in veno-arterial (VA) ECMO can make it more difficult. Continuous Positive Airway Pressure (CPAP) can help oxygenate the lungs. The ECMO circuit is the only source of oxygenation if mechanical ventilation is stopped while receiving ECMO support [104].

In VV ECMO, radial artery samples generally reflect systemic oxygenation [105]. In VA ECMO, the mix of native cardiac and ECMO flows can create a watershed area where gas tensions vary depending on the sampling site [106, 107]. Therefore, it is recommended to sample from both the right radial artery and post-oxygenator sites to confirm that PaCO2 targets are met and cerebral perfusion is adequately represented [27, 107].

Due to altered drug metabolism in critically ill ECMO patients, more time may be needed beyond five drug half-lives to rule out pharmacological confounders [103]. Continuous monitoring of hemodynamics, oxygen saturation, and serial ABGs (typically every 5 minutes) is key to ensuring test validity and patient safety [27].

During AT, ECMO patients are at risk of hypotension, hypoxia, and acidosis [27, 103]. Preparing in advance with appropriate vasoactive support and CO_2 management increases safety. If the patient becomes unstable, ancillary tests should be used instead [108, 109].

Whether ancillary testing is required varies by country. EEG and TCD are usually feasible [109]. CT angiography and cerebral scintigraphy require patient transport and may be less reliable due to ECMO flow dynamics. TCD tends to be reliable in VA ECMO if pulsatile flow remains [108].

9. Religious beliefs on brain death

9.1 Islamic views on death

Islamic theology posits that life and death are exclusively within the authority of Allah, as stated in the Qur'an: "It is He who gives life and causes death" (Qur'an 10:56).

The Hadith of the Prophet Muhammad, who said, "Sleep is the brother of death", helps to explain this Qur'anic command even more.

Some scholars posit that the persistent presence of a beating heart and other physiological functions in a brain-dead individual, especially if maintained artificially, indicates that the soul may not have completely exited, analogous to the state of sleep wherein the body remains operational despite the transient absence of complete consciousness.

The Islamic Fiqh Academy of the Organization of Islamic Cooperation and the Islamic Medical Association of North America have both recognized brain death as a valid indicator of death, contingent upon the fulfillment of rigorous diagnostic criteria.

9.2 Judaism and Christianity

Most mainstream Christian groups, including the Roman Catholic Church, which sees it as a valid sign of death when rigorously diagnosed, accept brain death. Jewish beliefs are more varied. Orthodox Judaism often requires the heart to stop beating, while Conservative and Reform Judaism may accept brain death in some cases.

9.3 Buddhism and Hinduism

In Hindu and Buddhist traditions, death is perceived as the exit of the soul and the termination of consciousness.

10. Future aspects in diagnosing brain death

No single specific test can confirm or refute the diagnosis of BD. A meticulous approach combining a thorough neurological clinical assessment, apnea test along with ancillary tests is currently adopted but do have their limitations. Future research should concentrate on developing a more precise and effective methods of diagnosing brain death, discovering new biomarkers, and developing advanced neurodiagnostic tools.

Machine learning coupled with neurological investigation, such as training and integration of EEG interpretation, radiological neuroimaging (computed tomography CT and MRI scans), and analysis through Artificial Intelligence (AI) algorithmic-based programs are promising [110, 111]. AI can look in depth at brain scans (CTs, MRIs) to measure blood flow or diagnose cellular edema.

Finding and establishing a novel biomarker that is both specific and sensitive to the irreversible brain cell death is underway [112–116]. Current biomarkers under study include:

a. Glial fibrillary acidic protein (GFAP): This promising novel biomarker is showing the potential to differentiate between brain death and serious brain cell injury.

b. Levels of >1.5 micrograms per liter have strongly predicted brain death.

c. Neuron Specific Enolase (SNE)

d. The S100 Calcium-Binding Protein Beta (S100b)

e. Ubiquitin carboxy-terminal hydrolase L1 (UCH-L1)

Current challenges in applying biomarkers include accessibility, requirement to have high specificity and high sensitivity regardless of any patient-related variable (age, gender, and medical condition), and the scarcity of well-designed trials that address the use and the utilization of these biomarkers.

11. Conclusion

The permanent cessation of all brain and brainstem activity is known as brain death. As critical care and organ transplants have improved, this concept has undergone significant change. The change from cardiopulmonary to neurological criteria for death has previously been impacted by clinical, ethical, and legal considerations. The terminology used, the diagnostic processes, and the addition of extra tests, however, continue to be contentious. A comprehensive clinical evaluation is required to determine brain death, which includes evaluating brainstem reflexes and apnea while ruling out conditions like metabolic issues or pharmacological side effects that could skew the results.

It is more challenging for certain groups of people, such as children, pregnant women, and those receiving extracorporeal membrane oxygenation (ECMO). This implies that various techniques are required to ensure the diagnosis is accurate. Accepting brain death is made even more difficult by religious and cultural beliefs, which highlights the significance of clinician collaboration and sensitivity to these concerns.

Future developments in biomarkers, artificial intelligence, and advanced neuroimaging could increase the precision and impartiality of brain death diagnosis. Standardization of international regulations is still crucial, though, to preserve moral integrity and minimize disparities. The diagnosis of brain death ultimately has significant ramifications for organ donation, patients, and their families. In addition to acknowledging diverse values and opinions, it necessitates rigorous adherence to evidence-based guidelines.

More research, education, and global consensus are required in this complex and evolving field to improve diagnostic criteria, address ethical concerns, and produce better outcomes.

Author details

Hana Elamin[1], Ahmad M. Obeidat[1], Ashish Kumar[1],
Mojahid Mohammed Khalid Alhussein[1], Mohammad Ataur Rahman[1], Zia Mahmood[1],
Fernando Ruiz Gonzalez[1], Sanghamitra Padhy[1], Prabu Bhuvanendran[1]
and Sohel M.G. Ahmed[1,2]*

1 Hamad Medical Corporation, Doha, Qatar

2 College of Medicine, Qatar University, Doha, Qatar

*Address all correspondence to: sohelm@yahoo.com

References

[1] Spears W, Mian A, Greer D. Brain death: A clinical overview. Journal of Intensive Care. 2022;**10**(1):16. DOI: 10.1186/s40560-022-00609-4

[2] Beck CS, Pritchard WH, Feil HS. Ventricular fibrillation of long duration abolished by electric shock. Journal of the American Medical Association. 1947;**135**:985-986. DOI: 10.1001/jama.1947.62890150005007a

[3] Bower AG et al. Investigation on the care and treatment of poliomyelitis patients. Annals of Western Medicine and Surgery. 1950;**4**:561-582. Available from: https://pubmed.ncbi.nlm.nih.gov/14777465/

[4] Belkin GS. Brain death and the historical understanding of bioethics. Journal of the History of Medicine and Allied Sciences. 2003;**58**:325-361. DOI: 10.1093/jhmas/jrg003

[5] Wertheimer P, Jouvet M, Descotes J. Diagnosis of death of the nervous system in comas with respiratory arrest treated by artificial respiration. La Presse Médicale. 1959;**67**:87-88. Available from: http://europepmc.org/abstract/MED/13633814

[6] Jouvet M. Diagnostic électrosouscorticographique de la mort du système nerveux central au cours de certains comas. Electroencephalography and Clinical Neurophysiology. 1959;**11**:805-808. DOI: 10.1016/00134694(59)901245

[7] Mollaret P, Goulon M. The depassed coma (preliminary memoir). Revue Neurologique (Paris). 1959;**101**:3-15

[8] Raymond R, Potts F, Bonazzi A. EEG as an aid in determining death in the presence of cardiac activity: Ethical, legal, and medical aspects. Electroencephalography and Clinical Neurophysiology. 1963;**15**:145-166'. Available from: https://www.scienceopen.com/document?vid=1c78d6c7-1c75-47c7-b536-d956a29c8684 [Accessed: May 14, 2025]

[9] Alderete J et al. Irreversible coma: A clinical, electroencephalographic and neuropathological study. Transactions of the American Neurological Association. 1968;**93**:16-20. Available from: http://europepmc.org/abstract/MED/5711010

[10] The Ad Hoc Committee of the Harvard Medical School to Examine the Definition of Brain Death. A definition of irreversible coma: Report of the ad hoc Committee of the Harvard Medical School to examine the definition of brain death. JAMA. 1968;**205**:337-340. DOI: 10.1001/jama.1968.03140320031009

[11] Anonymous. A way of dying. The Atlantic Monthly. 1957;**199**:53-57

[12] Joseph Garland MD. Life-in-death. New England Journal of Medicine. 1957;**256**(16):760-761. DOI: 10.1056/NEJM195704182561610

[13] Merrill JP et al. Successful homotransplantation of the human kidney between identical twins. JAMA. 1956;**160**:277-282. DOI: 10.1001/jama.1956.02960390027008

[14] Barnard CN. The operation: A human cardiac transplant: An interim report of a successful operation performed at Groote Schuur hospital, Cape Town. SAMJ: South African Medical Journal. 2017;**107**(12):1271-1274. Available

from: http://www.scielo.org.za/scielo.php?script=sci_arttext&pid=S0256-95742017001200004&lng=en&tlng=en [Accessed: May 13, 2025]

[15] Youngner SJ, Arnold RM. Philosophical debates about the definition of death: Who cares? The Journal of Medicine and Philosophy. 2001;**26**:527-537. DOI: 10.1076/jmep.26.5.527.3002

[16] Giacomini M. A change of heart and a change of mind? Technology and the redefinition of death in 1968. Social Science & Medicine. 1997;**44**:1465-1482. DOI: 10.1016/S02779536(96)002663

[17] Veatch RM. Brain death: Welcome definition... or dangerous judgment? Hastings Center Report. 1972;**2**:10-13. DOI: 10.2307/3561575

[18] The Conference of Medical Royal Colleges and their Faculties in the United Kingdom. Diagnosis of brain death. Statement issued by the honorary secretary of the conference of medical Royal Colleges and their faculties in the United Kingdom on 11 October 1976. BMJ. 1976;**2**:1187. DOI: 10.1136/bmj.2.6045.1187

[19] Pallis C. ABC of brain stem death. From brain death to brain stem death. BMJ. 1982;**285**:1487. DOI: 10.1136/bmj.285.6353.1487

[20] De Georgia MA. History of brain death as death: 1968 to the present. Journal of Critical Care. 2014;**29**:673-678. DOI: 10.1016/j.jcrc.2014.04.015

[21] The Quality Standards Subcommittee of the American Academy of Neurology. Practice parameters for determining brain death in adults. Neurology. 1995;**45**:1012-1014. DOI: 10.1212/WNL.45.5.1012

[22] Wijdicks EFM et al. Evidence based guideline update: Determining brain death in adults. Neurology. 2010;**74**:1911-1918. DOI: 10.1212/WNL.0b013e3181e242a8

[23] Shemie SD et al. International guideline development for the determination of death. Intensive Care Medicine. 2014;**40**:788-797. DOI: 10.1007/s0013401432427

[24] American Academy of Pediatrics. Report of special task force: Guidelines for determination of brain death in children. Pediatrics. 1987;**80**:298300. Available from: https://cir.nii.ac.jp/crid/1571698601324839168

[25] Nakagawa TA, Ashwal S, Mathur M, Mysore MR, Bruce D, Conway EE, et al. Guidelines for the determination of brain death in infants and children: An update of the 1987 task force recommendations. Critical Care Medicine. 2011;**39**(9):2139-2155. DOI: 10.1097/CCM.0b013e31821f0d4f

[26] Nakagawa TA et al. Guidelines for the determination of brain death in infants and children: An update of the 1987 task force recommendations—Executive summary. Annals of Neurology. 2012;**71**:573-585. DOI: 10.1002/ana.23552

[27] Greer DM et al. Determination of brain death/death by neurologic criteria: The world brain death project. JAMA. 2020;**324**:1078-1097. DOI: 10.1001/jama.2020.11586

[28] Bosnell R, Madder H. Concepts of brain death. Surgery-Oxford International Edition. 2011;**29**(7):289-294. DOI: 10.1016/j.mpsur.2011.04.001

[29] Snell RS. Clinical Anatomy by Regions. 10th ed. Philadelphia: Wolters Kluwer; 2018

[30] Fix JD. Neuroanatomy. Philadelphia, PA: Lippincott Williams & Wilkins; 2002

[31] Standring S. Gray's Anatomy: The Anatomical Basis of Clinical Practice. 41st ed. Edinburgh: Elsevier; 2015

[32] Nolte J. The Human Brain: An Introduction to its Functional Anatomy. 7th ed. Edinburgh: Elsevier; 2020

[33] Haines DE. Neuroanatomy: An Atlas of Structures, Sections, and Systems. 9th ed. Philadelphia: Wolters Kluwer; 2019

[34] Basinger H, Hogg JP. Neuroanatomy. Brainstem: StatPearls Publishing, Treasure Island (FL); 2025. Available from: http://europepmc.org/abstract/MED/31335017

[35] Machado C. Brain Death: A Reappraisal. New York: Springer; 2007. DOI: 10.1007/978-0-387-38977-6

[36] Mangat HS, Rosengart A. Coma, persistent vegetative state, and brain death. In: Hall JB, Schmidt GA, Kress JP, editors. Principles of Critical Care. 4th ed Chapter 88. New York, NY: McGraw-Hill Education; 2015

[37] Kumar AB. Coma and brain death. In: Bhardwaj A, Long MA, editors. A Practical Approach to Neuroanesthesia. Philadelphia, PA: Lippincott Williams & Wilkins; 2013. pp. 404-414

[38] Laureys S, Owen AM, Schiff ND. Function in brain death, coma, vegetative state, minimally conscious state and locked-in syndrome. The Lancet Neurology. 2004;**3**:537-546

[39] What is Brain Death. Available from: https://npistanbul.com/en/what-is-brain-death [Accessed: May 26, 2025]

[40] Agrawal D. Coma Vs Brain Death Vs Vegetative State. 2024. Available from: https://drdeepakaiims.com/coma-vs-brain-death-vs-vegetative-state [Accessed: May 26, 2025]

[41] Hutchinson PJ, Pickard JD. Brain death and the vegetative state. In: Warrell DA, Cox TM, Firth JD, editors. Oxford Textbook of Medicine. 5th ed. Oxford: Oxford University Press; 2010. DOI: 10.1093/med/9780199204854.003.240506

[42] Maiese K. Vegetative State and Minimally Conscious State (Unresponsive Wakefulness Syndrome). Rutgers University. Available from: https://www.rutgers.edu/content-url; 2024 [Accessed: May 24, 2024]

[43] Lewis A, Bakkar A, Kreiger-Benson E, et al. Determination of death by neurologic criteria around the world. Neurology. 2020;**95**(3):e299-e309. DOI: 10.1212/WNL.0000000000009888

[44] Wahlster S, Wijdicks EFM, Patel PV, et al. Brain death declaration: Practices and perceptions worldwide. Neurology. 2015;**84**(18):1870-1879. DOI: 10.1212/WNL.0000000000001540

[45] Sprung CL, Truog RD, Curtis JR, et al. Seeking worldwide professional consensus on the principles of end-of-life care for the critically ill: The consensus for worldwide end-of-life practice for patients in intensive care units (WELPICUS) study. American Journal of Respiratory and Critical Care Medicine. 2014;**190**(8):855-866. DOI: 10.1164/rccm.201403-0593CC

[46] Da Silva IR, Frontera JA. Worldwide barriers to organ donation. JAMA Neurology. 2015;**72**(1):112-118. DOI: 10.1001/jamaneurol.2014.3083

[47] Bernat JL. How much of the brain must die in brain death? The Journal of Clinical Ethics. 1992;**3**(1):21-26

[48] Gervais KG. Redefining Death. New Haven: Yale University Press; 1987

[49] Mohandas A, Chou SN. Brain death: A clinical and pathological study. Journal of Neurosurgery. 1971;**35**(2):211-218. DOI: 10.3171/jns.1971.35.2.0211

[50] Kung NH, Dhar R, Keyrouz SG. Diffuse leptomeningeal carcinomatosis mimicking brain death. Journal of the Neurological Sciences. 2015;**352**(1-2):132-134. DOI: 10.1016/j.jns.2015.03.045

[51] Rigamonti A, Basso F, Stanzani L, Agostoni E, Lauria G. Guillain-Barré syndrome mimicking brain death. Journal of the Peripheral Nervous System. 2009;**14**(4):316-319. DOI: 10.1111/j.1529-8027.2009.00244.x

[52] Vargas F, Hilbert G, Gruson D, Valentino R, Gbikpi-Benissan G, Cardinaud JP. Fulminant Guillain-Barré syndrome mimicking cerebral death: Case report and literature review. Intensive Care Medicine. 2000;**26**(5):623-627. DOI: 10.1007/s001340051213

[53] Moussouttas M, Chandy D, Dyro F. Fulminant acute inflammatory demyelinating polyradiculoneuropathy: Case report and literature review. Neurocritical Care. 2004;**1**(4):469-473. DOI: 10.1385/NCC:1:4:469

[54] Young GB. De-efferentation and de-afferentation in fulminant polyneuropathy: Lessons from the isolated brain. Canadian Journal of Neurological Sciences. 2003;**30**(4):305-306. DOI: 10.1017/S0317167100002997

[55] Liik M, Puksa L, Luus SM, Haldre S, Taba P. Fulminant inflammatory neuropathy mimicking cerebral death. BMJ Case Reports. 2012;**2012**:bcr1020114906

[56] Bakshi N, Maselli RA, Gospe SM, Ellis WG, McDonald C, Mandler RN. Fulminant demyelinating neuropathy mimicking cerebral death. Muscle & Nerve. 1997;**20**(12):1595-1597. DOI: 10.1002/(SICI)1097-4598(199712)20:12<1595::AID-MUS16>3.0.CO;2-#

[57] Martí-Massó JF, Suárez J, López de Munain A, Carrera N. Clinical signs of brain death simulated by Guillain-Barré syndrome. Journal of the Neurological Sciences. 1993;**120**(1):115-117. DOI: 10.1016/0022-510X(93)90034-V

[58] Ravikumar S, Poysophon P, Poblete R, Kim-Tenser M. A case of acute motor axonal neuropathy mimicking brain death and review of the literature. Frontiers in Neurology. 2016;**7**:63. DOI: 10.3389/fneur.2016.00063

[59] Bernard V, Van Pesch V, Hantson P. Guillain-Barré syndrome mimicking brain death pattern: A poorly reversible condition. Acta Neurologica Belgica. 2010;**110**(1):93-96

[60] Hantson P, Guérit JM, de Tourtchaninoff M, et al. Rabies encephalitis mimicking the electrophysiological pattern of brain death. European Neurology. 1993;**33**(3):212-217. DOI: 10.1159/000116939

[61] John J, Gane BD, Plakkal N, Aghoram R, Sampath S. Snake bite mimicking brain death. Cases Journal. 2008;**1**(1):16. DOI: 10.1186/1757-1626-1-16

[62] Dayal M, Prakash S, Verma PK, Pawar M. Neurotoxin envenomation mimicking brain death in a child: A case report and review of literature. Indian Journal of Anaesthesia. 2014;**58**(4):458-460. DOI: 10.4103/0019-5049.139008

[63] Freund B, Hayes L, Rivera-Lara L, et al. Adult intestinal colonization botulism mimicking brain death. Muscle & Nerve. 2017;**56**(4):E27-E28. DOI: 10.1002/mus.25689

[64] Joffe AR, Anton N, Blackwood J. Brain death and the cervical spinal cord: A confounding factor for the clinical examination. Spinal Cord. 2010;**48**(1):2-9. DOI: 10.1038/sc.2009.115

[65] Conference of Royal Colleges and Faculties of the United Kingdom. Diagnosis of brain death. The Lancet. 1976;**2**(7994):1069-1070

[66] Felton D, Carey JL, Boyer E, Neavyn MJ. Brain death and overdose. Clinical Toxicology. 2014;**52**:419

[67] López-Navidad A, Caballero F, Domingo P, et al. Early diagnosis of brain death in patients treated with central nervous system depressant drugs. Transplantation. 2000;**70**(1):131-135

[68] Morrow SA, Young GB. Selective abolition of the vestibular-ocular reflex by sedative drugs. Neurocritical Care. 2007;**6**(1):45-48. DOI: 10.1385/NCC:6:1:45

[69] Schmidt JE, Tamburro RF, Hoffman GM. Dilated nonreactive pupils secondary to neuromuscular blockade. Anesthesiology. 2000;**92**(5):1476-1480. DOI: 10.1097/00000542-200005000-00039

[70] Webb AC, Samuels OB. Reversible brain death after cardiopulmonary arrest and induced hypothermia. Critical Care Medicine. 2011;**39**(6):1538-1542. DOI: 10.1097/CCM.0b013e3182186687

[71] Larson MD, Muhiudeen I. Pupillometric analysis of the "absent light reflex". Archives of Neurology. 1995;**52**(4):369-372. DOI: 10.1001/archneur.1995.00540280051018

[72] Academy of Medical Royal Colleges. A Code of Practice for the Diagnosis and Confirmation of Death. London: Academy of Medical Royal Colleges; 2008

[73] Australian and New Zealand Intensive Care Society (ANZICS). The ANZICS Statement on Death and Organ Donation. 3rd ed. Melbourne: ANZICS; 2013

[74] Wijdicks EFM. Brain death worldwide: Accepted fact but no global consensus in diagnostic criteria. Neurology. 2002;**58**(1):20-25. DOI: 10.1212/WNL.58.1.20

[75] Shemie SD, Doig C, Dickens B, et al. Severe brain injury to neurological determination of death: Canadian forum recommendations. CMAJ. 2006;**174**(6):S1-S13

[76] Saposnik G, Bueri JA, Mauriño J, et al. Spontaneous and reflex movements in brain death. Neurology. 2000;**54**(1):221-223. DOI: 10.1212/WNL.54.1.221

[77] Saposnik G, Mauriño J, Saizar R, Bueri JA. Undulating toe movements in brain death. European Journal of Neurology. 2004;**11**(10):723-727. DOI: 10.1111/j.1468-1331.2004.00873.x

[78] Saposnik G, Mauriño J, Saizar R, Bueri JA. Spontaneous and reflex movements in 107 patients with brain death. The American Journal of Medicine. 2005;**118**(3):311-314. DOI: 10.1016/j.amjmed.2004.12.009

[79] Torbey MT. Neurocritical Care. 2nd ed. Cambridge: Cambridge University Press; 2019

[80] Nelson SE, Nyquist PA. Neurointensive Care Unit: Clinical Practice and Organization (Current Clinical Neurology). 1st ed. Cham: Springer; 2020

[81] Greer DM, Shemie SD, Lewis A, et al. Adult and pediatric brain death determination: The 2024 guidelines from the American Academy of Neurology, child neurology society, and Society of Critical Care Medicine. Neurology. 2024;**102**(14):678-690

[82] Wijdicks EFM. Brain Death. 3rd ed. Oxford: Oxford University Press; 2023

[83] Dobb GJ, Weekes JW. Clinical confirmation of brain death. Anaesthesia and Intensive Care. 1995;**23**(1):37-43. DOI: 10.1177/0310057X9502300125

[84] Wijdicks EFM. Determining brain death in adults. Neurology. 1995;**45**(5):1003-1011. DOI: 10.1212/wnl.45.5.1003

[85] Goudreau JL, Wijdicks EFM, Emery SF. Complications during apnea testing in the determination of brain death: Predisposing factors. Neurology. 2000;**55**(7):1045-1048. DOI: 10.1212/WNL.55.7.1045

[86] Nimmagadda U, Salem MR, Crystal GJ. Preoxygenation: Physiologic basis, benefits, and potential risks. Anesthesia & Analgesia. 2017;**124**(2):507-517

[87] Machado C, Perez J, Scherle C, Areu A, Pando A. Brain death diagnosis and apnea test safety. Annals of Indian Academy of Neurology. 2009;**12**(3):197-200

[88] Academy of Medical Royal Colleges (AoMRC). A Code of Practice for the Diagnosis and Confirmation of Death. London: AoMRC. Available from: https://www.aomrc.org.uk/wp-content/uploads/2025/01/Code_of_Practice_Diagnosis_of_Death_010125.pdf; 2025 [Accessed: May 10, 2025]

[89] Chang JJ, Tsivgoulis G, Katsanos AH, Malkoff MD, Alexandrov AV. Diagnostic accuracy of transcranial Doppler for brain death confirmation: Systematic review and meta-analysis. AJNR American Journal of Neuroradiology. 2016;**37**(3):408-414

[90] Sandroni C, Nolan JP, Andersen LW, Böttiger BW, Cariou A, Cronberg T, et al. ERC-ESICM guidelines on temperature control after cardiac arrest in adults. Intensive Care Medicine. 2022;**48**(3):261-269

[91] Frampas E, Videcoq M, de Kerviler E, Ricolfi F, Kuoch V, Mourey F, et al. CT angiography for brain death diagnosis. AJNR American Journal of Neuroradiology. 2009;**30**(8):1566-1570

[92] Shewmon DA. Recovery from “brain death”: A neurologist’s apologia. Linacre Quarterly. 1997;**64**:30-96

[93] Bernat JL. Controversies in defining and determining death in critical care. Nature Reviews Neurology. 2013;**9**(3):164-173. DOI: 10.1038/nrneurol.2013.12

[94] Joffe AR, Kolski H, Duff J, deCaen AR. A 10-month-old infant with reversible findings of brain death. Pediatric Neurology. 2009;**41**(5):378-382. DOI: 10.1016/j.pediatrneurol.2009.07.006

[95] Truog RD, Krishnamurthy K, Tasker RC. Brain death—Moving beyond consistency in the diagnostic criteria. JAMA. 2020;**324**(10):1045-1047. DOI: 10.1001/jama.2020.12241

[96] Suddaby EC, Schaeffer MJ, Brigham LE, Shaver TR. Analysis of

organ donors in the peripartum period. Journal of Transplant Coordination. 1998;**8**:35-39

[97] Slattery MM, Morrison JJ. Preterm delivery. Lancet. 2002;**360**(9344):1489-1497

[98] Esmaeilzadeh M, Dictus C, Kayvanpour E, Sedaghat-Hamedani F, Eichbaum M, et al. One life ends, another begins: Management of a brain-dead pregnant mother—A systematic review. BMC Medicine. 2010;**8**:74. DOI: 10.1186/1741-7015-8-74

[99] Moguillansky N, Mathelier M, Tuna IS. Brain dead and pregnant. Cureus. 2023;**15**(8):e44172. DOI: 10.7759/cureus.44172

[100] Wijdicks EFM, Varelas PN, Greer DM. There is no reversible brain death. Critical Care Medicine. 2011;**39**(9):2204-2205. DOI: 10.1097/CCM.0b013e318222724e

[101] Spanish Royal Decree 1723/2012, 2012. Regulating the Activities of Recovery, Clinical Use and Territorial Coordination of Human Organs Intended for Transplantation and Setting Quality and Safety Standards. Available from: https://www.boe.es/boe/dias/2012/12/29/pdfs/BOE-A-2012-15715.pdf [Accessed: January 3, 2018]

[102] Beam WB, Scott PD, Wijdicks EFM. The physiology of the apnea test for brain death determination in ECMO: Arguments for blending carbon dioxide. Neurocritical Care. 2019;**31**(2):395-397. (1)

[103] Shah V, Lazaridis C. Apnea testing on extracorporeal membrane oxygenation: Case report and literature review. Journal of Critical Care. 2015;**30**(4):784.e1-784.e5

[104] Veiga VC. Apnea test for the diagnosis of brain death in a patient undergoing extracorporeal membrane oxygenation. Revista Brasileira de Terapia Intensiva. 2020;**32**(3):468-473

[105] Marasco SF, Lukas G, McDonald M, McMillan J, Ihle B. Review of ECMO (extracorporeal membrane oxygenation) support in critically ill adult patients. Heart, Lung and Circulation. 2008;**17**(Suppl 4):S41-S47

[106] Hoeper MM. Extracorporeal membrane oxygenation watershed. Circulation. 2014;**130**:864-865

[107] Ihle JF. A protocol that mandates postoxygenator and arterial blood gases to confirm brain death on venoarterial extracorporeal membrane oxygenation. ASAIO Journal. 2019;**65**(3):e31-e33

[108] Bein T, Müller T, Citerio G. Determination of brain death under extracorporeal life support. Intensive Care Medicine. 2019;**45**(6):712-715

[109] Greer DM, Wang HH, Robinson LR, Wijdicks EFM. Determining brain death in adults: 2023 update of the American Academy of Neurology guidelines. Neurology. 2023;**100**(4):173-185

[110] Singh NM, Harrod JB, Subramanian S, Robinson M, Chang K, Cetin-Karayumak S, et al. How machine learning is powering neuroimaging to improve brain health. Neuroinformatics. 2022;**20**(4):943-964. DOI: 10.1007/s12021-022-09572-9

[111] Chau M, Vu H, Debnath T, Rahman MG. A scoping review of automatic and semi-automatic MRI segmentation in human brain imaging. Radiography. 2025;**31**(2):102878. DOI: 10.1016/j.radi.2025.01.013

[112] Lee D, Cho Y, Ko Y, Heo NH, Kang HG, Han S. Neuron-specific enolase level as a predictor of neurological outcome in near-hanging patients: A retrospective multicenter study. PLoS One. 2021;**16**(2):e0246898. DOI: 10.1371/journal.pone.0246898

[113] Lopes AN, Regner A, Simon D. The role of S100b protein biomarker in brain death: A literature review. Cureus. 2024;**16**(6):e62707. DOI: 10.7759/cureus.62707

[114] Juan JE-G, Murillo-Cabezas F, Gordillo-Escobar E, Rodríguez-Rodríguez A, Enamorado-Enamorado J, Revuelto-Rey J, et al. Title not provided. Journal of Neurotrauma. 2013;**30**(20):1762-1769

[115] Hellström S, Sajanti A, Jhaveri A, Srinath A, Bennett C, Cao Y, et al. Diagnostic and prognostic performance of urine ubiquitin carboxy-terminal hydrolase L1 across multiple acute brain injury types – A longitudinal prospective cohort study. Brain and Spine. 2025;**5**:104173. DOI: 10.1016/j.bas.2024.104173

[116] Butterfield DA. Ubiquitin carboxyl-terminal hydrolase L-1 in brain: Focus on its oxidative/nitrosative modification and role in brains of subjects with Alzheimer disease and mild cognitive impairment. Free Radical Biology and Medicine. 2021;**177**:278-286. DOI: 10.1016/j.freeradbiomed.2021.10.036

Chapter 10

Trends in Critical Care Medicine: Innovations Shaping the Future

Muhammad Saqib

Abstract

This chapter explores the transformative trends in critical care medicine, focusing on how emerging technologies and innovative practices are reshaping patient care in intensive care units (ICUs). It examines advancements in artificial intelligence, telemedicine, ECMO, and remote monitoring systems, discussing their impact on diagnostic accuracy, treatment efficiency, and overall patient outcomes. The chapter also highlights the integration of interdisciplinary approaches and the evolution of ICU design aimed at improving both clinical and psychological support. By analyzing current research, clinical trials, and real-world case studies from global centers of excellence, the chapter provides insights into future directions for critical care practices and strategies to overcome challenges such as resource constraints and workforce shortages. Ultimately, it underscores the need for continuous innovation to meet the dynamic demands of modern critical care.

Keywords: critical care, medical innovation, artificial intelligence, telemedicine, ECMO, remote monitoring, interdisciplinary care

1. Introduction

1.1 Overview of critical care medicine

Critical care medicine has evolved from a nascent field supporting postoperative patients to a sophisticated discipline that manages multi-organ failure, sepsis, and acute respiratory distress syndrome (ARDS), among other life-threatening conditions. Modern ICUs are characterized by continuous, high-resolution monitoring, integration of advanced therapeutics, and the use of cutting-edge technologies that allow for real-time decision-making. Today, our intensive care units are not merely places of reactive treatment—they are dynamic hubs of innovation that combine data analytics, personalized medicine, and interprofessional teamwork to provide the highest standard of care [1].

IntechOpen

2. Rationale for innovation in the ICU

The rationale for constant innovation in the ICU is multifaceted:

Complexity of illness: With patients presenting with increasingly complex clinical scenarios and multiple comorbidities, a one-size-fits-all approach is no longer sufficient.

Technological advancements: Breakthroughs in Artificial Intelligence (AI), telemedicine, and sensor technology have opened new avenues for continuous monitoring, early detection of deterioration, and personalized therapy.

Global health challenges: The COVID-19 pandemic starkly exposed the limitations of traditional critical care systems, highlighting the need for scalable, flexible, and technology-driven solutions.

Quality improvement: By reducing human error, standardizing interventions, and enabling proactive care, technological innovations have the potential to significantly improve patient outcomes, decrease ICU length of stay, and optimize resource utilization.

This chapter aims to provide a comprehensive review and in-depth analysis of the trends that are transforming critical care medicine. Specific objectives include:

- Describing the historical evolution of critical care.
- Detailing emerging technologies (AI, telemedicine, ECMO, and wearables) and their clinical applications.
- Exploring innovative ICU designs that emphasize patient-centered care.
- Discussing the role of precision medicine, pharmacogenomics, and biomarker-guided therapies.
- Examining the integration of big data and cybersecurity in modern ICUs.
- Addressing challenges and ethical dilemmas associated with advanced technologies.
- Presenting real-world case studies to illustrate the practical impact of these innovations.
- Outlining future directions, policy reforms, and global collaboration efforts.

Figure 1 shows a schematic overview of a modern ICU system.

An overview of key technologies in critical medicine is tabulated in **Table 1**.

Critical care medicine began in the 1950s with transformative innovations such as the heart-lung machine, which made open-heart surgery possible. Early ICUs were established to care for postoperative patients with limited technology—mechanical ventilation was rudimentary, and monitoring was intermittent and manual. As the field evolved, new tools like the pulmonary artery catheter enabled precise measurement of hemodynamic parameters, dramatically improving shock management. The transition from paper records to electronic health records (EHRs) in the 1990s further revolutionized the field by allowing for continuous data capture and analysis [2]. **Figure 2** shows the timeline of milestones in critical care medicine.

DOI: http://dx.doi.org/10.5772/intechopen.1010714

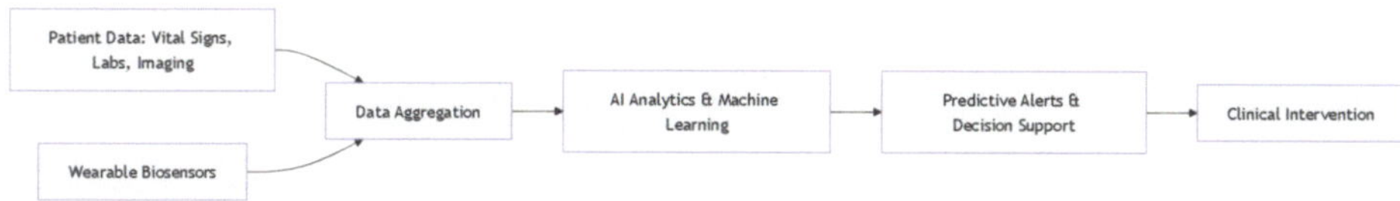

Figure 1.
Schematic overview of the modern ICU ecosystem. Description: This figure illustrates how various technologies—ranging from AI analytics and wearable biosensors to tele-ICU systems—are interconnected in a modern ICU, culminating in enhanced clinical interventions and improved patient outcomes (figure is author's own original work).

Technology	Key features	Clinical impact	Limitations
Artificial Intelligence	Real-time analytics, predictive algorithms, automated imaging analysis	Early sepsis detection and personalized treatment adjustments	Potential algorithm bias and continuous validation required
Tele-ICU Systems	HD video, remote EHR integration, real-time alerts	Increased specialist access and reduced inter-hospital transfers	Network and training challenges
ECMO	Adjustable flow, advanced oxygenators, refined anticoagulation protocols	Rescue therapy for severe ARDS and cardiac failure	High cost, resource-intensive, and risk of complications
Wearable Biosensors	Continuous, non-invasive monitoring, wireless data transmission	Early detection of deterioration and post-discharge monitoring	Integration with existing systems and accuracy limitations
Precision Medicine	Biomarker profiling, genomics integration, and tailored dosing algorithms	Personalized therapeutic strategies and optimized drug therapy	Complexity of data interpretation and high costs

Table 1.
Overview of key technologies in critical care medicine.

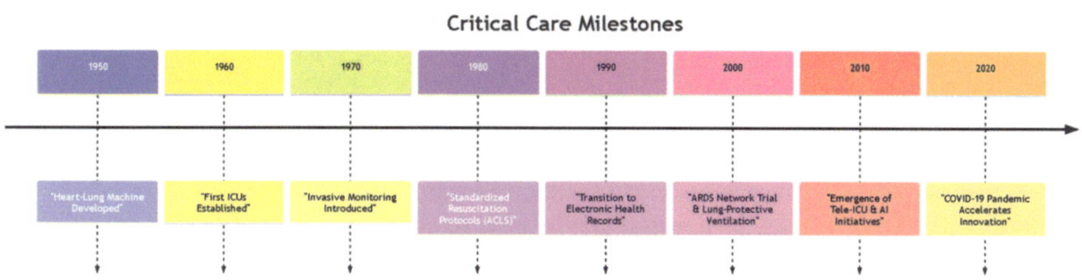

Figure 2.
Timeline of milestones in critical care medicine. Description: This figure is a timeline that visually represents key milestones in the development of critical care, highlighting how each innovation has built upon previous advances (figure is author's own original work).

Table 2 compares the historical versus the modern approaches in critical care.

Over the decades, key milestones have reshaped critical care:

Mechanical ventilation: Early ventilators evolved into modern devices implementing lung-protective strategies to minimize ventilator-induced lung injury [3].

Invasive monitoring: The introduction of devices such as central venous and pulmonary artery catheters revolutionized shock management.

Digital transformation: The transition to EHRs enabled the integration of vast patient data streams, paving the way for AI analytics.

Aspect	Historical approach	Modern approach
Monitoring	Intermittent and manual checks	Continuous and automated digital monitoring
Documentation	Paper-based records	Cloud-based EHRs and real-time data integration
Treatment protocols	Fixed and protocol-based interventions	Adaptive, data-driven, and AI-assisted personalized protocols
Team structure	Siloed and single-discipline focus	Interdisciplinary collaboration with simulation training

Table 2.
Historical versus modern approaches in critical care.

Clinical trials: Landmark studies like the ARDS Network [4], CESAR [5], and EOLIA [6] trials have provided evidence for best practices in ventilator management and ECMO utilization. ADRENAL trial [7] supported the notion that though steroids do not reduce mortality, they may still have secondary benefits, as listed in **Table 3**.

The landscape of ICU sedation has evolved significantly, initially exploring strategies like daily sedation holidays (Kress et al. [8]) and protocolized weaning (ABC [9]) to reduce ventilation time and ICU stay. Subsequent large trials, including SLEAP [10] and NONSEDA [11], refined our understanding, indicating the need for careful titration rather than complete avoidance. More recently, research has concentrated heavily on dexmedetomidine, with trials like MIDEX-PRODEX [12] comparing it to other agents and large studies such as SPICE-III [13] investigating its impact on mortality, collectively shaping current practice toward lighter, more individualized sedation goals. See **Table 3** for further details.

Fluid management in the ICU has undergone a significant evolution, driven by pivotal clinical trials that have challenged long-held beliefs. Moving beyond simple volume resuscitation, recent research highlights the crucial distinction between fluid types, strongly favoring balanced crystalloids over traditional saline to mitigate renal complications. Simultaneously, evidence supports the nuanced application of restrictive fluid strategies, particularly in conditions like ARDS, to improve pulmonary mechanics and reduce ventilator exposure [14–17]. These landmark studies (described further in **Table 3**) collectively underscore the need for an individualized, dynamic approach to fluid therapy guided by patient-specific factors and a clear understanding of the potential differential impacts of resuscitation fluids on organ function.

Landmark randomized controlled trials have profoundly reshaped our approach to red blood cell transfusion in the intensive care unit, largely favoring a more conservative strategy. Studies such as TRICC [18], TRISS [19], and RELIEVE [20] have provided robust evidence demonstrating that maintaining a lower hemoglobin threshold (typically around 7 g/dL) is non-inferior to a higher threshold (often >10 g/dL) regarding mortality in most critically ill patients, particularly those without active bleeding or acute coronary syndromes. This evidence base has justifiably driven a significant shift toward more restrictive transfusion practices, minimizing unnecessary exposures while maintaining equivalent outcomes for the majority of our patients.

Global health crises, such as the H1N1 and COVID-19 pandemics, have accelerated innovation in critical care. The COVID-19 crisis, in particular, exposed limitations in ICU capacity and resource allocation, prompting the rapid adoption of tele-ICU systems, ECMO expansion, and AI-based monitoring tools. These challenges spurred a global collaboration that has permanently reshaped critical care protocols and accelerated regulatory and funding support for advanced technologies [21].

Trial	Intervention	Key outcomes	Clinical implications
ARDS network trial	Lower tidal volume ventilation (LTVV)	Reduced mortality, decreased ventilator-induced lung injury (VILI)	Adopt lung-protective ventilation protocols as standard care.
CESAR trial	ECMO referral vs. standard ventilation	Improved survival in ECMO-referred patients	Established ECMO as a viable rescue therapy for severe ARDS in specialized centers.
EOLIA trial	Early ECMO initiation in severe ARDS	Mixed mortality results; significant crossover to ECMO in the control group	Refines patient selection and timing for ECMO; highlights benefit potential upon use.
ADRENAL trial	Hydrocortisone vs. placebo in ventilated patients	No reduction in 3-month mortality	Supports hydrocortisone for faster recovery/resource use, not routine survival benefit.
Kress et al.'s trial	Daily interruption of sedation (DSI)	Significantly reduced time on ventilator (4.9 vs. 7.3 days) and ICU LOS (6.4 vs. 9.9 days)	DSI improves outcomes, particularly when baseline sedation is deep.
ABC trial	Protocolized SATs/SBTs (wake/wean)	Improved ventilator-free days and shorter ICU LOS, lower mortality, and higher self-extubation	Wake-and-wean protocols are beneficial but require vigilant monitoring for self-extubation.
SLEAP trial	DSI vs. light and continuous sedation	No difference in extubation time or other outcomes	DSI offers no additional benefit over maintaining sensible light sedation.
NONSEDA trial	Primary avoidance of sedation	No change in mortality, vent days, or ICU LOS, higher self-extubation, and crossover	Complete no-sedation strategy increases risks and is not universally superior.
MIDEX-PRODEX trial	Dexmedetomidine vs. propofol or midazolam	Shorter ventilation vs. midazolam, similar vs. propofol, and non-inferior otherwise	Dexmedetomidine is a comparable sedative, potentially better for ventilation time than midazolam.
SPICE-III trial	Dexmedetomidine as the main sedative vs. others	No 90-day mortality difference, small increase in ventilator-free days	Dexmedetomidine as a primary sedative does not impact mortality; marginal vent-free day gain.
SAFE trial	4% Albumin vs. 0.9% saline for resuscitation	Similar 28-day mortality, less fluid used with albumin	Albumin is a safe alternative to saline for resuscitation and may reduce fluid load.
SALT and SALT-ED trials	Balanced crystalloids vs. 0.9% saline	Lower Major Adverse Kidney Events (MAKE30) with balanced crystalloids	Prefer balanced crystalloids over saline, especially for patients at renal risk.
SPLIT trial	0.9% Saline vs. plasma-lyte 148	No difference in AKI, RRT, or mortality (in less severe cohort)	Initial data on crystalloid choice; findings less conclusive than larger trials.
TRICC trial	Restrictive (Hb <7) vs. liberal (Hb <10) RBC transfusion (non-bleeding ICU)	No 30-day mortality difference	Supports safety/efficacy of restrictive RBC transfusion in many critical patients.

Trial	Intervention	Key outcomes	Clinical implications
TRISS trial	Restrictive vs. liberal RBC transfusion in septic shock	No 90-day mortality difference	Validates restrictive RBC transfusion safety in the septic shock population.
RELIEVE trial (TBI)	Liberal (Hb ≤10) vs. restrictive (Hb ≤7) RBC transfusion in TBI with anemia	No difference in 6-month unfavorable neurologic outcome or mortality	Liberal transfusion in TBI did not improve overall neurologic outcome; balance functional gain vs. ARDS risk.

Abbreviations: ARDS: Acute Respiratory Distress Syndrome, DSI: Daily Sedation Interruption, ECMO: Extracorporeal Membrane Oxygenation, Hb: Hemoglobin, ICU LOS: Intensive Care Unit Length of Stay, LTVV: Lower Tidal Volume Ventilation, MAKE30: Major Adverse Kidney Events within 30 days, RBC: Red Blood Cell, RRT: Renal Replacement Therapy, SATs: Spontaneous Awakening Trials, SBTs: Spontaneous Breathing Trials, TBI: Traumatic Brain Injury, VILI: Ventilator-Induced Lung Injury.

Table 3.
Summary of key clinical trials impacting ICU practices.

3. Emerging technologies in critical care

AI systems now continuously process data from vital signs, laboratory values, and imaging to predict patient deterioration. Deep learning models identify subtle changes—such as incremental rises in lactate or shifts in heart rate

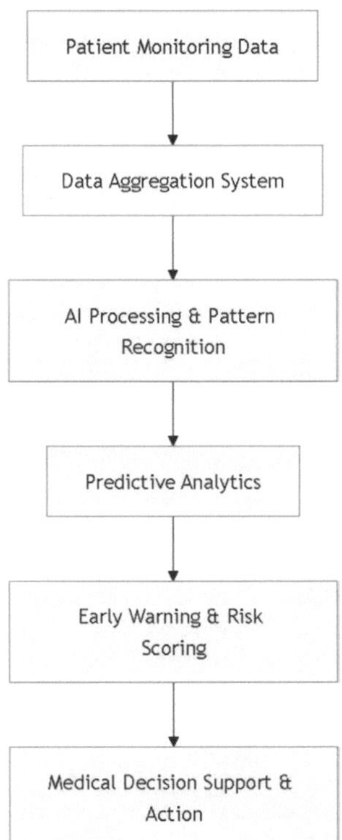

Figure 3.
AI data pipeline in the ICU. Description: This figure illustrates the process of acquiring patient data, aggregating it, processing it through AI algorithms, and generating real-time decision support that leads to timely clinical interventions (figure is author's own original work).

Application	Data sources	Predicted outcomes	Performance indicators
Sepsis early detection	Vital signs, lab values, and EHR data	Early identification of sepsis	Sensitivity ~85%, Specificity ~80%
Automated imaging analysis	Chest X-rays and CT scans	Detection of pneumonia and ARDS	Comparable to expert radiologists
Personalized ventilator adjustments	Continuous physiological data and patient history	Optimized ventilation settings	Reduced adverse events and lung injury rates

Table 4.
Key AI applications in the ICU.

variability—that may indicate impending sepsis. Early-warning systems trigger alerts, enabling timely interventions that have been associated with reductions in ICU mortality and length of stay [22].

Advanced algorithms analyze imaging data (e.g., chest X-rays and CT scans) with remarkable speed and accuracy. These tools assist in diagnosing conditions like pneumonia and ARDS, often delivering results that match expert radiologist interpretations. By standardizing image analysis, AI reduces diagnostic variability and expedites clinical decision-making [23].

Personalized decision support integrates patient data—including demographic information, EHR inputs, and genomic profiles—to recommend individualized treatment plans. These systems dynamically adjust ventilator settings, fluid management, and medication dosing based on real-time data, thus minimizing adverse events and optimizing patient care [24]. **Figure 3** shows an AI data pipeline in the ICU.

Table 4 shows key AI applications in the ICU.

4. Telemedicine and remote monitoring

Tele-ICU systems comprise multiple interconnected components:

- *Bedside monitors*: Capture continuous data from patients.
- *Data transmission networks*: Secure, high-speed channels that relay data to remote centers.
- *Remote command centers*: Equipped with high-definition video conferencing, integrated EHR access, and centralized dashboards.
- *AI-enhanced alert systems*: Prioritize and flag critical events for immediate intervention [25].

Figure 4 shows the tele-ICU system architecture.

5. Clinical outcomes, cost-effectiveness, and global deployment

Tele-ICU systems have demonstrated improved clinical outcomes:

- *Reduced ICU mortality*: Studies report a 10–15% reduction [26].

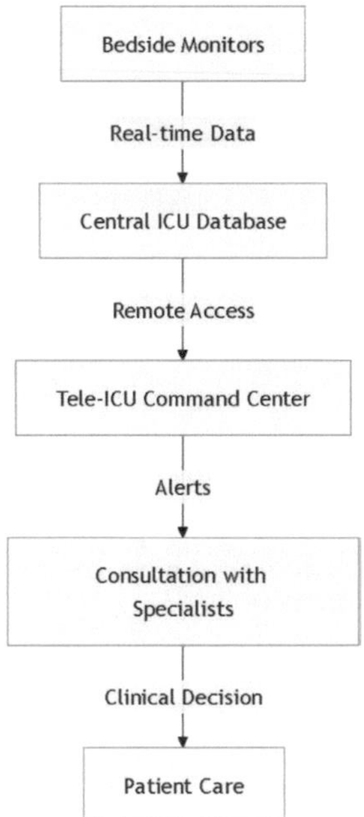

Figure 4.
Tele-ICU system architecture. Description: This figure shows the flow of data from bedside monitors to a remote command center where real-time dashboards and AI alerts facilitate timely intervention by remote specialists (figure is author's own original work).

Outcome measure	Improvement (%)	Key observations
ICU mortality	10–15% reduction	Early remote intervention saves lives
ICU length of stay	20–25% reduction	Faster, more efficient patient management
Inter-hospital transfers	60–70% reduction	Significant cost savings and reduced transfer risks

Table 5.
Clinical outcomes from tele-ICU implementations.

- *Shortened ICU length of stay*: Up to 25% reduction in stay duration [27].
- *Cost savings*: Decreased inter-hospital transfers and efficient resource allocation lower overall costs. These benefits make tele-ICU systems particularly attractive for deployment in regions with limited access to specialized care [28].

Table 5 shows the clinical outcomes from tele-ICU implementations.

6. Extracorporeal membrane oxygenation (ECMO)

6.1 Technological evolution and circuit advances

ECMO technology has advanced considerably:
Adjustable flow rates: Tailor oxygen delivery based on patient requirements.

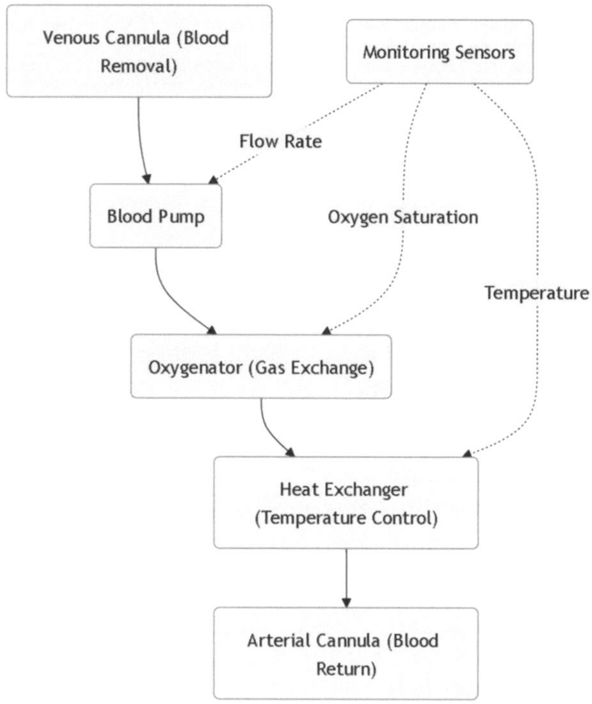

Figure 5.
Anatomy of an ECMO circuit. Description: This figure is an annotated diagram showing the major components of an ECMO circuit, including cannulae, pump, oxygenator, heat exchanger, and integrated monitoring sensors (figure is author's own original work).

Advanced oxygenators: Use state-of-the-art membrane materials for efficient gas exchange.

Refined anticoagulation protocols: Reduce bleeding and thrombotic complications [29].

Portability: New designs allow for more compact and portable systems, broadening clinical applications.

Figure 5 shows the anatomy of an ECMO circuit.

7. Clinical applications, patient selection, and management protocols

ECMO is used as a rescue therapy in severe ARDS and cardiogenic shock. Patient selection criteria include:

- Reversibility of the underlying condition.
- Absence of contraindications (e.g., irreversible brain injury).
- Reasonable likelihood of recovery. Clinical management involves continuous monitoring of oxygenator function, adjustment of flow rates, and strict anticoagulation protocols.

Table 6 shows the comparison of ECMO studies in clinical studies.

Study	Patient population	Survival rate (%)	Common complications
CESAR trial [5]	Severe ARDS patients	Approximately 63%	Bleeding, thromboembolism
EOLIA trial [6]	Refractory ARDS	35–46%	Increased thrombocytopenia
Recent studies [30]	Mixed critical illnesses	Variable, trend toward improved outcomes	Circuit-related issues, infection risk

Table 6.
Comparison of ECMO outcomes in clinical studies.

Despite its potential, ECMO is resource-intensive. Challenges include high costs, the need for specialized teams, and risks such as bleeding, thrombus formation, and infections. Future directions focus on:

- Miniaturizing ECMO devices.
- Enhancing circuit safety with real-time digital monitoring.
- Developing protocols for broader, safe deployment in pre-hospital and resource-constrained settings.

8. Wearable and smart devices

Wearable biosensors continuously capture patient data non-invasively using advanced optical and electronic sensors. These devices measure heart rate, oxygen saturation, body temperature, and activity levels, transmitting data wirelessly for analysis [31]. **Figure 6** shows an example of a wearable biosensor device.

The continuous data streams from wearable devices are fed into AI systems for real-time analysis. These systems detect patterns such as gradual temperature increases or abnormal heart rate variability that may indicate early deterioration, enabling remote monitoring and prompt intervention [32].

Wearable devices extend the continuum of care beyond the ICU. By monitoring patients after discharge, these devices help detect complications early, reducing readmission rates and facilitating tailored rehabilitation programs [33].

Table 7 shows parameters monitored by wearable devices in critical care.

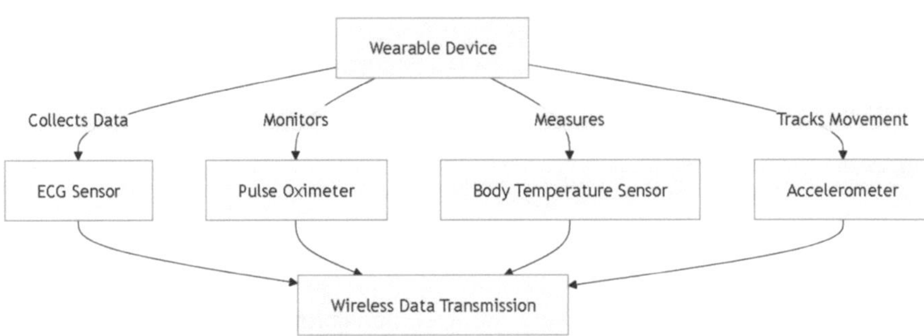

Figure 6.
Example of a wearable biosensor device. Description: This figure illustrates a wearable biosensor device with components labeled for ECG, pulse oximetry, temperature monitoring, and movement detection, along with wireless data connectivity (figure is author's own original work).

Parameter	Measurement technique	Clinical significance
Heart rate	Optical sensors, ECG	Detection of arrhythmias and cardiac performance
Oxygen saturation (SpO_2)	Pulse oximetry	Assessment of respiratory function
Body temperature	Thermistor	Early detection of infection
Mobility and activity	Accelerometer	Monitoring recovery progress and rehabilitation

Table 7.
Parameters monitored by wearable devices in critical care.

9. Innovations in ICU design and patient-centered care

9.1 The ICU of the future

The design of future ICUs emphasizes both technological integration and patient comfort. Smart environmental control systems automatically adjust lighting, noise, and temperature based on patient needs. Studies have demonstrated that such adjustments can reduce the incidence of delirium and promote better sleep, which is critical for recovery. Moreover, modular ICU layouts allow rapid expansion during patient surges, ensuring that critical care capacity is maintained even during crises [34]. **Figure 7** shows the conceptual design of a smart ICU.

Table 8 shows the comparison of a traditional ICU versus a smart ICU.

9.2 Patient-centered approaches

Modern ICU care extends beyond physiological stabilization to include psychological and emotional support. Non-pharmacologic interventions such as live music

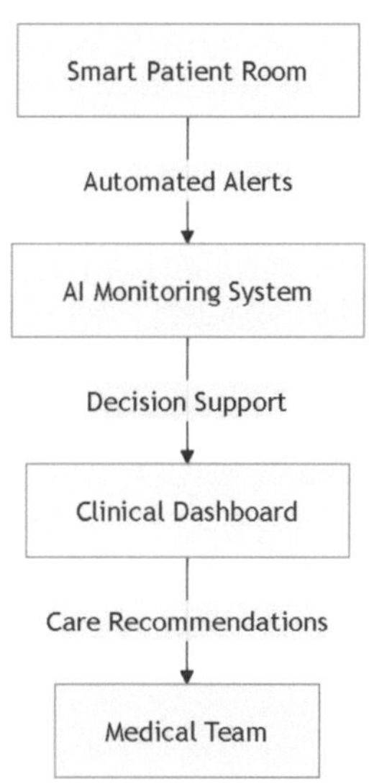

Figure 7.
Conceptual design of a smart ICU. Description: This figure is a conceptual rendering showing modular patient rooms, a centralized monitoring station, and adaptive environmental controls that work together to optimize the ICU environment (figure is author's own original work).

Feature	Traditional ICU	Smart ICU
Environmental control	Manual adjustments	Automated, sensor-driven adaptive systems
Patient monitoring	Standalone monitors	Integrated, continuous digital dashboards
Layout	Fixed design	Modular and reconfigurable design
Data integration	Fragmented data sources	Unified EHR with real-time analytics

Table 8.
Comparison of traditional ICU vs. smart ICU.

therapy, art therapy, and VR relaxation sessions help reduce anxiety, lower sedative use, and improve overall patient well-being. Clinical studies have demonstrated that these interventions can reduce patient agitation and improve sleep quality [1].

9.3 Family-centered rounds and communication

Incorporating family-centered rounds into daily ICU care enhances communication and ensures that patient care aligns with family and patient values. In these rounds, family members actively participate in discussions, ask questions, and provide insights into the patient's baseline, thereby facilitating more personalized care decisions [35].

9.4 Holistic recovery, rehabilitation, and post-ICU care

A comprehensive recovery strategy integrates medical treatment with nutritional support, physiotherapy, and psychological counseling. Early mobilization programs and post-ICU rehabilitation, often guided by wearable technology, help reduce the incidence of post-intensive care syndrome (PICS) and promote long-term recovery [36] . **Figure 8** shows the components of patient-centered care in the ICU.

Table 9 shows the impact of patient-centered interventions.

9.5 Interdisciplinary teamwork and training

Effective critical care is achieved through interdisciplinary collaboration. Daily rounds now involve intensivists, pharmacists, respiratory therapists, nutritionists, physiotherapists, and mental health professionals, ensuring that all aspects of patient care are addressed comprehensively. This teamwork results in faster, more coordinated interventions and reduced errors [37, 38].

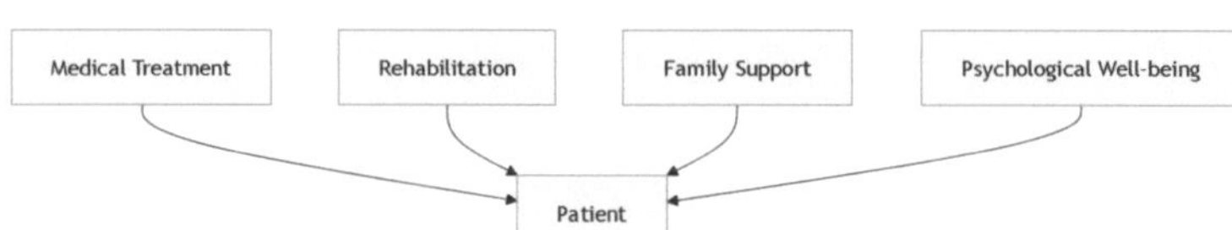

Figure 8.
Components of patient-centered care in the ICU. Description: This figure outlines the integration of medical treatment, non-pharmacologic interventions, family-centered rounds, and rehabilitation, all contributing to improved patient outcomes and psychological well-being (figure is author's own original work).

Intervention	Outcome improvement	Key benefits
Music therapy	Reduced agitation and pain	Lower sedative use, enhanced mood
VR relaxation sessions	Improved sleep, reduced delirium	Enhanced comfort and relaxation
Family-centered rounds	Increased patient and family satisfaction	Better communication and care alignment

Table 9.
Impact of patient-centered interventions.

9.6 Simulation and virtual reality training

Simulation-based training and VR platforms allow ICU teams to rehearse complex procedures, manage emergencies, and refine communication skills in a safe, controlled environment. Regular training sessions improve coordination and preparedness, contributing to a reduction in medical errors and enhanced patient outcomes [39–41].

9.7 Integrated communication platforms

Modern communication platforms facilitate real-time data sharing and collaboration among ICU staff. Secure messaging, interactive dashboards, and automated alert systems ensure that every team member is updated continuously, leading to more effective and efficient patient care [42].

Figure 9 shows the workflow diagram of multidisciplinary ICU rounds.

Table 10 shows the outcomes of interdisciplinary team approaches.

9.8 Precision medicine and pharmacogenomics in the ICU

Precision medicine tailors treatment to the individual patient. By integrating clinical data with genomic, proteomic, and metabolomic information, clinicians can develop personalized treatment plans that optimize therapeutic efficacy and reduce adverse events. This approach enables dynamic adjustment of interventions based on the patient's unique biological profile [43].

Pharmacogenomics examines how genetic variations influence drug response. In the ICU, this can guide the dosing of high-risk medications such as antibiotics, sedatives, and vasopressors. Genetic profiling helps predict which patients are at risk for adverse drug reactions, allowing clinicians to customize dosing regimens and avoid potentially harmful side effects [44].

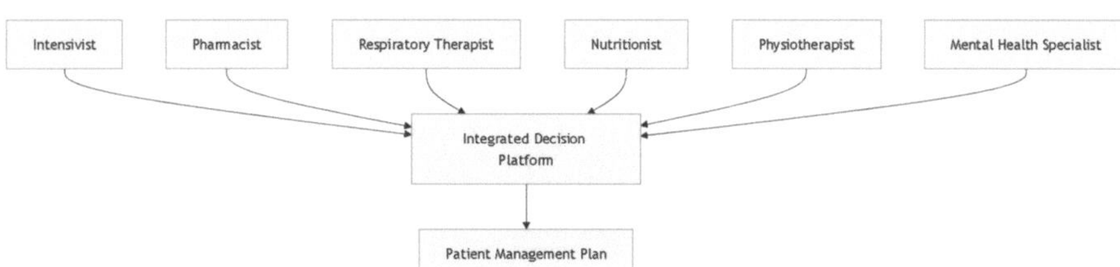

Figure 9.
Workflow diagram of multidisciplinary ICU rounds. Description: This figure depicts a workflow of interdisciplinary rounds, showing how various specialists collaborate via *an integrated communication platform (figure is author's own original work).*

Outcome	Improvement (%)	Observations
Reduction in medical errors	20–30%	Enhanced communication reduces mistakes
ICU length of stay	15–20%	Timely, coordinated interventions shorten stays
Patient satisfaction	High	Improved holistic care and communication

Table 10.
Outcomes of interdisciplinary team approaches.

Biomarkers such as procalcitonin, NGAL, and cell-cycle arrest proteins are critical in the early detection of organ dysfunction. Rapid biomarker assays allow clinicians to initiate targeted interventions, such as fluid resuscitation or renal replacement therapy before clinical deterioration becomes irreversible [45, 46].

Figure 10 shows the integration of genomic and biomarker data into personalized ICU care.

Table 11 shows the examples of biomarkers in critical care.

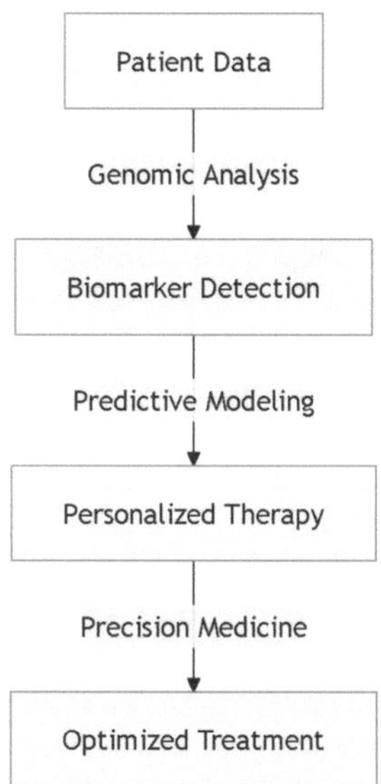

Figure 10.
Integration of genomic and biomarker data into personalized ICU care. Description: This figure shows how patient data is integrated with biomarker analysis and digital twin simulation to generate a personalized treatment plan (figure is author's own original work).

Biomarker	Clinical relevance	Intervention trigger
Procalcitonin	Bacterial infection, sepsis diagnosis	Early initiation of antibiotic therapy
NGAL	Early detection of acute kidney injury	Adjust fluid management, consider RRT
Cell-cycle arrest markers	Prediction of organ dysfunction	Intensify monitoring, preemptive interventions

Table 11.
Examples of biomarkers in critical care.

10. Big data, Cybersecurity, and health information technology

10.1 Integration of big data analytics in critical care

Big data analytics allow us to harness vast amounts of clinical data to derive insights that improve patient care. Integrating data from EHRs, wearable devices, laboratory systems, and imaging modalities provides a comprehensive view of patient health. Advanced analytics help in predicting adverse events, optimizing resource allocation, and tailoring individualized care plans [47, 48].

Cloud-based platforms facilitate real-time data sharing and integration across various healthcare systems. Interoperability standards ensure that data from disparate sources is harmonized, providing clinicians with a unified view of the patient's condition. This integration is critical for effective decision-making and collaboration across disciplines [49].

With increasing digitization, protecting patient data is paramount. Robust cybersecurity measures—including encryption, access control, and continuous network monitoring—are essential to safeguard sensitive information. Cybersecurity protocols ensure the integrity and confidentiality of data, maintaining trust and compliance within the digital ICU environment [50, 51].

Figure 11 shows the cybersecurity framework for a digital ICU.

Table 12 shows the key components of big data integration in critical care.

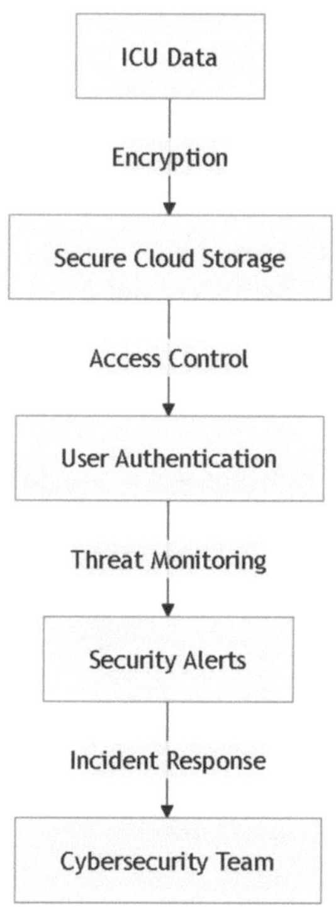

Figure 11.
Cybersecurity framework for a digital ICU. Description: This figure outlines a cybersecurity framework that secures patient data from acquisition to cloud storage and continuous monitoring, ensuring compliance and data integrity (figure is author's own original work).

Component	Function	Clinical benefit
Data aggregation	Collects data from multiple sources	Comprehensive patient overview
Cloud computing	Enables real-time data access and sharing	Enhanced collaboration and faster decision-making
Interoperability standards	Harmonizes data from diverse systems	Streamlined workflows, reduced errors
Cybersecurity protocols	Protects data integrity and privacy	Maintains trust and regulatory compliance

Table 12.
Key components of big data integration in critical care.

11. Challenges and ethical considerations

11.1 Resource limitations and global disparities

The deployment of advanced critical care technologies is often limited by high costs, specialized training needs, and infrastructure deficits. In high-income countries, access to ECMO, AI, and tele-ICU systems is relatively widespread, yet workforce shortages remain. Middle- and low-income regions face significant challenges in adopting these technologies due to limited funding and infrastructure [52].

Table 13 shows the comparison of critical care resources by region.

11.2 Ethical dilemmas in AI and advanced technologies

Integrating AI and digital technologies into critical care raises several ethical issues:

- *Algorithmic bias*: AI systems must be continually validated to prevent biases that could lead to inequitable treatment.
- *Data privacy and consent*: Ensuring patient data is protected through robust encryption and adherence to privacy standards.
- *Clinical autonomy*: AI should act as a support tool and not replace the clinician's judgment.
- Transparency: Patients and families must be informed about the role of AI in their care, ensuring informed consent.

Figure 12 shows the ethical considerations in AI-integrated critical care.

Region	Availability of advanced technologies	Major challenges
High-income countries	High – widespread access to ECMO, AI, and tele-ICU systems	Workforce shortages, high operational costs
Middle-income countries	Moderate – limited tele-ICU and basic ECMO	Budget constraints, infrastructure gaps, and training needs
Low-income countries	Low – primarily basic monitoring equipment	Severe infrastructure deficits, limited funding, and expertise

Table 13.
Comparison of critical care resources by region.

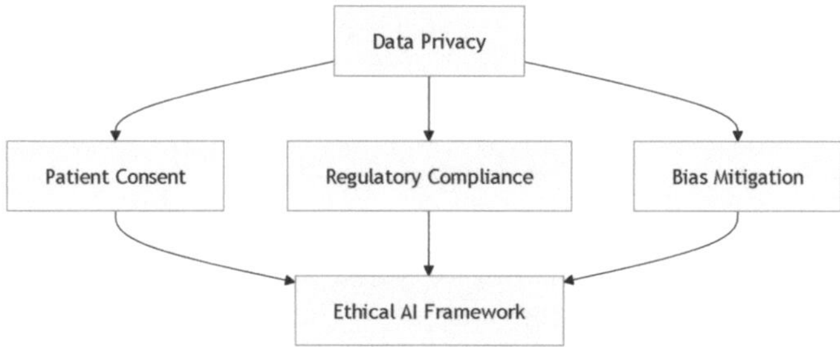

Figure 12.
Ethical considerations in AI-integrated critical care. Description: This figure illustrates the critical ethical aspects of integrating AI into the ICU, including data privacy, bias mitigation, clinical oversight, and transparency with patients and families (figure is author's own original work).

Criterion	Considerations	Decision pathway
Quality of life	Baseline health status, patient values	Family consultations and ethics committee review
Clinical prognosis	Severity of illness, comorbidities	Multidisciplinary team evaluation
Resource availability	ICU capacity, cost of interventions	Standardized triage protocols

Table 14.
Ethical framework for end-of-life decision-making in the ICU.

11.3 End-of-life decisions and equitable resource allocation

Advanced critical care technologies can prolong life but also complicate decisions regarding quality of life and resource allocation. Clinicians must balance aggressive interventions against the potential for prolonged suffering, particularly in patients with a poor prognosis. Equitable triage protocols and the integration of palliative care are essential to ensure that treatment decisions respect patient dignity and are based on ethical principles.

Table 14 shows the ethical framework for end-of-life decision-making in the ICU.

12. Next-generation technologies: Nanomedicine, regenerative therapies, and digital twins

The future of critical care lies in the integration of next-generation technologies:

- *Nanomedicine*: Research is underway to develop nanoparticle-based drug delivery systems that target specific tissues, thereby minimizing systemic side effects and maximizing therapeutic efficacy [53].

- *Regenerative medicine*: Stem cell therapies and 3D bioprinting are being explored to repair or replace damaged organs. These regenerative approaches could dramatically alter the prognosis for patients with end-stage organ failure [54].

- *Digital twins*: The development of digital twin technology—virtual models of patients based on real-time data—allows clinicians to simulate various treatment strategies and predict outcomes, facilitating truly personalized care [55].

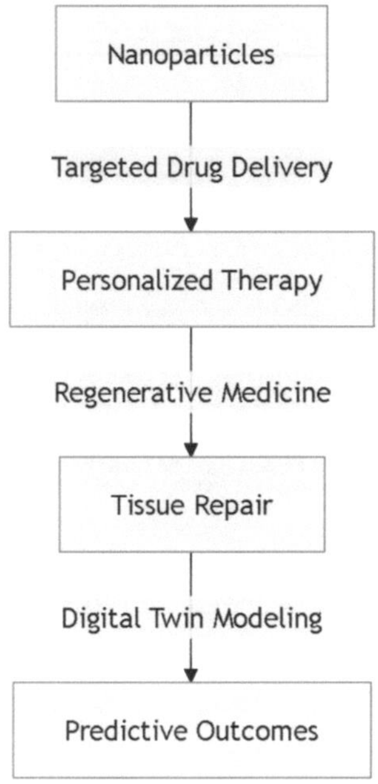

Figure 13.
Integration of nanotechnology, regenerative medicine, and digital twin technology. Description: This figure illustrates how nanoparticle drug delivery, regenerative medicine, and digital twin simulations converge to provide personalized, precision critical care (figure is author's own original work).

Figure 13 shows the integration of nanotechnology, regenerative medicine, and digital twin technology.

13. Policy, system reforms, and workforce development

For the successful integration of advanced technologies, systemic reforms are essential:

- *Funding and subsidies*: Establish public–private partnerships and government grants to support high-cost technology deployment in underserved areas.

- *Standardization of clinical guidelines*: Develop unified protocols and quality assurance programs for technologies such as ECMO, AI, and tele-ICU systems.

- *Workforce training*: Invest in simulation-based training, continuous education, and certification programs to prepare healthcare professionals for the evolving technological landscape.

- *Regulatory frameworks*: Update regulations to address data privacy, AI transparency, and interoperability, ensuring patient safety and ethical use of technology.

Table 15 outlines policy recommendations for integrating advanced technologies into critical care.

DOI: http://dx.doi.org/10.5772/intechopen.1010714

Recommendation	Key components	Expected outcome
Funding and subsidies	Public-private partnerships and targeted grants	Broader accessibility in low-resource settings
Standardization protocols	National/international guidelines for quality assurance programs	Consistent and safe technology implementation
Workforce development	Simulation training, continuous education, and certification programs	Enhanced clinical competency and reduced errors
Regulatory oversight	Updated data privacy laws, AI validation standards, interoperability mandates	Increased patient trust and improved system performance

Table 15.
Policy recommendations for integrating advanced technologies into critical care.

14. Global collaboration and knowledge sharing

- *Data sharing networks*: Expand international registries and databases to facilitate the rapid dissemination of clinical data and best practices.
- *Multicenter clinical trials*: Conduct global clinical trials to validate new technologies across diverse patient populations.

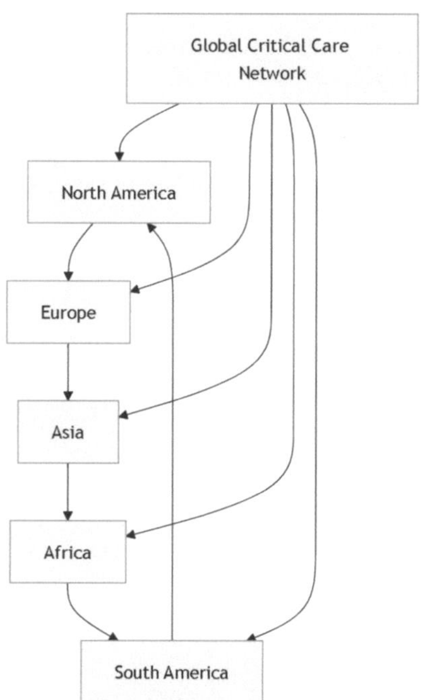

Figure 14.
Global map of critical care collaborations. Description: This figure shows a global map with interconnected nodes representing critical care collaborations and data-sharing networks among continents (figure is author's own original work).

Benefit	Description	Impact on patient care
Shared Data and Protocols	Unified international registries and guidelines	Accelerated innovation and improved outcomes
Multicenter Trials	Diverse patient populations, standardized data collection	Enhanced validity and clinical applicability
Knowledge Dissemination	Open-access research platforms	Equitable access to cutting-edge practices

Table 16.
Benefits of global collaboration in critical care.

- *Open-access research platforms*: Establish platforms that allow free access to research findings and clinical protocols, ensuring equitable dissemination of knowledge.
- *Collaborative consortia*: Form multinational research consortia to share expertise, resources, and funding, accelerating innovation and improving patient outcomes globally.

Figure 14 shows the global map of critical care collaborations.
Table 16 shows the benefits of global collaboration in critical care.

15. Conclusion

Critical care medicine is undergoing a transformative evolution driven by technological innovation, data integration, and a patient-centered approach. Advances in AI, telemedicine, ECMO, wearable biosensors, and precision medicine have redefined our capacity to predict, prevent, and manage life-threatening conditions. These

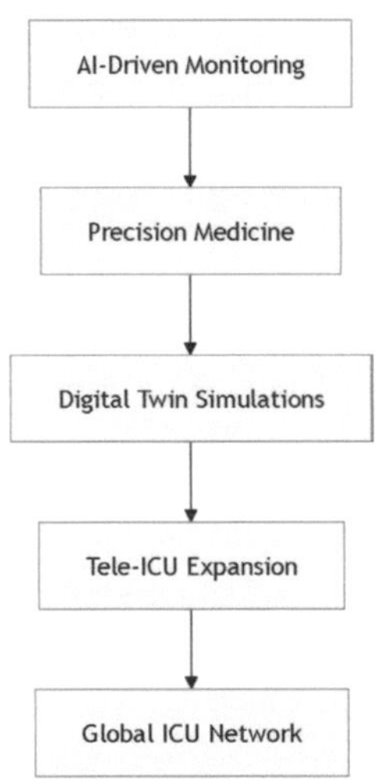

Figure 15.
Vision for the future ICU. Description: This figure represents the ideal future ICU, where advanced monitoring, digital twin technology, smart environmental controls, global collaborations, and integrated teams converge to deliver personalized and optimal critical care (figure is author's own original work).

innovations have led to significant improvements in survival rates, reduced complications, and enhanced overall quality of care.

However, challenges persist. Resource disparities, ethical dilemmas, cybersecurity issues, and the need for updated regulatory frameworks require ongoing attention. By investing in workforce training, fostering global collaboration, and standardizing protocols, we can ensure that the benefits of these advanced technologies extend to all patients, regardless of geographic or economic boundaries.

Looking ahead, the integration of next-generation technologies such as nanomedicine, regenerative therapies, and digital twins promises to usher in a new era of precision critical care. Our vision for the future ICU is one where personalized, data-driven, and compassionate care converge to provide optimal outcomes for every critically ill patient.

Figure 15 shows the vision for the future ICU.

In summary, this chapter provides an exhaustive exploration of the trends shaping modern critical care medicine. By embracing innovation, leveraging advanced technologies, and fostering interdisciplinary collaboration, we are paving the way for a future in which the ICU becomes a dynamic, responsive, and truly patient-centered environment.

A.Glossary of key terms

Artificial Intelligence (AI): Computer systems that simulate human intelligence to process data, learn from it, and support clinical decision-making.

Telemedicine: The remote diagnosis and treatment of patients using telecommunications technology.

ECMO: Extracorporeal Membrane Oxygenation, a technology that provides prolonged cardiac and respiratory support.

Wearable Biosensors: Devices that continuously and non-invasively measure physiological parameters.

Precision Medicine: An approach that tailors medical treatment based on individual genetic, biomarker, and clinical information.

Digital Twin: A virtual model of a patient that is used to simulate and predict responses to various treatments.

B.Descriptions of figures and tables

Figure 1: Schematic overview of the modern ICU ecosystem, showing integration of AI, tele-ICU, ECMO, and wearable biosensors.

Figure 2: Timeline of milestones in critical care medicine from the 1950s to the present.

Figure 3: Flowchart of the AI data pipeline from data acquisition to clinical decision support.

Figure 4: Diagram of tele-ICU system architecture showing the flow from bedside monitors to remote command centers.

Figure 5: Annotated diagram of an ECMO circuit with key components.

Figure 6: Illustration of a wearable biosensor device with labeled sensors and connectivity modules.

Figure 7: Rendered conceptual design of a smart ICU with modular layouts and adaptive environmental controls.

Figure 8: Diagram of patient-centered care components including non-pharmacologic interventions, family involvement, and rehabilitation.
Figure 9: Workflow diagram of multidisciplinary ICU rounds, illustrating team communication.
Figure 10: Diagram integrating genomic and biomarker data into personalized ICU care.
Figure 11: Cybersecurity framework for a digital ICU showing key security measures.
Figure 12: Diagram of ethical considerations in AI integration in critical care.
Figure 13: Conceptual diagram depicting integration of nanomedicine, regenerative therapies, and digital twin technology.
Figure 14: Global map showing interconnected critical care collaborations and data-sharing networks.
Figure 15: Visionary illustration of the future ICU integrating advanced monitoring, digital twin simulations, smart controls, and global collaborations.
Table 1: Overview of key technologies in critical care.
Table 2: Comparative summary of historical versus modern critical care approaches.
Table 3: Summary of key clinical trials impacting ICU practices.
Table 4: Key AI applications in the ICU.
Table 5: Clinical outcomes from tele-ICU implementations.
Table 6: Comparison of ECMO outcomes in clinical studies.
Table 7: Parameters monitored by wearable devices in the ICU.
Table 8: Comparison of traditional ICU versus smart ICU.
Table 9: Impact of patient-centered interventions.
Table 10: Outcomes of interdisciplinary team approaches.
Table 11: Examples of biomarkers in critical care.
Table 12: Key components of big data integration in critical care.
Table 13: Comparison of critical care resources by region.
Table 14: Ethical framework for end-of-life decision-making in the ICU.
Table 15: Policy recommendations for integrating advanced technologies.
Table 16: Benefits of global collaboration in critical care.

This comprehensive chapter provides an in-depth exploration of the evolution, current innovations, and future directions in critical care medicine. By combining advanced technologies with a patient-centered, interdisciplinary approach, the future of the ICU is set to be more responsive, precise, and compassionate. With continued global collaboration, rigorous training, and supportive policy reforms, we can overcome current challenges and ensure that every critically ill patient receives the highest standard of care.

The integration of AI, telemedicine, ECMO, wearable biosensors, precision medicine, and robust health IT is transforming the ICU into a dynamic ecosystem. As we move forward, these advancements will not only save lives but also improve the quality of life for survivors, ultimately redefining critical care medicine for the twenty-first century.

DOI: http://dx.doi.org/10.5772/intechopen.1010714

Author details

Muhammad Saqib
Khyber Medical College, Peshawar, Pakistan

*Address all correspondence to: muhammadsaqib.drkmc@gmail.com

References

[1] Padte S, Samala Venkata V, Mehta P, Tawfeeq S, Kashyap R, Surani S. 21st century critical care medicine: An overview. World Journal of Critical Care Medicine. 2024;**13**(1):90176. DOI: 10.5492/wjccm.v13.i1.90176

[2] Vincent JL. Critical care--where have we been and where are we going? Critical Care (London, England). 2013; **17 Suppl 1**(Suppl. 1):S2. DOI: 10.1186/cc11500

[3] Slutsky AS. History of mechanical ventilation. From vesalius to ventilator-induced lung injury. American Journal of Respiratory and Critical Care Medicine. 2015;**191**(10):1106-1115. DOI: 10.1164/rccm.201503-0421PP

[4] Brower RG, Matthay MA, Morris A, Schoenfeld D, Thompson BT, Wheeler A. Ventilation with lower tidal volumes as compared with traditional tidal volumes for acute lung injury and the acute respiratory distress syndrome. The New England Journal of Medicine. 2000;**342**(18):1301-1308. DOI: 10.1056/nejm200005043421801

[5] Peek GJ, Clemens F, Elbourne D, Firmin R, Hardy P, Hibbert C, et al. CESAR: Conventional ventilatory support vs extracorporeal membrane oxygenation for severe adult respiratory failure. BMC Health Services Research. 2006;**6**:163. DOI: 10.1186/1472-6963-6-163

[6] Combes A, Hajage D, Capellier G, Demoule A, Lavoué S, Guervilly C, et al. Extracorporeal membrane oxygenation for severe acute respiratory distress syndrome. The New England Journal of Medicine. 2018;**378**(21):1965-1975. DOI: 10.1056/NEJMoa1800385

[7] Venkatesh B, Finfer S, Cohen J, Rajbhandari D, Arabi Y, Bellomo R, et al. Adjunctive glucocorticoid therapy in patients with septic shock. The New England Journal of Medicine. 2018;**378**(9):797-808. DOI: 10.1056/NEJMoa1705835

[8] Kress JP, Pohlman AS, O'Connor MF, Hall JB. Daily interruption of sedative infusions in critically ill patients undergoing mechanical ventilation. The New England Journal of Medicine. 2000;**342**(20):1471-1477. DOI: 10.1056/nejm200005183422002

[9] Girard TD, Kress JP, Fuchs BD, Thomason JWW, Schweickert WD, Pun BT, et al. Efficacy and safety of a paired sedation and ventilator weaning protocol for mechanically ventilated patients in intensive care (awakening and breathing controlled trial): A randomised controlled trial. The Lancet. 2008;**371**(9607):126-134. DOI: 10.1016/S0140-6736(08)60105-1

[10] Mehta S, Burry L, Cook D, Fergusson D, Steinberg M, Granton J, et al. Dailysedationinterruptioninmechanically ventilated critically ill patients cared for with a sedation protocol: A randomized controlled trial. Journal of the American Medical Association. 2012;**308**(19):1985-1992. DOI: 10.1001/jama.2012.13872 %J JAMA

[11] Olsen HT, Nedergaard HK, Strøm T, Oxlund J, Wian KA, Ytrebø LM, et al. Nonsedation or light sedation in critically ill, mechanically ventilated patients. The New England Journal of Medicine. 2020;**382**(12):1103-1111. DOI: 10.1056/NEJMoa1906759

[12] Jakob SM, Ruokonen E, Grounds RM, Sarapohja T, Garratt C, Pocock SJ, et al.

Dexmedetomidine vs midazolam or propofol for sedation during prolonged mechanical ventilation: Two randomized controlled trials. Journal of the American Medical Association. 2012;**307**(11):1151-1160. DOI: 10.1001/jama.2012.304 %J JAMA

[13] Shehabi Y, Howe BD, Bellomo R, Arabi YM, Bailey M, Bass FE, et al. Early sedation with dexmedetomidine in critically ill patients. The New England Journal of Medicine. 2019;**380**(26):2506-2517. DOI: 10.1056/NEJMoa1904710

[14] Finfer S, Bellomo R, Boyce N, French J, Myburgh J, Norton R. A comparison of albumin and saline for fluid resuscitation in the intensive care unit. The New England Journal of Medicine. 2004;**350**(22):2247-2256. DOI: 10.1056/NEJMoa040232

[15] Self WH, Semler MW, Wanderer JP, Wang L, Byrne DW, Collins SP, et al. Balanced crystalloids versus saline in noncritically ill adults. The New England Journal of Medicine. 2018;**378**(9):819-828. DOI: 10.1056/NEJMoa1711586

[16] Semler MW, Self WH, Wanderer JP, Ehrenfeld JM, Wang L, Byrne DW, et al. Balanced crystalloids versus saline in critically ill adults. The New England Journal of Medicine. 2018;**378**(9):829-839. DOI: 10.1056/NEJMoa1711584

[17] Young P, Bailey M, Beasley R, Henderson S, Mackle D, McArthur C, et al. Effect of a buffered crystalloid solution vs saline on acute kidney injury among patients in the intensive care unit: The SPLIT randomized clinical trial. Journal of the American Medical Association. 2015;**314**(16):1701-1710. DOI: 10.1001/jama.2015.12334 %J JAMA

[18] Hébert PC, Wells G, Blajchman MA, Marshall J, Martin C, Pagliarello G, et al. A multicenter, randomized, controlled clinical trial of transfusion requirements in critical care. Transfusion requirements in critical care investigators, Canadian critical care trials group. The New England Journal of Medicine. 1999;**340**(6):409-417. DOI: 10.1056/nejm199902113400601

[19] Holst LB, Haase N, Wetterslev J, Wernerman J, Guttormsen AB, Karlsson S, et al. Lower versus higher hemoglobin threshold for transfusion in septic shock. The New England Journal of Medicine. 2014;**371**(15):1381-1391. DOI: 10.1056/NEJMoa1406617

[20] Turgeon AF, Fergusson DA, Clayton L, Patton MP, Neveu X, Walsh TS, et al. Liberal or restrictive transfusion strategy in patients with traumatic brain injury. The New England Journal of Medicine. 2024;**391**(8):722-735. DOI: 10.1056/NEJMoa2404360

[21] Thomson WR, Puthucheary ZA, Wan YI. Critical care and pandemic preparedness and response. British Journal of Anaesthesia. 2023;**131**(5):847-860. DOI: 10.1016/j.bja.2023.07.026

[22] McGaughey J, Fergusson DA, Van Bogaert P, Rose L. Early warning systems and rapid response systems for the prevention of patient deterioration on acute adult hospital wards. The Cochrane Database of Systematic Reviews. 2021;**11**(11):Cd005529. DOI: 10.1002/14651858.CD005529.pub3

[23] Khalifa M, Albadawy M. AI in diagnostic imaging: Revolutionising accuracy and efficiency. Computer Methods and Programs in Biomedicine Update. 2024;**5**:100146. DOI: 10.1016/j.cmpbup.2024.100146

[24] Alexiuk M, Elgubtan H, Tangri N. Clinical decision support tools in the electronic medical record. Kidney

International Reports. 2024;**9**(1):29-38. DOI: 10.1016/j.ekir.2023.10.019

[25] Watanabe T, Ohsugi K, Suminaga Y, Somei M, Kikuyama K, Mori M, et al. An evaluation of the impact of the implementation of the Tele-ICU: A retrospective observational study. Journal of Intensive Care. 2023;**11**(1):9. DOI: 10.1186/s40560-023-00657-4

[26] Sadaka F, Palagiri A, Trottier S, Deibert W, Gudmestad D, Sommer SE, et al. Telemedicine intervention improves ICU outcomes. Critical Care Research and Practice. 2013;**2013**:456389. DOI: 10.1155/2013/456389

[27] Zang K, Chen B, Wang M, Chen D, Hui L, Guo S, et al. The effect of early mobilization in critically ill patients: A meta-analysis. Nursing in Critical Care. 2020;**25**(6):360-367. DOI: 10.1111/nicc.12455

[28] Vranas KC, Slatore CG, Kerlin MP. Telemedicine coverage of intensive care units: A narrative review. Annals of the American Thoracic Society. 2018;**15**(11):1256-1264. DOI: 10.1513/AnnalsATS.201804-225CME

[29] Dorsey M, Phillips K, James L, Kelley E, Duff E, Lewis T, et al. Decreased bleeding and thrombotic complications on extracorporeal membrane oxygenation support following an updated anticoagulation protocol. JTCVS Open. 2025;**23**:199-209. DOI: 10.1016/j.xjon.2024.11.019

[30] Kingren MS, Starr ME, Saito H. Divergent sepsis pathophysiology in older adults. Antioxidants and Redox Signaling. 2021;**35**(16):1358-1375. DOI: 10.1089/ars.2021.0056

[31] Erdem A, Eksin E, Senturk H, Yildiz E, Maral M. Recent developments in wearable biosensors for healthcare and biomedical applications. TrAC Trends in Analytical Chemistry. 2024;**171**:117510. DOI: 10.1016/j.trac.2023.117510

[32] Tsvetanov F. Integrating AI Technologies into Remote Monitoring Patient Systems. 2024;**70**(1):54

[33] Angelucci A, Greco M, Cecconi M, Aliverti A. Wearable devices for patient monitoring in the intensive care unit. Intensive Care Medicine Experimental. 2025;**13**(1):26. DOI: 10.1186/s40635-025-00738-8

[34] Tronstad O, Flaws D, Patterson S, Holdsworth R, Fraser JF. Creating the ICU of the future: Patient-centred design to optimise recovery. Critical Care. 2023;**27**(1):402. DOI: 10.1186/s13054-023-04685-2

[35] Secunda KE, Kruser JM. Patient-centered and family-centered care in the intensive care unit. Clinics in Chest Medicine. 2022;**43**(3):539-550. DOI: 10.1016/j.ccm.2022.05.008

[36] Brockman A, Krupp A, Bach C, Mu J, Vasilevskis EE, Tan A, et al. Clinicians' perceptions on implementation strategies used to facilitate ABCDEF bundle adoption: A multicenter survey. Heart and Lung: The Journal of Critical Care. 2023;**62**:108-115. DOI: 10.1016/j.hrtlng.2023.06.006

[37] Xie A, Barany EA, Tanner EK, Blakeney EA, Bahouth MN, Hanson GC, et al. Interprofessional collaboration and patient/family engagement on rounds in a comprehensive stroke center: A mixed-methods study. Quality Management in Health Care. 2024;**33**(4):231-238. DOI: 10.1097/qmh.0000000000000437

[38] Yumoto T, Hongo T, Obara T, Ageta K, Aokage T, Tsukahara K, et al. Evolution and effects of ad hoc multidisciplinary team meetings in

the emergency intensive care unit: A five-year analysis. Journal of Clinical Medicine. 2024;**13**(15). DOI: 10.3390/jcm13154324

[39] Elendu C, Amaechi DC, Okatta AU, Amaechi EC, Elendu TC, Ezeh CP, et al. The impact of simulation-based training in medical education: A review. Medicine. 2024;**103**(27):e38813. DOI: 10.1097/md.0000000000038813

[40] Seam N, Lee AJ, Vennero M, Emlet L. Simulation training in the ICU. Chest. 2019;**156**(6):1223-1233. DOI: 10.1016/j.chest.2019.07.011

[41] Barsness KA. Achieving expert performance through simulation-based education and application of mastery learning principles. Seminars in Pediatric Surgery. 2020;**29**(2):150904. DOI: 10.1016/j.sempedsurg.2020.150904

[42] Quinn M, Forman J, Harrod M, Winter S, Fowler KE, Krein SL, et al. Electronic health records, communication, and data sharing: Challenges and opportunities for improving the diagnostic process. Diagnosis (Berlin, Germany). 2019;**6**(3):241-248. DOI: 10.1515/dx-2018-0036

[43] Lazăr A, Georgescu AM, Vitin A, Azamfirei L. Precision medicine and its role in the treatment of sepsis: A personalised view. Journal of Critical Care Medicine (Universitatea de Medicina si Farmacie din Targu-Mures). 2019;**5**(3):90-96. DOI: 10.2478/jccm-2019-0017

[44] Zhou S, Skaar DJ, Jacobson PA, Huang RS. Pharmacogenomics of medications commonly used in the intensive care unit. Frontiers in Pharmacology. 2018;**9**:1436. DOI: 10.3389/fphar.2018.01436

[45] Póvoa P, Salluh JIF. Biomarker-guided antibiotic therapy in adult critically ill patients: A critical review. Annals of Intensive Care. 2012;**2**(1):32. DOI: 10.1186/2110-5820-2-32

[46] Heilmann E, Gregoriano C, Schuetz P. Biomarkers of infection: Are they useful in the ICU? Seminars in Respiratory and Critical Care Medicine. 2019;**40**(4):465-475. DOI: 10.1055/s-0039-1696689

[47] Sanchez-Pinto LN, Luo Y, Churpek MM. Big data and data science in critical care. Chest. 2018;**154**(5):1239-1248. DOI: 10.1016/j.chest.2018.04.037

[48] Behdani AM, Lai J, Kim C, Basalelah L, Halsey T, Donohoe KL, et al. Optimizing pharmacogenomic decision-making by data science. PLOS Digital Health. 2024;**3**(2):e0000451. DOI: 10.1371/journal.pdig.0000451

[49] Sachdeva S, Bhatia S, Al Harrasi A, Shah YA, Anwer K, Philip AK, et al. Unraveling the role of cloud computing in health care system and biomedical sciences. Heliyon. 2024;**10**(7):e29044. DOI: 10.1016/j.heliyon.2024.e29044

[50] Burke W, Stranieri A, Oseni T, Gondal I. The need for cybersecurity self-evaluation in healthcare. BMC Medical Informatics and Decision Making. 2024;**24**(1):133. DOI: 10.1186/s12911-024-02551-x

[51] Niki O, Saira G, Arvind S, Mike D. Cyber-attacks are a permanent and substantial threat to health systems: Education must reflect that. Digital Health. 2022;**8**:20552076221104665. DOI: 10.1177/20552076221104665

[52] Shetty VU. Mobile critical care in resource-limited settings: An unmet need. Annals of Global Health. 2024;**90**(1):59. DOI: 10.5334/aogh.4506

[53] Amin KWK, Deák Á, Csanády M Jr, Szemerédi N, Szabó D, Turcsányi Á, et al. pH-triggered hydrogel nanoparticles for efficient anticancer drug delivery and bioimaging applications. Pharmaceutics. 2024;**16**(7). DOI: 10.3390/pharmaceutics16070931

[54] Wang X, Zhang D, Singh YP, Yeo M, Deng G, Lai J, et al. Progress in organ bioprinting for regenerative medicine. Engineering. 2024;**42**:121-142. DOI: 10.1016/j.eng.2024.04.023

[55] Papachristou K, Katsakiori PF, Papadimitroulas P, Strigari L, Kagadis GC. Digital twins' advancements and applications in healthcare, towards precision medicine. Journal of Personalized Medicine. 2024;**14**(11). DOI: 10.3390/jpm14111101